Databook for Clinical Pharmacology

Databook for Clinical Pharmacology

Dr. Tapan Kumar Chatterjee
M. Pharm. (J.U), Ph.D (J.U.), FIC (Cal.).
Ex. Research Scientist (UGC),
Department of Pharmceutical Technology,
Jadavpur University, Kolkata.
Director,
Clinical Research Centre (CRC),
Department of Pharmaceutical Technology,
Jadavpur University, Kolkata.
Associate Professor,
Division of Pharmacology,
Department of Pharmaceutical Technology,
Jadavpur University, Kolkata.

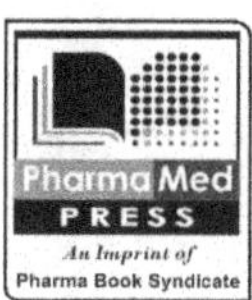

PharmaMed Press
An imprint of Pharma Book Syndicate
A unit of BSP Books Pvt. Ltd.
4-4-309/316, Giriraj Lane,
Sultan Bazar, Hyderabad - 500 095.

Published by

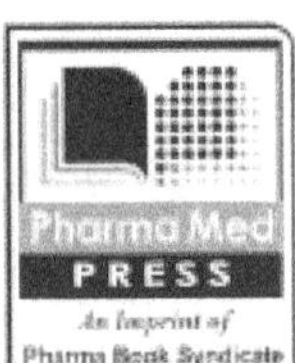

PharmaMed Press
An imprint of Pharma Book Syndicate
A unit of BSP Books Pvt. Ltd.
4-4-309/316, Giriraj Lane, Sultan Bazar, Hyderabad - 500 095.
Phone: 040-23445605, 23445688; Fax: 91+40-23445611
E-mail: info@pharmamedpress.com

ISBN: 978-93-85433-63-4 (HB)

PRELUDE

With the emergence of toxic drugs for the treatment of wide spectrum of human diseases, a basic understanding of clinical and pharmacokinetic data along with drug-drug interactions, ADR are essential for medical and pharmaceutical students as well as clinicians.

Dr. Tapan Kumar Chatterjee, faculty member of Jadavpur University has made a commendable work in bringing out this compilation entitled **" Databook for Clinical Pharmacology.** In this book, Dr. Chatterjee has included clinical data to give essential background information, which complement the kinetic data of several drugs. He has also included in this book the important chapters on drug-drug interactions and ADR in a rather exhaustive manner.

The book will be a useful tool for medical and pharmacy students, medical practitioners, pharmacologists and toxicologists. I hope, the readers will find this book very interesting and beneficial.

Prof. A. N. Basu
Ex. *Vice-Chancellor*
Jadavpur University
Kolkata – 700 032

PREFACE

When I was on the career of study and research work, I confess that I badly needed the aid of a databook on clinical data etc. I have, therefore, been provoked to compile this databook to deliver substantial aid to researchers who might be interested to carry on the research work in clinical field. It has been a long time since I initially conceived the idea of bringing out a compendium of clinical, pharmacokinetic data, drug interactions and adverse drug rection (ADR) as I felt such publication would immensely benefit medical and pharmacology students both at undergraduate and post-graduate level beside being essential companion for the practicing doctors, pharmacologists and toxicologists. The idea was sustained and followed up by hectic work involving searching for and finally collating the relevant data from various research-papers and other similar sources after necessary evaluation. This book will be a strong tool to do pharmacovigilance.

Today, all my efforts stand vindicated as the book entitled **"Databook for Clinical Pharmacology"** is ready for the readers. In this connection, it may not be out of place to mention that a conscious effort has been made to include essential clinical material for the necessary background information and to complement the kinetic data (Pharmacokinetic). The book also includes the important chapters on drug-drug interactions and ADR in a most exhaustive manner.

The data book has been segregated into four chapters. **Chapter I** comprises clinical data of hundreds of drugs. **Chapter II** assembles the pharmacokinetic data of several drugs. The **Chapter III** elaborates the drug-drug interactions of many drugs in a most appropriate manner and the **Chapter IV** included the Adverse Drug Reactions (ADR) of the drugs. The book has separately included reference section.

While every reasonable effort has been made to keep the data free of mistakes, these will nonetheless be there. Myself cannot be urged to accept any responsibility in the event of any error or omission creeping. I should be extremely grateful to those bringing these mistakes to my notice immediately so that necessary corrections could take place at the earliest. In a fast changing world existing ideas and theories are continuously replaced by new ones. The clinical pharmacology cannot remain immune to this changing scenario and influx of new ideas. I am prepared to welcome any such new suggestions in this regard. The effort being only a glimpse of the vast 'field' that lies beyond, I am fully aware of the limitations of the scope of my work.

The idea of writing the collection would have largely remained a distant dream but for a constant inspiration from Prof. A. N. Basu, ex. Vice Chancellor of our University who despite his busy schedule and the grave responsibility was extremely nice to write a foreword for this book and provided the necessary encouragement and support to ensure that the book finally sees the light of the day. There was also unstinted help and support from other faculty members of our University whose major presence in the overall effort can never be overemphasised.

A special thanks goes to Prof. T.K. Maity, Head of the Department, Deptt. of Pharmaceutical Technology, Prof. B. Mukherjee, Prof. A. Banerjee, Dr. A. Samanta, Prof. B. Sa, Dr. T. Sen, Dr. P. Halder, Dr. S. Dewenjee, Senior faculty members of the Department of Pharmaceutical Technology, Jadavpur University.

Databook is the result of enormous encouragement received from my family. Moral support of my wife (Lisa) and daughter (Anuja) have been a fortunate thing for writing this book. My late father (who wrote more than 80 informative articles in journals) is one of my role models as an author.

Miss. Soumita Goswami, *M.Pharm (Clinical)* has provided the desired help with her skill for typing and secretarial support. The job is extermely painstaking and I would not belittle her effort recording my appreciation for it.

I am grateful to my publisher "BSP Books Pvt.Ltd." and to their editorial staff for their co-operation, encouragement and valuable suggestions. I hope the databook will be useful for the students, researchers and teachers. Suggestions and comments are always welcome from any part.

It would have been impossible to complete this Databook without the invaluable assistance of Sri Hari Home, Sri Saumen Karan, Sri Saswata Banerjee, Mr. Souvick Debnath, Mr. Biswajit Ruidas, Mr. Biswaroop Sengupta and Sumanta Das who kindly laid hands in correction of the manuscript and helped in preparation of sketches. I must thanks them for all assistance rendered to me in this venture.

It is a databook to read, keep and refer to again and again.

Dr. Tapan Kumar Chatterjee
Jadavpur University
Kolkata – 700 032
JULY, 2014

LIST OF CONTRIBUTORS

Dr. (Mrs.) M. Uma Maheswari, M.Pharm, Ph.D
Assistant Professor,
Department of Pharmacology,
College of Pharmacy,
Sri Ramkrishna Institute of Paramedical Sciences,
Coimbator, Tamilnadu, India.

Dr. A. T. Sivashanmugam, M. Pharm, Ph.D
Assistant Professor,
Department of Pharmacology,
College of Pharmacy,
Sri Ramkrishna Institute of Paramedical Sciences,
Coimbator, Tamilnadu, India.

Dr. D. Chattopadhyay, M.Sc, Ph.D
Deputy Director,
ICMR Viral Unit,
ID & BG Hospital, GB-4 Ist Floor,
57 Dr. Suresh Chandra Banerjee Road Beleghata
Kolkata – 700 010, India.

Dr. Pinaki Dutta, MBBS (Cal), DNB, FRAS Fccs, CCEBDM, CCGDM
Consultant Physician,
Speacial Interefest in Cardiology and Diabetology,
AMRI Hospitals, Kolkata.

Mr. Biswajit Das, M. Pharm
UGC Research Fellow and Lecturer
Department of Pharmaceutical Technology,
Jadavpur University, Kolkata - 700 032

Miss. Soumita Gosweami, M.Pharm (Clinical)
Course Co-ordinator, Clinical Research Centre (CRC),
Jadavpur University, Kolkata - 700 032

Dr. Subrojyoti Bhowmick, MBBS (Cal) (Gold Medalist), MD (Pharmacology), FIAMS, Fellow British
Medical Journal
Medical Superintendent (Academics, Quality & Research) & Consultant
Clinical Pharmacologist
Peerless Hospital & B.K. Roy Research Centre, Kolkata
Ethics Committee Member,
Jadavpur Univeristy.

Contents

Introduction

A scientific group of world Health Organization (WHO) has defined a drug as "any substance or product that is used or intended to be used to modify or explore physiological systems or pathological states for the benefit of the recipient" (Technical report no. 34 of WHO 1996). **Paul Martini** (1889-1964) was first who used the term **"clinical pharmacology"**. Clinical pharmacology comprises all aspects of the scientific study of drugs in human. Its objective is to optimize drug therapy and it is justified in so far as it is put to the practical use. Clinical pharmacology finds appearance in performance with other clinical specialities. Therapeutic accomplishment with drugs is becoming more and more dependent on the user having at least an outline understanding of both pharmacokinetics and pharmacodynamics.

Pharmacodynamics: Finding out what drugs do to the body and how. This includes not just the cellular and molecular aspects, but also more relevant clinical measurements. **Pharmacokinetics** - what happens to the drug while in the body. This involves the body systems for handling the drug, usually divided into the following classification:

- *Absorption*
- *Distribution*
- *Metabolism*
- *Excretion*

Clinical pharmacology is the science of drugs and their clinical use. It is underpinned by the basic science of pharmacology, with added focus on the application of pharmacological principles and methods in the real world. It has a broad scope, from the discovery of new target molecules, to the effects of drug usage in whole population.

Clinical pharmacology connects the gap between medical practice and laboratory science. The main objective is to promote the safety of prescription, maximise the drug effects and minimise the side effects. It is important that there be association with clinical pharmacists skilled in areas of drug information, medication, safety and other aspects of pharmacy practice related to clinical pharmacology. Clinical pharmacologists are physicians, pharmacists and scientists whose focus is developing and understanding new drug therapies. Clinical pharmacologists work in a variety of settings in academia, industry and government. In the laboratory setting they study biomarkers, pharmacokinetics, drug metabolism and genetics. In the office setting they design and evaluate clinical trials, create and implement regulation guidelines for drug use, and look at drug utilization on local and global scales. In the clinical setting they work directly with patients, participate in experimental studies, and investigate adverse reactions and interactions.

Clinical Pharmacology, in theory, has been practiced for centuries through observing the effects of herbal remedies and early drugs on humans. Most of this work was done through trial and error. In the early 1900s, scientific advances allowed scientists to combine the study of physiological effects with biological effects. This led to the first major breakthrough when scientists used clinical pharmacology to discover insulin. Since that discovery clinical pharmacology has expanded to be a multidisciplinary field and has contributed to the understanding of drug interaction, therapeutic efficacy and safety in humans. Over time clinical pharmacologists have been able to make more exact measurements and personalize drug therapies

Clinical pharmacologists usually have a rigorous pharmaceutical and scientific training which enables them to evaluate evidence and produce new data through well designed clinical studies. Clinical pharmacologists must have access to enough outpatients for clinical care, teaching and education, and research as well be supervised by medical specialists. Their responsibilities to patients include, but are not limited to analyzing adverse drug effects, therapeutics, and toxicology including reproductive toxicology, cardiovascular risks, perioperative drug management and psycho-pharmacology.

A doctor can only do rational prescription   using the right medication, at the right dose, using the right route and frequency of administration for the patient, and stopping the drug appropriately. For that the doctor should know about the clinical data, pharmacokinetics data, adverse drug reactions (ADR), and drug interactions of the drugs.

CHAPTER I

CLINICAL DATA TEXT

Dose

Clinically the expression dose is self-explanatory. Throughout prescription of proper dose for any patient, so many things must be well thought-out. Some antibiotics are obtainable in tablet, capsule or suspension form for oral route. So doctors should prefer the formulation suitable for the patients. It is significant because it influences the bioavailability of the drug. For instance, bioavailability of digoxin is 62 when given in oral route on the other hand, the bioavailability of digoxin elixir administered orally is 0.08. In the following tables, in case of dose it is oral route. And when another route is more usual, this has been indicated in tables.

Therapeutic Concentration

Following absorption, drug reaches the plasma or blood to produce therapeutic effect. The concentration that needs to be reached for drug to exert a significant therapeutic benefit without any side effect is called therapeutic concentration.

Penetration to CNS

The majority of the drugs are either weak acid or weak base and remain in non-ionized and lipid soluble form. Presence of hydrocarbon chain, steroid nucleus, benzene ring or halogen favor lipid solubility. On the other hand, water solubility is favored by the possession of alcohol (–OH), amide (–CONH$_2$), carboxyl group (–COOH), and conjugated products. Within any closely related series of compounds more lipid soluble will show better penetration to the central nervous system (CNS). Lipid soluble drugs can pass through the blood brain barrier(BBB). CSF/PI is the ratio which indicate the ability of drug to penetrate the CNS.

Lactation

Breast-feeding mothers may deliver substantial amount of some drugs to her child whose ability to handle the foreign compound is very low. So, this parameter is extremly important and this parameter is depend on the time of sampling breast milk in relation to drug administration. (Table 1.1)

T$_{1/2}$ in Renal and Hepatic failure

Understanding in renal failure case, or decrease in renal function with age, can be related to creatinine clearance.

In some case of hepatic disease, increased bioavailability can be observed. This is due to the reduction of first-pass effect diseased liver. (Table 1.2)

Risk in Pregnancy

During first timester, many drugs are known to damage the developing fetus, resulting malformations. There are some drugs which can exert toxic effects during second and third timester, giving rise to retarded growth and poor functional development of certain tissues.

Table 1.1 Concentration of Various Drugs in Maternal Blood and Breast Milk under Normal pH Conditions

Drug Levels (Units/100 ML)			
Drug Administered (Therapeutic Dosage)	**Plasma or Serum (pH 7.4)**	**Milk (pH 7.0)**	**Administered Drug Appearing in Milk (%day)**
Aspirin	1-5 mg	1-3 mg	0.5
Bishydroxycourmarin	11-16.5 mg	0.2 mg	0.5
Chloral hydrate	0-3 mg	0-1.5 mg	0.6
Chloramphenicol	2.5-5 mg	1.5-2.5 mg	1.3
Chlorpromazine	0.1 mg	0.03 mg	0.07
Colistin Sulfate	0.3-0.5 mg	0.05-0.09 mg	0.07
Cycloserine	1.5-2 mg	1-1.5 mg	0.6
Diphenylhydantoin	0.3-4.5 mg	0.6-1.8 mg	1.4
Erythromycin	0.1-0.2 mg	0.3-0.5 mg	0.1
Ethanol	50-80 mg	50-80 mg	0.25
Ethyl biscoumacetate	2.7-14.5 mg	0-0.17 mg	0.1
Folic acid	3 µg	0.07 µg	0.1
Imipramine hydrochloride	0.2-1.3 mg	0.1 mg	0.1
Iodine 131	0.002 µc	0.13 µc	2-5
Isoniazid	0.6-1.2 mg	0.6-1.2 mg	0.75
Kanamycin sulfate	0.5-3.5 mg	0.2 mg	0.05
Lincomycin	0.3-1.5 mg	0.05-0.2 mg	0.025
Lithium carbonate	0.2-1.1 mg	0.07-0.4 mg	0.12
Meperidine hydrochloride	0.07-0.1 mg	Trace (<0.1 mg)	<0.1
Methotrexate	3 µg	0.3 µg	0.01
Nalidixic acid	3-5 mg	0.4 mg	0.05
Novobiocin	1.2-5.2 mg	0.3-0.5 mg	0.15
Penicillin	6-120 µg	1.2-3.6 µg	0.03
Phenobarbital	0.6-1.8 mg	0.1-0.5 mg	1.5
Phenylbutazone	2-5 mg	0.2-0.6 mg	0.4
Pyrilamine maleate	-	0.2 mg	0.6
Pyrimethamine	0.7-1.5 mg	0.3 mg	0.3
Quinine sulfate	0.7 mg	0.1 mg	0.05
Rifampicin	0.5 mg	0.1-0.3 mg	0.05
Streptomycin sulfate	2-3 mg	1-3 mg	0.5
Sulfapyridine	3-13 mg	3-13 mg	0.12
Tetracycline hydrochloride	80-320 µg	50-260 µg	0.03
Thiouracil	3-4 mg	9-12 mg	5

Table 1.2 Drugs whose Dosage Regimen should be Changed in Various Degrees of Renal Impartment

Mild Impairment	Moderate Impairment	Severe Impairment
Acetohexamide	Acetazolamide	Acetaminophen*
Cefazolin	Acetasalicycic acid	Acetazolamide*
Chlorpropamide	Acetohexamide *	Amphotericin B
Clofibrate	Allopurinol	Azathioprine
Colistimethate	Aminosalicylic ac id *	Cephalexin
Gentamicin	Amoxicillin	Cephalothin
Kanamycin	Ampicillin	Colchicine
Methadone	Carbenicillin	Digitoxin
Streptomycin	Chlordiazepoxide	Diphenhydramine
Tetracycline	Chlorpropamide*	Fthaccrynic acid*
Vancomycin	Cyctophosphamide	Glutethimide
	Digoxin	Hydralazine
	Ethambutol	Lincomycin
	Flucytosine	Methicillin
	Gertamicin	Neostigmine
	Gold sodium thiromalate*	Nitrofurantoin
	Guanethidine	Penicillin G
	Insulin	Phenformin*
	Lithium carbonate*	Phenobarbital
	Meprobamate	Quinine
	Mercurials*	Spironolactone*
	Methenamine mandalate*	Sulfamethoxazole-trimethoprim *
	Methotrexate	Thiazides*
	Methyldopa	Triamterene*
	Minocyc line	Tolbutamide
	Neomycin	
	Ouabain	
	Penicillamine	
	Pentamidine	
	Phenazopyridine	
	Phenylbutazone*	
	Primidone	
	Phenothiazines	
	Probenecid*	
	Procainamide	
	Propylthiouracil	
	Sultamethoxazole-trimethoprim	
	Sulfisoxazole	
	Trimethadone	

Table 1.3 Potential Bioequivalency Problems of Some Drugs

Acetazoiamide	Hydrochlorothiazide	Promethazine
Acetyldigitoxin	Hydroflumethiazide	Propylthiouracil
Alseroxylon	Imipramine	Pyrimethamine
Aminophyllin	Isoproterenol	Quinethiazide
Aminosalicylic acid	Liothyronine	Quinidine
Bendroflumethiazide	Menadione	Rauwolfia serpentin
Benzthiazide	Mephenytoin	Rescinnamine
Betamethasone	Methazolamide	Reserpine
Bishydroxycoumarin	Methyclothiazide	Salicylazosulfapyridine
Chlorambucil	Methylprednisolone	Sodium sulfoxone
Chlorodiazepoxide	Methyltestosterone	Spironolactone
Chlorothiazide	Nitrofurantoin	Sulfadiazine
Chloropromazine	Oxtriphylline	Sulfadimethoxine
Cortisone acetate	Para-aminosalicylic acid	Sulfamerazine
Deserpidine	Para-methadione	Sulfaphenazole
Dexamethasone	Perphenazine	Sulfasomidine
Dichlorphenamide	Phenacemide	Sulfasoxazole
Dienestrol	Phensuximide	Theophylline
Diethylstilbestrol	Phenylaminosalicylate	Thioridazine
Dyphylline	Phenytoin	Tolbutamide
Ethinyloestradiol	Phytonadione	Triamcinolone
Ethosuximide	Polythiazide	Trichlormethiazide
Ethotoin	Prednisolone	Triethyl melamine
Ethoxzolamide	Primidone	Trifluoperazine
Fludrocortisone	Probenecid	Triflupromazine
Fluphenazine	Procainamide	Trimeprazine
Fluprednisolone	Prochlorperazine	Trimethadione
Hydralazine	Promazine	Uracil mustard Warfarin

CLINICAL DATA

Drugs	Dose mg/day	Therapeutic cons. mg/L	Penetration to CNS	Lactation	T ½ in Renal Failure	T ½ in Hepatic Failure	Risk in Pregnancy
Abacavir (Nucleoside reverse transcriptase inhibitor, Antiviral)	600	2.3-2.9 µg/dl	High	CI	0.8-1.5	-	CI
Abciximab (Platelet aggregation inhibitor)	10 mcg/min for 12 hrs.			CI			CI
Acarbose (Antidiabetic)	50 mg t.i.d	-	-	CI	-	-	CI
Acebutolol (β-adrenoreceptor antagonist)	400	0.2-2	Low	>1	+	0	3
Aceclofenac (Antiinflammatory)							
Acedapsone (Antileprotic)	300 mg			CI			CI
Acetazolamide (Antiepileptic)	250-1000	10-15		CI	Avoid		SP
Acetohexamide (Antidiabetic)	250-1500	20-60					
Acetylcysteine (Mucolytic agent)	600	0.4-4					
Acrosoxacin (Quinolone antibiotic)	300						SP
Actinomycin (Antineoplastic)	1000	10-12	0				
Acyclovir (Antiviral)	1000-2000	10		CI	+		CI
Adrenaline (Sympathomimetic)	0.5 iv.im 0.2-0.5 sc	0.4-4					
Albendazole (Anthelmintic)	400-800	1	0.4	CI			P, CI

Drugs	Dose mg/day	Therapeutic cons. mg/L	Penetration to CNS	Lactation	T ½ in Renal Failure	T ½ in Hepatic Failure	Risk in Pregnancy
Alfentanil (Anaesthetic)	0.03/kg iv				+		
Alfuzosin (Urogential, Antispasmodic)	10		-	CI	3-5		CI
Allopurinol (Antigout)	100-900	1.4-2.6		SP	+		SP
Alphaxalone (General anaesthetic)	IV				+		
Alprazolam (Anxiolytic)	0.75-1.5	0.01-0.02		CI	0	+	3.CI
Alprenolol (β-adrenoreceptor Antagonist)	100	0.05-0.1	High	CI	0	+	3
Amantadine (Antiviral)	100-400	0.1-1.0	+	CI	+	SP	CI
Amidopyrine (Analgesic)							SP
Amifloxacin (Quinolone antibiotic)	2400	8			+		CI
Amikacin (Antibacterial)	1000 im/iv	15-25		CI	+		2,3, SP
Amiloride (Diuretic)	10-20				Avoid		2,3
Aminocaproic acid (Anticoagulant)	12000-18000	100-400					
Aminoglutethimide (Antineoplastic)	upto 1000						
Amiodarone (Antiarrhythmic)	600-12000	0.5-2.5	Low	CI	0		2,3
Amitriptyline (Tricyclic antidepressant)	50-100	0.1-0.2		(CI)	0		SP

Drugs	Dose mg/day	Therapeutic cons. mg/L	Penetration to CNS	Lactation	T ½ in Renal Failure	T ½ in Hepatic Failure	Risk in Pregnancy
Amlodipine (Calcium channel blocker)	5-10			(SP)			CI
Amodiaquine (Anti protozoal)	1200	0.3-0.7					SP
Amoxicillin (Antibacterial)	80-90 MG		High	COMPATIBLE	0.7-1.4 HRS		B
Amoxycillin (Antimicrobial)	750-1000	6-15	+	(SP)	+		SP
Amphotericin B (Antifungal)	2.5 MG/KG		LESS	CI	<24HRS		B
Amphotericin (Antifungal)	800	CI		(CI)			SP
Ampicillin (Antibacterial)	250-500 MG EVERY 6HRS		HIGH	C	1-1.8HRS		B
Ampicillin (Antibiotic)	1000-8000	7-14	+	(CI)	+		SP
Amrinone (Inotropic agent)	10 mg/kg			(SP)			SP
Amsacrine (Antineoplastic)	90-120/ sq.m						
Amylobarbitone (Barbiturate)	100-200	2-12	+			+	CI
Androgen (Hormone)	90 mg		high	CI	10-100 mins		X
Antipyrine (Anti inflammatory & decongestant. drug)	10 mg/kg iv					+	
Aspirin (NSAID, Antiplatelet, Anticoagulant, Fibrinolytic)	75-300	150-300 SA		(CI)	+		CI
Astemizole (Antiallergic)	10		Low	(CI)			P, CI

Drugs	Dose mg/day	Therapeutic cons. mg/L	Penetration to CNS	Lactation	T ½ in Renal Failure	T ½ in Hepatic Failure	Risk in Pregnancy
Atenolol (β-adrenoreceptor antagonist)	50-100	0.2-0.6	Low	(CI)	+	0	3, SP
Atracurium (Non-depolarizing neuromuscular blocker)	400-500 µg/kg iv			SP	+		SP
Atropine (Antispasmodic)	0.6-1.2 mg iv	0.003		SP			SP
Aurothiomalate (Antigout)	50/week im	3-5		Avoid	Avoid		CI
Azapropazone (Antiinflammatory)	600-1200	34-54		SP	+	+	SP
Azathioprine (Antineoplastic)	1-5/kg	0.05-0.08		CI	+		CI
Azelastin (Antiinflammatory, Antiallergy)	8	0.01		SP			SP
Azlocillin (Antibiotic)	2000-6000 iv			SP			
Aztreonam (Antibacterial)	< 4000 im, iv	5-10	+	SP	+	+	CI
Bacampicillin (Antibacterial)	800-2400						
Baclofen (Anaesthetic/neuro muscular blocker)	15-60		Low	CI			P
Bacmecillinam (Antibiotic)	1200-1600	2-4					
Bamethan (Calcium antagonist)	100	0.04-0.12					
Beclomethasone (Corticosteroid)	200 MCG	0.025%					

Drugs	Dose mg/day	Therapeutic cons. mg/L	Penetration to CNS	Lactation	T ½ in Renal Failure	T ½ in Hepatic Failure	Risk in Pregnancy
Bedomethasone (Corticosteroid)	0.3-0.4 inhale			(Cl)			P
Bendrofluazide (Diuretic)	5-10	0.07-0.1					3
Benorylate (Analgesic)	4000-8000	120 SA			+		SP
Benoxaprofen (Antiinflammatory)	100	4				+	
Benperidol (Antipsychotic)	0.25-1.5						SP
Benzylpenicillin (Antibacterial)	0.51 MCG	3-6 MCG	Low		30MINS		
Benzylpenicillin (Antibiotic)	600-2400	12		SP	+		
Betahistine (Antiemetic, Antivertigo)	24-48			(SP)			SP
Betamethasone (Corticosteroid)	0.5-5			(SP)			SP
Betaxolol (β-adrenoreceptor antagonist)	10-40	0.005-0.02		(SP)	0	0	3, CI
Bethanidine (Antihypertensive)	30-200	0.02-0.5					3
Bevantolol (β-adrenoreceptor antagonist)	200-400				+	0	3
Bezafibrate (Lipid lowering agent)	600				+		CI
Bifonazole (Antifungal)	1%tropical						
Biperiden (Antiparkinson)	2-6	0.004-0.006					

Drugs	Dose mg/day	Therapeutic cons. mg/L	Penetration to CNS	Lactation	T ½ in Renal Failure	T ½ in Hepatic Failure	Risk in Pregnancy
Bisoprolol (β-adrenoreceptor antagonist)	5-10			(SP)			CI
Bleomycin (Antineoplastic)	10-60/w	0.15	0	(CI)	+		P
Bopindolol (β-adrenoreceptor antagonist)	1-2	0.006				+	
Bretylium (Antiarrhythmic)	15.0/kg im	1-2			+		
Bromazepam (Anxiolytic)	3-18	0.1-0.2					3
Bromhexine Mucolytic agent)	24-64	0.01-0.14					
Bromocriptine (Antiparkinson)	10-40	0.001-0.004		CI	0		CI
Brompheniramine (Antiallergic)	12-32	0.012-0.017					
Budesonide (Corticosteroid)	100-200 µg inhalation/day			SP			SP
Bufuralo (β-adrenoreceptor antagonist)	30-60	0.01-0.1					3
Bumetanide (Cardiovuscular agent)	1-2	0.03		SP			SP
Bupivacaine (Anaesthetic)	150 epidural	1-2		CI			SP
Buprenorphine (Opioid analgesic/ antimigraine)	600-1200 µg	0.0005-0.0009		SP			SP
Bupropion (Antidepressant, Smoking cessation aid)	150-300	141± 19 ng/dl	Yes	-	11±1		SP

Drugs	Dose mg/day	Therapeutic cons. mg/L	Penetration to CNS	Lactation	T ½ in Renal Failure	T ½ in Hepatic Failure	Risk in Pregnancy
Buserelin (Hormone)	<2 nasal	0.1		SP			
Busulphan (Antineoplastic)	2-4	0.05-0.08		CI	0		CI
Butobarbitone (Barbituratesc)	100-200	2-15					CI
Butriptyline (Antidepressant)	75-150	0.024-0.11					CI
Cadralazine (Antihypertensive)	30	0.25					
Caffeine (CNS stimulant)				CI, avoid			
Capecitabine (Antineoplastic)	2.5 g/m²	6.6 ± 6 µg/dl	Low	CI	1.3		CI
Capreomycin (Antitubercular)	20 mg/kg im	30		SP			SP
Captopril (Antihypertensive)	25-100	0.15		SP			P, CI
Carbamazepine (Antiepileptic)	800-1200	4-12		SP	+		CI
Carbenicillin (Antibiotic)	1000-2000 im	50		(CI)	+	+	
Carbenoxolone (Antiulcer)	100-300						
Carbimazole (Thyroid agent)	30-60	0.5-3.4		SP			SP
Carbocisteine (Mucolytic)	1500	8					
Carboplatin (Antineoplastic)	400/sq.m			CI	+		P,CI
Carisoprodol (Skeletal muscle relaxant)		10-30		CI			SP

Drugs	Dose mg/day	Therapeutic cons. mg/L	Penetration to CNS	Lactation	T ½ in Renal Failure	T ½ in Hepatic Failure	Risk in Pregnancy
Carmustine (Antineoplastic)	200/sq.m		Good				
Carprofen (Antiinflammatory)	50-100						
Carteolol (β-adrenoreceptor antagonist)	15-30	0.005-0.01					3
Cefaclor (Antibacterial)	1000-4000	10-15		SP	+		SP
Cefadroxil (Antibacterial)	1000-2000			SP	+		SP
Cefapirin (Antibacterial)	1000 im	16-24		SP	+		
Cefazaflur (Antibacterial)	1000 im	25					
Cefazedone (Antibacterial)	6000 im						
Cefbuperazone (Antibacterial)	1000 iv						
Cefixime (Antibacterial)	400	1-2		SP	+		SP
Cefmenoxime (Antibacterial)	1000-4000 im				+		
Cefmetazole (Antibacterial)	30 mg/kg.im	90			+		
Cefonicid (Antibacterial)	1000 im	67-126					
Cefoperazone (Antibacterial)	1000-2000 im	65-97		SP		+	SP
Ceforanide (Antibacterial)	500-1000 im	38-70			+		
Cefotaxime (Antibacterial)	<1200 im	12-25	*+	SP	+		SP

Drugs	Dose mg/day	Therapeutic cons. mg/L	Penetration to CNS	Lactation	T ½ in Renal Failure	T ½ in Hepatic Failure	Risk in Pregnancy
Cefotetan (Antibacterial)	1000-2000 im	65-90		SP			
Cefoxitin (Antibacterial)	<1200 im	30		SP	<0.05	+	
Cefpodoxime (Antibacterial)	100-800	1-3		SP			SP
Cefroxadine (Antibacterial)	1000 iv	01					
Cefsulodin (Antibacterial)	1000-4000 im				+		
Cefsumide (Antibacterial)							
Ceftazidime (Antibacterial)	3000-4000 im		*+		+		
Ceftizoxime (Antibacterial)	1000-8000 im	40-160	0.2	SP	+		SP
Cefuroxime (Antibacterial)	1000-3000 im		*+	SP	+		SP
Celiprolol (β-adrenoreceptor antagonist)	600	0.05-0.4			+	0	3
Cephacetrile (Antibacterial)						3	
Cephalexin (Antibacterial)	1000-2000	6-50		(Cl)	+		P, (Cl)
Cephaloridine (Antibacterial)		0.1-15		SP			SP
Cephalothin (Antibacterial)	<12000 iv				+		
Cephamandole (Antibacterial)	<12000 iv	0.5-5	*+		+		
Cephazolin (Antibacterial)	<4000 im, iv	0.1-50		SP	+		SP

Drugs	Dose mg/day	Therapeutic cons. mg/L	Penetration to CNS	Lactation	T ½ in Renal Failure	T ½ in Hepatic Failure	Risk in Pregnancy
Cephradine (Antibacterial)	1000-4000	0.5-10	*+	SP	+		
Chloral hydrate (Hypnotic)	500-2000	Hydrolyses					CI
Chlorambucil (Antineoplastic)	0.03-0.1/kg			CI			CI
Chloramphenicol (Antibacterial)	2000	10-20	+	CI	0	+	CI
Chlormethiazole (Hypnotic)	320-800 iv	0.1-2.8				+	
Chlormezanone (Hypnotic)	600-800	2.5-3.4		SP			SP
Chloroquine (Antimalarial)	500/week	0.02-0.2		CI	+		CI
Chloroquine (Antimalarial)	Topical	0.3-1.3					
Chlorothiazide (Diuretic)	500-2000	0.5-1.4					3
Chlorpheniramine (Antiallergic)	12-16	0.01-0.23		SP	0		SP
Chlorpromazine (Antipsychotic/Anti nausea/antivertigo)	40-150	0.002-0.12	+	CI	0	0	3, SP
Chlorpropamide (Antidiabetic)	100-500	30-250		SP			SP
Chlorprothixine (Antipsychotic)	60-200	0.01					SIP
Chlortetracycline (Antibacterial)	1000-2000						CI
Chlorthalidone (Diuretic)	25-50	0.2-1.4			CI		3, CI
Ciclacillin (Antbiotic)	1000-2000				+		

Drugs	Dose mg/day	Therapeutic cons. mg/L	Penetration to CNS	Lactation	T ½ in Renal Failure	T ½ in Hepatic Failure	Risk in Pregnancy
Cilazapril (Antihypertensive)	2.5	0.-04			+	+	
Cimetidine (H_2 antagonist)	800	0.26-0.80	0.2	CI	+	+	P, (CI)
Cinnarizine (Antivertigo)	90-225	0.0.8		SP			SP
Cinoxacin (Antibiotic)	1000	15			+		CI
Ciprofloxacin (Antibiotic)	500-1500	2-3	Low	CI	0	+	CI
Cisplatin (Antineoplastic)	<120 sq.m/4w		0	CI	+		CI
Clavulanic acid (Antibacterial)		2-3					
Clemastine (Respiratory agent)	2	0.002		CI			SP
Clindamycin (Antibiotic)	600-1200	0.5		SP		+	SP
Clobazam (Antiepileptic)	20-30	0.3-0.5		CI			3 P - (CI)
Clofazimine (Antileprotic)	50-300	0.1	+	CI			P, (CI)
Clofibrate (Lipid lowering agent)	100-1500	100			+		CI
Clomipramine (Antidepressant)	30-150	0.1-0.5		SP			SP
Clomocycline (Antibiotic)	510-1360	1-2					CI
Clonazepam (Anticonvulsant)	4-8	0.01-0.07		SP	0		SP
Clonidine (Antihypertensive)	0.1	0.001-0.004		CI			CI

Drugs	Dose mg/day	Therapeutic cons. mg/L	Penetration to CNS	Lactation	T ½ in Renal Failure	T ½ in Hepatic Failure	Risk in Pregnancy
Cloxacillin (Antibiotic)	2000	7-14	+	SP	0		SP
Clozapine (Antiepileptic/ Antipsychotic)	100-500	0.1-1		CI			CI
Codeine (Analgesic)	120-240, 42-360	0.11-0.23		CI	0		Avoid
Colaspase (Antineoplastic)	100 µg/kg.iv						
Colchicine (Antigout)	1-10	0.0003-0.0024		SP	+	-	CI
Colistin (Antibacterial/GI antiinfective)	6 mega-units	1-5	0	CI	+		CI
Cortisone (Corticosteroid)	25-50					0	SP
Cycloserin (Antitubercular)	25-1000	22-34	+	CI	Avoid		SP
Cyclosporin (Immunosuppressant agent)	14-18/kg			CI	0	+	P, (CI)
Cydobarbitone (Barbiturates)	100-400	2-10					CI
Cydophosphamide (Antineoplastic)	2-6/kg	1-6	0.5	CI	+		CI
Cyproheptadine (Appetite stimulant/ Antiallergy)	32			CI			SP
Cyproterone (Hormone)	100	0.1-0.15					CI
Cytarabin (Antineoplastic)	2-4/kg	0.05-0.1	+	CI	0		CI

Drugs	Dose mg/day	Therapeutic cons. mg/L	Penetration to CNS	Lactation	T ½ in Renal Failure	T ½ in Hepatic Failure	Risk in Pregnancy
Dacarbazine (Antineoplastic)	2-5/kg		Low	SP			SP
Danazol (Hormone)	200-400			CI			P, CI
Dapsone (Antileprotic)	200/week			SP			SP
Daunorubicin (Antineoplastic)	30-60/sq.m		0	CI			P, (CI)
Debrisoquine (Antihypertensive)	10-120	0.02-0.18					3
Demeclocycline (Antibiotic)	600	2-3		CI			P, CI
Desipramine (Antidepressant)	75-200	0.02-0.88			0		CI
Dexamethasone (Corticosteroid)	0.5-9			SP			SP
Dexamphetamine (CNS stimulant)	10-60	<0.1		Avoid			
Dextromethorphan (Antitussive)	40-50	0.001-0.008			+	+	3
Dextropropoxyphene (Respiratory agent)	260	0.05-0.75		CI	+	+	P, (CI)
Dezocine (Analgesic)	5-20 iv	0.005-0.02					
Diamorphine (Analgesic)	5-60 sc	Metabolized to Morpphine					
Diazepam (Sedative)	10-30 iv	0.1-2.5	Yes	CI	0	+	3 P-(CI)
Diazoxide (Antihypertensive)	300-900	15-50					
Diclofenac (Antiinflammatory)	75-150	0.8-2		CI	0		P, (CI)

Drugs	Dose mg/day	Therapeutic cons. mg/L	Penetration to CNS	Lactation	T ½ in Renal Failure	T ½ in Hepatic Failure	Risk in Pregnancy
Dicloxacillin (Antibiotic)	500	10-18			0		
Dicyclomine (Antispasmodic)	30-60						1
Didanosine (Antiviral)	400	1.5 ± 0.7 μg/dl	-	CI	1.4 ± 0.3		SP
Diethylpropion (Monoamineoxidase inhibitor)	75	0.007					
Diflunisal (Analgesic)	500-1000	66-183	Low		+		SP
Digitoxin (Cardiac glycoside)	500-1000	0.3-1.3					CI
Digoxin (Cardiac glycoside)	1-1.5	0.001-0.002		CI	+		P, (CI)
Dihydralazine (Antihypertensive)	150						
Dihydrocodeine (Analgesic)	120-180	0.07-0.15					SIP
Dihydroergotamine (Antimigraine)	3 im	0.0002-0.001		CI	+ (CI)	+ (CI)	P - CI
Dilevalol (β-adrenoreceptor antagonist)	4000	0.02					
Dilevalol (β-adrenoreceptor antagonist)	4000	0.02					
Diltiazem (Calcium antagonist)	180-360			CI	0	+ (SP)	P - CI
Diltiazem (Calciumchannel antagonist)	180-360			CI	0	+ (SP)	P - CI
Diphenylpyraline (Respiratory agent)	10-20						

Drugs	Dose mg/day	Therapeutic cons. mg/L	Penetration to CNS	Lactation	T ½ in Renal Failure	T ½ in Hepatic Failure	Risk in Pregnancy
Diphenylpyraline (Sedative antihistaminic)	10-20						
Dipyridamole (Anticoagulant)	300-800	0.1-1.5		CI			P (CI)
Dipyridamole (Anticoagulant)	300-800	0.1-1.5		CI			P (CI)
Dipyridamole (Anticoagulant)	300-800	0.1-1.5		CI			P (CI)
Distigmine (Acetylcholinesterage inhibitor)	20						
Distigmine (Misc Drug)	20						
Distigmine (Vasodilator)	20						
Disulfiram (Antabuse)	100-200	0.4		CI	+ (SP)	+ (SP)	P - CI
Dobutamine (Adrenergic Agonist)	iv infusion						P (CI)
Dobutamine (Cerebral vasodilator)	iv infusion						P (CI)
Dobutamine (Sympathomimetic)	iv infusion						P (CI)
Domperidon (Antiemetic)	40-120	0.04		SP	0.25	+ (SP)	P - CI
Domperidon (Antinausea/antivertigo)	40-120	0.04		SP	0.25	+ (SP)	P - CI
Dopamine (Sympathomimetic)	iv infusion						P, (CI)
Dopexamine (Adrenergic Agonist)	0.18/kg inf	100					

Drugs	Dose mg/day	Therapeutic cons. mg/L	Penetration to CNS	Lactation	T ½ in Renal Failure	T ½ in Hepatic Failure	Risk in Pregnancy
Dopexamine (Vasodilator Drug)	0.18/kg inf	100					
Dothiepin (Antidepressant)	75-150	0.02-0.06		CI			P, CI
Doxapram (Respiratory agent)	20				+ (SP)	+ (SP)	P, (CI)
Doxazosin (Antihypertensive)	8-16	0.008		CI	+ (SP)	+ (SP)	P, (CI)
Doxepin (Antidepressant)	30-300	0.05-0.15		CI	0		P, (CI)
Doxorubicin (Antineoplastic)	20-30/sq.m	0.01		CI	+	+	P, (CI)
Doxycycline (Antibiotic)	50-100	1.5-3		CI	0	+ (CI)	P, CI
Droperidol (Antipsychotic)	30-120			SP	+ (SP)	+ (SP)	SP
d-Tubocurarine Skeletal muscle relaxant)		0.6-1.2			+		
Dihydrogesterone (Hormone)	20-30			SP	+ (SP)	+ (SP)	CI
Edrophonium (Anticholinesterase)	10 mg/ml iv	<0.15					
Enalapril (Antihypertensive)	5-40	0.04		CI		+ (SP)	P, CI
Encainide (Antiarrhythmic)	75-200	0.02			+	+	
Enoxacin (Antibiotic)	200-600	1-4			+		CI
Epirubicin (Antineoplastic)	70-90/sq.m			CI	+ (SP)	+CI	CI

Drugs	Dose mg/day	Therapeutic cons. mg/L	Penetration to CNS	Lactation	T ½ in Renal Failure	T ½ in Hepatic Failure	Risk in Pregnancy
Ergotamine (Antimigraine)	6	0.0001-0.001		CI	+ (CI)	+ (CI)	P - CI
Erythromycin (Antibiotic)	1000-4000	2-6		(C/I)	+ (SP)	+	P (CI)
Esmolol (β-adrenoreceptor antagonist)	0.3/kg/min	2		CI	+ (SP)		P, (C)
Estramustine (Antineoplastic)	560-1120						
Ethacrynic acid (Cardiovascular agent)	50-150					Avoid	P, (CI)
Ethacrynic acid (Diuretic)	50-150					Avoid	P, (CI)
Ethambutol (Antitubercular)	1200-1800	3-6	+	CI	+	Perform liver tests regularly	P, (CI)
Ethanol (Alcohol)		1000		SP			
Ethosuximide (Antiepileptic)	500-2000	40-100		Avoid			1
Etidocaine (Anaesthetic)	400 infit	1-1.5					
Etintidine (Antispasmodic)	300	2.1					
Etomidate (Anaesthetic)	0.3/kg iv						
Etoposide (Antineoplastic)	50-100/sq.m	1-20	+	CI	+	0	P, CI
Famotidine (H$_2$ antagonist)	20-40	0.01-0.1	<0.1	-2 (CI)	+	+ (SP)	P, (CI)
Felodipine (Calcium antagonist)	10-20	0.002-0.01		CI	+ (SP)	+ (SP)	P, CI

Drugs	Dose mg/day	Therapeutic cons. mg/L	Penetration to CNS	Lactation	T ½ in Renal Failure	T ½ in Hepatic Failure	Risk in Pregnancy
Fenbufen (Antiinflammatory)	600-900	8		SP			SP
Fenfluramine (Monoamineoxidase inhibitor)	60-120	0.05-0.15	+				
Fenoprofen (Antiinflammatory)	600-2400	20-30					SP
Fenoterol (Respiratory agent)	0.2-0.4 inhale						
Fentanyl (Anaesthetic)	0.05/kg iv			(CI)	+ (SP)	+ (SP)	P, (CI)
Flecainide (Antiarrhythemic)	200-400	0.12-0.80			+		
Floxuridine (Antineoplastic)	< 30 I kg		+				
Flucloxacillin (Antibiotic)	1000-2000	5-15			+		
Fluconazole (Antifungal)				Avoid			P, CI
Flucytosine (Antifungal)	2000	30-40			+		CI
Fludrocortisone (Corticosteroid)	0.1-0.3			SP			SP
Flufenamic acid (Antiinflammatory)	600						SP
Flumazenil (Benzodiazepine antagonist)	2 iv	0.05					
Flunitrazepam (Hypnotic)	1-2	0.01		Low		0	
Fluorouracil (Antineoplastic)	12/kg iv				0		

Drugs	Dose mg/day	Therapeutic cons. mg/L	Penetration to CNS	Lactation	T ½ in Renal Failure	T ½ in Hepatic Failure	Risk in Pregnancy
Flupenthixol (Antipsychotic)	6-18			CI			SP
Fluphenazine (Antipsychotic)	2.5-10	0.0002-0.004		CI			P, (CI)
Flurazepam (Anxiolytic)	15-30	0.06 met		CI	0		P, (CI)
Flurbiprofen (NSAID)	150-300	9-17		CI			P, (CI)
Fluspirilene (Antipsychotic)	2 im						SP
Flutamide (Antineoplastic)	750	0.05-0.18		CI			P, (CI) 3
Foscarnet (Antiviral)	0.1/kg/min						
Fosfomycin (Antibiotic)	2500	40					
Frusemide (Diuretic)	20-80	1.8-5.0		SP	+	+	SP
Fusidic acid (Antifungal)	1500	30	0	SP	0		SP
Gallopamil (Calcium antagonist)	100						
Ganciclovir (Antiviral)	5-10 /kg iv	20-45 µmol/l	0.7	CI			CI
Gemfibrozil (Antilipid drug)	300-200			CI	0		CI
Gentamicin (Antibiotic)	140-350 l m	4-10	Low	SP	+		P, (CI) 2,3
Glibenclamide (Antidiabetic)	5-15	0.17-0.36		CI			P, CI
Gliclazide (Antidiabetic)	40-320	0.7-4.9		CI			P, CI

Drugs	Dose mg/day	Therapeutic cons. mg/L	Penetration to CNS	Lactation	T ½ in Renal Failure	T ½ in Hepatic Failure	Risk in Pregnancy
Glipizide (Antidiabetic)	2.5-30			CI			P, CI
Gliquidone (Antidiabetic)	15-180						
Glutethimide (Anaesthetic)		0.2-0.8					
Glyceryltrinitrate (Antianginal)	0.3-1 sublingual	0.001-0.002		SP			SP
Glycopyrronium (Antispasmodic)	3-12			SP			SP
Glymidine (Antidiabetic)	500-2000						
Goserelin (Hormone)	0.1 sc	0.001		CI	+		CI
Guanabenz (Antihypertensive)	16-32	0.002-0.003					
Guanadrel (Antihypertensive)	400						
Guanethidine (Antihypertensive)	20-100						
Guaniacine (Antihypertensive)	2-4						
Haloperidol (Antipsychotic)	1.5-20	0.0008-0.033		CI	0		SP
Hydralazine (Antihypertensive)	50-100	0.1-0.2			+		1,2
Hydrochlorothiazide (Diuretic)	25-200	0.05-0.15		CI	Avoid		CI
Hydrocortisone (Corticosteroid)	10-30			SP		+	SP

Drugs	Dose mg/day	Therapeutic cons. mg/L	Penetration to CNS	Lactation	T ½ in Renal Failure	T ½ in Hepatic Failure	Risk in Pregnancy
Hydroflumethiazide (Diuretic)	25-50	0.17-0.6					3
Hydroxy progesterone (Hormone)	<5001 week im			CI			CI
Hydroxychloroquine (DMARD)	1200	0.003-0.2		CI	+		SP
Hydroxyurea (Antineoplastic)	20-30 /kg			CI	+		P/CI
Hydroxizine (Anxiolytic)	200-400	0.07-0.09		CI			P, CI
Hyoscine (Antinausea/ Antispasmodic)	80			SP			SP
Ibuprofen (Antiinflammatory)	600-2400	20-30		SP	0	0	SP
Idoxuridine (Antiviral)	0.1% topical						
Ifosfamide (Antineoplastic)	<6000 I sq.m			CI			P, CI
Imipramine (Antidepressant)	75-2000	0.01-0.11		SP	0		SP
Indapamide (Diuretic/ Antihypertensive)	2.5	0.02-0.05		CI			P, (CI) 3
Indomethacin (Antiinflammatory)	50-200	0.3-0.6	+	SP	0		P, CI
Indoramin (Antihypertensive)	50-200	0.08-0.22					
Insulin (Hormone)	<80 units im						SP
Ipratropium (Anticholinergic)	0.04 inhale			CI			P, (CI)

Drugs	Dose mg/day	Therapeutic cons. mg/L	Penetration to CNS	Lactation	T ½ in Renal Failure	T ½ in Hepatic Failure	Risk in Pregnancy
Iproniazid (Monoaminoxidase inhibitor)	25-150						P, (CI)
Isocarboxazid (Monoaminoxidase inhibitor)	10-30						
Isoniazid (Antitubercular)	<200	3-10		SP	0	+	SP
Isoprenaline (Sympathomimetic)	5-40/day						
Isosorbide dinitrate (Antianginal)	30-240	0.02-0.1		CI			P, (CI)
Isosorbide-mononitrate (Antianginal)	20-120	0.34-0.68		CI			P, (CI)
Isoxsuprine (Vasodilator)	10-80						P, (CI)
Isradipine (Calcium channel blocker)	2.5-10				+	+	C
Itraconazole (Antifungal)	100-400	0.5 µg/ml		CI	0	0	P, CI
Ivermectin (Antiparasitic)	150-200 µg/kg	38 ± 5 µg/dl	N0	CI	56 ± 7		CI
Kanamycin (Antibiotic)	1000 im	20-25	Low	CI	+		P, (CI) 2,3
Ketaconazole (Antifungal)	200-400	7		CI	0		P, CI
Ketamine (Anaesthetic)	2.0/kg iv		+				P, (CI)
Ketanserin (Antihypertensive)	40-80			CI			

Drugs	Dose mg/day	Therapeutic cons. mg/L	Penetration to CNS	Lactation	T ½ in Renal Failure	T ½ in Hepatic Failure	Risk in Pregnancy
Ketazolam (Anxiolytic)	15-60	C 0.0004					3
Ketoprofen (Antiinflammatory)	100-200	6-14		CI	+		P, (CI)
Ketorolac (Antiinflammatory)	10	0.9		CI	+	0	P, (CI)
Labetalol (β-adrenoreceptor antagonist)	200-400	0.05-0.1	Low	CI	0	+	3
Lamivudine (Antiretroviral)	300	0.8 ± 1.2 μg/ml	-	CI	9.1 ± 5		SP
Lanatoside C (Cardiotonic)	1.5-2	0.0005-0.001					
Lesuride (Dopamine agonist)		0.0001					
Levamisole (Anthelmintic)				CI			P, CI
Levobutalol (β-adrenoreceptor antagonist)	2% eye soln.	0.2-0.3		CI			P, (CI)
Levodopa (Antiparkinson)	125-1000	1		CI	0		P, (CI)
Levolorphan (Analgesic)	1-2 iv	0.02					
Lidoflazine (Calcium antagonist)	120-360	0.12		CI			P, (CI)3
Lignocaine (Local anaesthetic)	200 iv	1-6		SP	0	+	(CI)
Lincomycin (Antibacterial)	1500-2000	1-3		CI	+		(CI)
Liothyronine (Thyroid agent)	0.1	0.001-0.002					

Drugs	Dose mg/day	Therapeutic cons. mg/L	Penetration to CNS	Lactation	T ½ in Renal Failure	T ½ in Hepatic Failure	Risk in Pregnancy
Lisinopril (Antihypertensive)	10	0.04		CI			P, CI
Lithium (Antipsychotic)	250-2000	0.6-1.2 µmol/l		CI	+		(CI)
Lofepramine (Antidepressant)	140-210	C0.003		CI			
Lomefloxacin (Antibacterial)	200-800	1-2		CI	+		(CI)
Loperamide (Antispasmodic)	16	0.002		CI			(CI)
Loratidine (Antiallergic)	5-10	0.003		CI	0	0	(CI)
Lorazepam (Anxiolytic)	4 iv	0.05-0.24	<1	CI	+	+	(CI) 3
Lorcainide (Antiarrhythmic)	100-400	0.15-0.40					
Lormustine (Antineoplastic)	00-130/sq.m		+	CI			CI
Lornoxicam (Antiinflammatory)	4	0.3					
Lymecycline (Antibiotic)	300	1.4					CI
Mebendazole (Anthelmintic)	100-200			CI			CI
Mecillinam (Antibiotic)	400 im	6-12	low	SP	+		
Meclizine (Anti nausea)	75-150						SP
Medazepam (Anxiolytic)	15-30	0.14-0.26					
Medifoxamine (Antidepressant)	200-1000	0.2-1.4					

Drugs	Dose mg/day	Therapeutic cons. mg/L	Penetration to CNS	Lactation	T ½ in Renal Failure	T ½ in Hepatic Failure	Risk in Pregnancy
Medroxy progesterone (Hormone)	2.5-10			CI			P, CI
Mefenamic acid (Antiinflammatory)	500-1500	0.3-2.4		low	0		SP
Mefloquin (Antimalariall)	250/week	0.4-1		CI			P, (CI)
Mefruside (Diuretic)	25-50	0.07-0.13					
Melphalan (Antineoplastic)	0.2-0.3/kg			CI	0		P, (CI)
Mepacrine (Antineoplastic)	100						
Mepenzolate (Antispasmodic)	100-200			SP			
Mepivacaine (Anaesthetic)	<1000 infilt	0.4					
Meprobamate (Hypnotic)	1200-1600	5-20			+		3
Meptazinol (Analgesic)	600-1600	0.01-0.1					
Mepyramine (Respiratory agent)	300						
Mercaptopurine (Antineoplastic)	2.5/kg			CI		+	CI
Mesalazine (Antiinflammatory)	2400	0.1-10		SP			
Metaraminol (Cardiovascular agent)	15-100 iv						CI
Metformin (Antidiabetic)	1500-3000	0.59-1.3					
Methadone (Respiratory agent)	6-12	0.05-1		0.5	+		

Drugs	Dose mg/day	Therapeutic cons. mg/L	Penetration to CNS	Lactation	T ½ in Renal Failure	T ½ in Hepatic Failure	Risk in Pregnancy
Methaqualone (Hypnotic)	150-300			Avoid	+		
Methicillin (Antibiotic)	<12000 iv	10	Low	SP	+		
Methocarbamol (Muscle relaxant)	100 mg/ml iv, im			(CI)	+ CI	+ CI	(CI)
Methohexitone (Anaesthetic)	40 iv	2-5					
Methotrexate (Antineoplastic)	5-10-25/week		Low	P	Avoid		CI
Methotrimeprazine (Antipsychotic)	25-50	0.05-0.14					SP
Methyl phenobarbitone (Barbiturate)	100-600	2-3					CI
Methyldopa (Antihypertensive)	250-750	1-5		(CI)	+	+ SP	
Methylprednisolone (Corticosteroid)	4-48				+ SP		SP
Methyltestosterone (Hormone)	5-80	0.02-0.04					CI
Methyprylone (Barbiturate)	200-400	10-20					
Methysergide (Analgesic)	2-6	0.04					CI
Metoclopramide (Antinausea)	30	0.04-0.06		Avoid	+	+	SP
Metolazone (Antihypertensive)	2.5-10	0.01			+ SP	+ SP	3
Metoprolol (β-adrenoreceptor antagonist)	100-400	0.05-0.1	High	CI	0	0	3

Drugs	Dose mg/day	Therapeutic cons. mg/L	Penetration to CNS	Lactation	T ½ in Renal Failure	T ½ in Hepatic Failure	Risk in Pregnancy
Metronidazole (Antiprotozoal)	1000-2000	1-3		CI			(CI)
Mexiletine (Antiarrhythmic)	600-800	0.75-2.0		CI	+	+ SP	(CI)
Mezlocillin (Antibiotic)	6000-8000 iv	45	low	P	+	+	
Mianserin (Antidepressant)	30-200	0.03-0.09		CI		+ SP	P, (CI)
Miconazole (Antifungal)	1000	1		(CI)		+	(CI)
Midazolam (Anxiolytic)	2.5-7.5 iv			(CI)	0	+	(CI)
Midodrine (Antihypertensive)	40						
Minocycline (Antibiotic)	100-200	1-4	+	CI	0		P, CI
Minoxidil (Vasodilator, Hair growth promotor)	5-10			(CI)			(CI)
Misonidazole (Antineoplastic)	<5000/sq.m						
Mitomycin (Antineoplastic)	2/sq.m iv			CI	+		CI
Mitotane (Antineoplastic)	6-15/kg						
Mitoxantrone (Antineoplastic)	12/sq.m iv		0	CI			CI
Moclobemide (Monoamine oxidase inhibitor/Antidepressant)	200-600	1		CI		+	CI
Molindone (Anxiolytic)	50-100						

Drugs	Dose mg/day	Therapeutic cons. mg/L	Penetration to CNS	Lactation	T ½ in Renal Failure	T ½ in Hepatic Failure	Risk in Pregnancy
Monosialo ganglioside (Nerve growth factor)	100 iv	40					
Moricizine (Antiarrhythmic)	300-1500	0.5-1.7					
Morphine (Analgesic)	60-120	0.05		2.5 CI	+		CI
Mustine (Antineoplastic)	0.4/kg iv			(CI)			(CI)
Nabilone (Antiemetic)	2-4						SIP
Nabumetone (Antiinflammatory)	1000			(CI)	0	+	(CI)
Nadolol (β-adrenoreceptor antagonist)	80-240	0.04-0.1	Low	CI	+	0	3
Naftidrofuryl (Cerebral vasodilator)	400 iv						
Nalbuphine (Analgesic)	40-160 sc	0.015					
Nalidixic acid (Antibacterial)	2000-4000	20-50		(CI)	Avoid +		(CI)
Naproxen (Antiinflammatory)	500-000	23-51		(CI)	0	+	P,CI,SP
Natamycin (Antifungal)	7.5 inhale			(CI)			(CI)
Nefopam (Analgesic)	90-270	0.07-0.15		(CI)			P CI
Neomycin (Antibiotic)	6000	4-10		(CI)			(CI) 2,3
Neostigmine (Cholinergic drug)	75-300			(CI)	+		(CI)

Drugs	Dose mg/day	Therapeutic cons. mg/L	Penetration to CNS	Lactation	T ½ in Renal Failure	T ½ in Hepatic Failure	Risk in Pregnancy
Netilmicin (Antibiotic)	280-420 im	4		(CI)	+		(CI)
Nicardipine (Calcium antagnoist)	30-90						CI
Nicotinic acid (Anticoagulant)	300-6000	4-18		CI		+	CI
Nicoumalone (Anticoaqulant)	1-8	0.02-0.07					CI
Nifedipine (Calcium antagonist)	10-60			CI	0	+	(CI)
Nilvadipine (Calcium antagonist)	2-6						
Nimesulide (COX-2 inhibitor, NSAID)	200		-	SP			CI
Nimodipine (Calcium antagonist)	90-120	0.05	Low	CI	+	+	(CI)
Nisoldipine (Calcium antagonist)	30-60				0	+	
Nitrazepam (Hypnotic)	5-10	0.08-0.1	0.2	(CI)			(CI)
Nitrendipine (Calcium channel blocker)	40			CI	0	+	(CI)
Nitrofurantoin (Antibacterial)	300			(CI)	+	+	(CI)
Nizatidine (Antiulcer)	150-300	1-3				+	
Noradrenaline (Sympathomimetic)	Rapid iv						CI
Norethisterone (Hormone)	5-25			(CI)		+	CI

Drugs	Dose mg/day	Therapeutic cons. mg/L	Penetration to CNS	Lactation	T ½ in Renal Failure	T ½ in Hepatic Failure	Risk in Pregnancy
Norlloxacin (Antibacterial)	400	1-2		CI	+		P, CI
Nystain (Antifungal)	1.5-4 M units						(CI)
Oestradiol (Hormone)	2						CI
Ofloxacin (Antibacterial)	200-400	2-6		CI	+		P,CI
Omalizumab (Anti-IgE antibodies) **Omeprazole** (Antiulcer)	150-375 mg 2/4 weeks 20-40	1		SP	0		SP
Ondansetron (Antiemetic)				SP			SP
Orciprenaline (Respiratory agent)	80	0.002-0.01		(CI)			(CI)
Orphenadrine (Antiparkinson)	150 mg			SP			SP
Oxamniquine (Anthelmintic)	15-30/kg						
Oxazepam (Hypnotic)	45-120	0.5-2.0		(CI)	+	0	3 (CI)
Oxprenolol (β-adrenoreceptor antagonist)	80-480	0.04-0.1	High	SP	0		3
Oxybutynin (Antispasmodic)	5-10 mg			SP			SP
Oxypentifylline (Bronchodilator)	800-1200	1.5					
Oxyphenbutazone (NSAID)				(CI)			(CI)
Oxytetracycline (Antibacterial)	1000-2000	1.2-3.4		CI	+		CI

Drugs	Dose mg/day	Therapeutic cons. mg/L	Penetration to CNS	Lactation	T ½ in Renal Failure	T ½ in Hepatic Failure	Risk in Pregnancy
Pamidronate Hormones & related drugs	60-90 mg over 2-4 hours, iv	2		CI			CI
Papaverine (Anti spasmodic drug)		0.6					
Paracetamol (Analgesic & antipyretic)	2000-4000	10-20		avoid	+	+	
Paraldehyde (Antiepileptic)	5-10 ml im	30-100					
Paroxetine (Antidepressant)	20	0.008-0.05		SP			SP
PAS (Antitubercular)	12000	1-2	-	CI	-	-	-
Pefloxacin (Antibacterial)	400-1200	1-10	<1	CI	0	+	CI
Pemoline (Monoamine oxidase inhibitor)	40-120	0.8-1.2					
Penbutolol (β-adrenoreceptor antagonist)	40-80	0.05-0.2					3
Penicillamine (Antigout)	125-1500	1.7-5.6		CI	Avoid		CI
Pentaerythritol trinitrate (Antihypertensive)	40-240			SP			(CI)
Pentazocine (Analgesic)	100-300	0.05-0.2				0	SP
Pentobarbitone (Barbiturate)	100-200	1-4				0	+	
Pentoxifylline (Vasodilator)	1200	1		(CI)			(CI)

Drugs	Dose mg/day	Therapeutic cons. mg/L	Penetration to CNS	Lactation	T ½ in Renal Failure	T ½ in Hepatic Failure	Risk in Pregnancy
Pergolide (Dopamine antagonist)	Upto 5	1-2					
Pericyazine (Antipsychotic)	15-30						3
Perindopril (Antihypertensive)	4	0.06		CI			CI
Perinorm (Antiemetic agent)	100						
Perphenazine (Antipsychotic)	12	0.0003-0.025					SP
Pethidine (Analgesic)	300-900	0.2-0.8			+	+	SP
Phenelzine (Monoamine oxidase inhibitor)	45-60	0.002-0.05					
Phenindamine (Respiratory Agent)	100-200						
Phenindione (Anticoagulant)	50-150			CI			P -CI
Pheniramine (Antiallergic)	150	0.01-0.19		SP			SP
Phenobarbitone (Barbiturates)	60-180	2-30		(CI)	+		(CI)
Phenoxy Mepenicillin (Antibiotic)	500-3000	3-6					
Phentermine (Monoamineoxidase inhibitor)	15-30	0.1					
Phenylbutazone (Antiinflammatory		40-150					
Phenylephrine (Sympathomimetic)	5 im, sc	0.001					CI

Drugs	Dose mg/day	Therapeutic cons. mg/L	Penetration to CNS	Lactation	T ½ in Renal Failure	T ½ in Hepatic Failure	Risk in Pregnancy
Phenytoin (Antiepileptic/ Antiarrhythmic)	150-600	10-20		SP	0		(CI) 1,3
Pholcodine (Respiratory Agent)	60	0.02					
Pimozide (Antipsychotic)	20-60	0.004		SP			SP
Pindolol (β-adrenoreceptor (antagoinst)	15-45	0.05-0.15	Fair		+	0	3
Piperacillin (Antibiotic)	<20000 iv	30-40			+		(CI)
Piperazine (Anthelmintic)	2000			SP			(CI)
Pipothiazine (Antipsychotic)	20 depot 4w	0.018-0.058					3
Pirbuterol (Respiratory Agent)	30-60						
Piretanide (Diuretic)	6-12						3
Piroxicam (Antiinflammatory)	20-40	9-16		CI	+		CI, SP
Pirprofen (Antiiinflammatory)	1200	20-40			+		
Pivampicillin (Antibiotic)	1000-2000						
Plvmecillinam (Antibiotic)	1200-1600	5					
Pizotifen (Analgesic)	1.5						
Polymixin B (Antibacterial)	180000 units		0	SP			SP

Drugs	Dose mg/day	Therapeutic cons. mg/L	Penetration to CNS	Lactation	T ½ in Renal Failure	T ½ in Hepatic Failure	Risk in Pregnancy
Polythiazide (Diuretic)	1-4	0002-0.007					3
Practolol (β-adrenoreceptor antagonist)	5 iv	1.5-5	Fair		+		3
Prazepam (Hypnotic)	10-60	0.2-0.4					3
Praziquantel (Anthelmintic)	5-10 /kg			(CI)			(CI)
Prazosin (Antihypertensive)	1-20	0.001-0.007		SP			1, (CI)
Prednisolone (Corticosteroid)	2.5-60	0.65		SP		+	SP
Prenalterol (Cerebral Vasodilator)	5-10 iv	0.05					
Primaquine (Antiprotozoal)	15-45	0.13-0.18					(CI)
Primidone (Antiepilepic)	500-1000	5-12		(CI)	+		(CI)
Probenecid (Antigout)	500-2000	20-150		SP	Avoid		SP
Probucol (Anticoagulant)	500-1000						CI
Procainamide (Antiarrhythmic)	1000	3-12			+		
Procarbazine (Antineoplastic)	50-300		+				CI
Prochlorperazine (Antipsychotic)	25-100	0.0008		CI			CI
Procyclidine (Antiparkinson)	10-30	0.15-0.63		SP			SP
Progabide (Antiepileptic)	1800						

Drugs	Dose mg/day	Therapeutic cons. mg/L	Penetration to CNS	Lactation	T ½ in Renal Failure	T ½ in Hepatic Failure	Risk in Pregnancy
Progesterone (Hormone)	50 im			SP			CI
Promethazine (Antiemetic)	25-75	0.002-0.018		CI			(CI)
Propafenone (Antiarrhythmic)	450-900	0.4-4.0		SP			SP
Propanolol (β-adrenoreceptor antagonist)	160-320	0.05-0.1	High	(SP)	0	+	(CI) 3
Propantheline (Antispasmodic)	45			SP			SP
Propofol (General Anaesthetic)	2.5/kg	0.1		CI	0		CI
Propylthiouracil (Thyroid agent)	200-600	1.6-7.5		(CI)	+		CI
Protriptyline (Antidepressant)	15-60	0.11-0.38			0		(CI)
Pyrantel (Anthelmintic)	5-10/kg				0		(CI)
Pyrazinamide (Antitubercular)	2000-3000	134	+	(CI)			CI
Pyridostigmine (Parasympatho mimetic	300-1200	0.05-0.1		SP	+		SP
Pyrimethamine (Antiprotozoal)	25/week	0.21-0.43			0		SP
Quazepam (Hypnotic)	10-25	0.1					
Qubian (Cardiac glycoside)	1 iv	0.0005			+		
Quinaibarbitone (Barviturates)	50-100	2-10	+		0		CI

Drugs	Dose mg/day	Therapeutic cons. mg/L	Penetration to CNS	Lactation	T ½ in Renal Failure	T ½ in Hepatic Failure	Risk in Pregnancy
Quinapril (Antihypertensive)	5						
Quinidine (Antiarrhythmic/ Antimalarial)	800-1600	2-6		SP	0	+	SP
Quinine (Antimalarial)	1800	3-7	+	SP	+		CI
Ramipril (Antihypertensive)	5-20	0.001-0.005		CI	+	+	CI
Ranitidine (H_2 receptor antagonist)	300	0.31-0.82	<0.1	SP	+	+	SP
Reproterol (Respiratory Agent)	30-60						
Reserpine (Antihypertensive)	100-500 µg	0.0004-0.0006			Avoid		
Rifampicin (Antibacterial)	600	0.5-10	+	SP	0	+	SP
Rimiterol (Respiratory Agent)	0.2-0.5 inhale	0.001					
Rizatriptan (Antimigraine)	10	20 ± 4.9µg/dl	Yes	SP	2.2		SP
Rosiglitazone (Antidiabetic)	4	598 ± 117µg/dl	-	CI	3-4		CI
Roxatidine (Antiulcer)	25-150	0.1-0.80		CI			SP
Salbutamol (Bronchodilator)	6-32	0.01					SP
Salicylate (Analgesic)	20% toical						
Salsalate (Antiinflammatory)	<4000	20				+	SP

Drugs	Dose mg/day	Therapeutic cons. mg/L	Penetration to CNS	Lactation	T ½ in Renal Failure	T ½ in Hepatic Failure	Risk in Pregnancy
Secbutobarbitone (Barbiturateas)	50-100						
Selegiline (Antiparkinson)	5-10			(CI)			(CI)
Semustine (Antineoplastic)	200/sq.m				Avoid		
Sodium cromoglycate (Mast Cell stabilizer)	40-80	0.006-0.012		SP			
Sotalol (β-adrenoreceptor antagonist)	160-600	0.5-4	0.1	SP	+	0	SP
Spectinomycin (Antibacterial)	2000 im	100					
Spironolactone (K sparing diuretic)	100-400	0.2			Avoid		SP
Streptomycin (Antibacterial/ Antitubercular)	1000 im	40-50		(CI)			SP
Streptozocine (Antineoplastic)	1000/sq.m/w		0		+		
Sufentanil (General anaesthetic)	0.08/kg iv						
Sulfacetamide (Antibacterial)	60 GM			CI	7-12.8 h		C
Sulfadoxin (Antiprotozoal)	500/week						
Sulfametopyrazine (Antibacterial)	2000 weekly	0.1-0.80				0	3
Sulfaurea (Antibacterial)	3000						3
Sulindac (Antiinflammatory)	200-400	5			0	+	SP

Drugs	Dose mg/day	Therapeutic cons. mg/L	Penetration to CNS	Lactation	T ½ in Renal Failure	T ½ in Hepatic Failure	Risk in Pregnancy
Sulipride (Antipsychotic)	400-2400	0.18-0.32					SP
Sulphadiazine (Antibacterial)	6000-9000	19-40	+	(Cl)			(Cl) 3
Sulphadimidine (Antibacterial)	2000-4000	50-100			+		3,C/1
Sulphaguanidine (Antibacterial)	9000-12000	15-40					3
Sulphamethoxazole (Antibacterial)	2000-3000	28-45			+		Cl
Sulphinpyrazone (Antigout)	100-600	6-17			Avoid		SP
Sulphsalazine (Antigout/ Antiinflammatory)	1500-3000	5-45		Cl			SP
Sumatriptan (Antimigraine)	50-300			SP			SP
Sutamicillin (Antibiotic)	250						
Tacrine (Immunosuppressant)	25-50	0.01		Cl			SP
Talampicillin (Antibiotic)	750-1500						
Tamazepam (Anxiolytic)	20-40	0.9	0.05				
Tamoxifen (Antineoplastic/ Antiestrogen)	20-40			Cl			Cl
Tenoxicam (Antiinflammatory)	20	2		(Cl)			(Cl)
Terbutaline (Antiasthmatic/ Uterine relaxant	1-15	0.002-0.005		(Cl)			(Cl) 3

Drugs	Dose mg/day	Therapeutic cons. mg/L	Penetration to CNS	Lactation	T ½ in Renal Failure	T ½ in Hepatic Failure	Risk in Pregnancy
Testosterone (Androgenic hormone)	40-160 im			CI			CI
Tetrabenazine (Antiparkinson)	25-200	0.015		CI			SP
Tetracycline (Antibiotic)	1000-2000	1-5	low	CI	+		CI
Tetrahydro cannabinol (Hallucinogen)	inhale	0.05	low	CI			CI
Thalidomide (Immunomodulator)	100-300	2 ± 0.6 µg/ml	Yes	CI	6.2 ± 2.6		CI
Theophylline (Bronchodilator)	180-1000	10-15		SP	0		SP
Thiabendazole (Anthelmintic)	50/kg				0		
Thioguanine (Antineoplastic)	2-2.5/kg		0	CI			CI
Thiopentone (Ultra short acting barbiturate)	100-150 iv			SP			SP
Thioridazine (Antipsychotic)	150-800	0.05-0.5		SP			SP
Thiotepa (Antineoplastic)	60 im			CI			CI
Thyroxine (Hormone)	0.05-0.3	0.05-0.12					
Tiaprofenic acid (Antiinflammatory)	600	19-73					SP
Ticarcillin (Antibiotic)	<20000 iv	20-30			+		

Drugs	Dose mg/day	Therapeutic cons. mg/L	Penetration to CNS	Lactation	T ½ in Renal Failure	T ½ in Hepatic Failure	Risk in Pregnancy
Ticlopidine (Anticoagulant)	500-1000	10-20		CI			SP
Timolol (β-adrenoreceptor antagonist)	10-60	0.005-0.01		CI	0		(CI) 3
Tinidazole (Antiprotozoal)	2000 mg			CI			CI
Tobramycin (Antibiotic)	210-350 im/iv	4-10	Low	SP	+		CI
Tocainide (Antiarrhythemic)	1200	5-7			+	+	
Tolazamide (Antidiabetic)	100-1000						
Tolbutamide Oral hypoglycaemic agent)	250-3000			SP			SP
Tolmetin (Antiinflammatory)	600-1800	8-79		SP			SP
Topotecan (Antineoplatic)	1.5 mg/m²	5.9 ± 0.8 μg/dl	High	CI	3.5-4.1		CI
Torasemide (Diuretic)	10-20			CI			CI
Tranexamic acid (Haemostatic)	4000-6000	10-50		SP			SP
Tranylcypromine (Monoamine oxidase inhibitor)	10-20	0.04					
Trazadone (Antidepressant)	200-600	0.7		SP			CI
Triamcinolone (Corticosteroid)	4-48			SP			SP
Triamterene (K sparing diuretic)	150-300	0.13-0.15		CI	Avoid		SP

Drugs	Dose mg/day	Therapeutic cons. mg/L	Penetration to CNS	Lactation	T ½ in Renal Failure	T ½ in Hepatic Failure	Risk in Pregnancy
Triazolam (Anxiolytic)	0.13-0.25				0		3
Trifluoperazine (Antipsychotic/ Neuroleptic)	15-20	0.001-0.004		CI			SP
Trimeprazine (Respiratory agent)	30-40	0.008-0.017		CI			
Trimethoprim (Antibacterial)	400	3-10			+		1,CI
Trimipramine (Antidepressant)	50-300 mg			CI			
Tripolidine (Respiratory agent)	7.5-15	0.004-0.017		CI			
Urapidil (Antihypertensive)	30-120	0.1-0.2	Yes		+		
Vancomycin (Antibacterial)	500-2000	10-40		SP	+	+	SP
Vecuronium (Non-depolarizing muscle relaxant)	80-100 µg/kg			SP	0	+	SP
Venlafaxine (Antidepressant)	75	167 ± 55 µg/dl	High	CI	10.3 ± 4.3	10.3 ± 4.3	CI
Verapamil (Calcium channel antagonist)	120-480	0.25		SP	0	+	SP
Vidarabine (Antiviral)	10/kg. iv	0.4			+		SP
Vigabartrin (Antiepileptic)	2000				Avoid		
Viloxazine (Antidepressant)	300-400	cl.3					CI
Vinblastine (Antineoplastic)	3.7 mg/sq.m of BSA		0	CI	0		CI

Drugs	Dose mg/day	Therapeutic cons. mg/L	Penetration to CNS	Lactation	T ½ in Renal Failure	T ½ in Hepatic Failure	Risk in Pregnancy
Vincristine (Antineoplastic)	1.4 mg/sq.m of BSA		0	CI	0		CI
Vindesine (Antineoplastic)	3 mg.sq.m of BSA		0				
Warfarin (Anticoagulant)	2-10	1-3		SP			CI
Xipamide (Diuretic)	20-40	5		(CI)		0	CI, 3
Zafirleukast (Leukotreine receptor antagonist) **Zalepon** (Hypnotic)	20 t.i.d 20	26 ± 4 µg/dl	High	CI	1.1	-	CI
Zidovudine (Antiretroviral)	500-600		CI	CI			SP
Zolpidem (Hypnotic)	10	76-139 µg/dl	High	CI	1.9	-	CI
Zopiclone (Anxiolytic)	5-10			CI		+	P, (CI)
Zuelopenthixol (Antipsychotic)	20-150						SP

0 = no response. + = positive response. - = negative response. CI - contraindication, P - precaution, SP - special precaution.

1 - first timester, 2 - second timester and 3 - third timester.

BSA = Body Surface Area

CHAPTER II

PHARMACOKINETIC DATA TEXT

Ionization Constant (pKa)

Majority of the drugs are of organic in nature and contain acidic or basic group capable of ionization, and the pKa is an utterance of the strength of the group. For example, the hydrochloric acid is a strong acid because it is absolutely dissociated into hydrogen ion (H^+) and chloride ion (Cl^-).

$$H^+ + Cl^- \rightleftharpoons HCl \text{ [a strong acid]}$$

Where as a fraction of an acidic drug is present in undissociated form (HA) and ionized form (both A^- and H^+).

$$HA \rightleftharpoons H^+ + A^-$$

Acidic drugs are *ampicillins, aspirin, disodium chromoglycate, fusemide, phenobarbitone, sulphonamide* etc. And basic drugs are *allupurinol, amphetamine, chlorprosmazine, imipramine*, and *morphine propranol* etc. The extent to which a drug molecule in solution behaves as an acid or base depends not only on its own nature, but also on local hydrogen ion concentration.

The pKa of a drug is the pH at which the concentration of ionized and nonionized forms are equal.

The low pKa means that it is a strong acid, while high pKa means it is a strong base. The Anderson Hasselbalch equation, for an acid,

$$\log(\text{ionized/unionized}) = pH - pKa$$

For a base,

$$\log(\text{ionized/unionized}) = pKa - pH$$

Can be used to calculate the degree of ionization of a particular group at a given pH and help to predict whether a drug will easily cross membranes be absorbed, metabolized or excreted. Drugs cross membrances more easily in their unionized forms.

Unionized acids are lipid-soluble, but the dissociated ions are not. Therefore, an acid drug like salicylic acid is better absorbed in the stomach (because gastric pH is low and dissociation will be poor) than the intestine (where pH is high and dissociation will be high). So, the basic drug like quinine will be better absorbed in the intestine than in the stomach. [Table 2.1]

Table 2.1 pKa Values of Drugs in Common Use

Drug	Nature	pKa
Acetazolamide	Acid	7.2
Allopurinol	Base	9.4
Amiloride	Base	8.7
Aminocaproic acid	Ampholyte	4.4, 10.7
Aminopyrine	Base	5.0
Aminosalicylic acid	Acid	3.2
Amitriptyline	Base	9.4
Amphetamine	Base	9.8
Amphotericin B	Ampholyte	5.5, 10.0
Ampicillin	Acid	2.5, 7.2
Amylobarbital	Acid	7.7
Antipyrine	Base	1.4

Drug	Nature	pKa
Apomorphine	Base	7.2, 8.9
Aspirin	Acid	3.5
Atropine	Base	9.8
Barbital	Acid	7.8
Benzylpenicillin	Acid	2.8
Betahistine	Base	3.5, 9.7
Bishydroxycoumarin	Acid	5.7
Bupivacaine	Base	8.1
Burimamide	Base	7.5
Butobarbital	Acid	7.9
Caffeine	Base	0.8
Carbenicillin	Acid	2.6, 2.7
Cephalexin	Acid	5.2, 7.3
Cephalothin	Acid	2.5
Chlorambucil	Base	8.0
Chlordiazepoxide	Base	4.6
Chlormethiazole	Base	3.2
Chloroquine	Base	8.4, 10.8
Chlorpheniramine	Base	9.2
Chlorpromazine	Base	9.3
Chlorpropamide	Acid	4.8
Chlortetracycline	Base	3.3, 7.4, 9.3
Clindamycein	Base	6.9
Cloxacillin	Acid	2.7
Codeine	Base	6.0
Cyclizine	Base	8.2
Cyclobarbital	Acid	7.3
Cytarabine	Base	4.3
Dapsone	Acid	1.2-2.5
Demethylchlortetracycline	Base	7.2, 9.4
Desipramine	Base	9.5
dextromoramide	Base	7.0
Dextropropoxyphene	Base	6.3
Diamorphine	Base	7.6
Diazepam	Base	3.3
Dicoumarol	Acid	5.7
Dihydrocodeine	Base	8.8
Diphenhydramine	Base	8.3
Diphenylhydantoin	Acid	8.3
Disodium Cromoglycate	Acid	2.0
Doxycycline	Ampholyte	3.4, 7.7, 9.7
Droperidol	Base	7.6
Emetine	Base	5.8, 6.6
Ephedrine	Base	9.6

Drug	Nature	pKa
Ergometrine	Base	7.3
Ergonovine	Base	7.3
Erythromycin	Base	8.8
Eserine	Base	8.5
Ethacrynic acid	Acid	3.5
Ethambutol	Base	6.5, 9.0
Ethosuximide	Acid	9.3
Ethyl biscoumacetate	Acid	3.1
Fenfluramine	Base	9.9
Flucloxacillin	Acid	2.7
5-Fluorouracil	Base	8.1
Frusernide	Acid	3.7
Heroin	Base	7.6
Hexobarbital	Acid	8.2
Homatropine	Base	9.7
Hydrochlorothiazide	Acid	7.9, 9.2
Hyoscine	Base	8.1
Ibuprofen	Acid	4.4
Imipramine	Base	9.5
Indoramin	Base	7.8
Iprindole	Base	8.2
Isoprenaline	Base	8.6
Isoxsurpine	Base	8.0, 9.8
Levallorphan	Base	45
Levodopa	Amino acid	2.3, 8.7, 9.9
Lignocaine	Base	7.9
Lincomycin	Base	7.6
Lorazepam	Ampholyte	1.3, 11.5
Lysergide	Base	3.3, 7.8
Mecamylamine	Base	11.2
Mefenamic	Acid	4.2
Mepacrine	Base	7.7, 10.3
Meperidine	Base	8.7
Metaraminol	Base	8.6
Methadone	Base	8.6
Methicillin	Acid	2.8
Methohexital	Acid	7.9, 8.3
Methotrexate	Acid	4.8, 5.5
Methotrimeprazine	Base	9.2
Methoxamine	Base	4.8
Methylamphetamine	Base	10.0
Morphine	Base	7.9, 8.1, 9.9
Nalidixic acid	Acid	6.7
Nalorphine	Base	7.8
Nitrazepam	Base	3.2, 10.8
Nitrofurantoin	Acid	7.2
Novobiocin	Acid	4.3, 9.1
Orciprenaline	Base	8.9, 11.8
Orphenadrine	Base	8.4

Drug	Nature	pKa
Oxazepam	Ampholyte	1.7, 11.6
Oxyphenbutazone	Acid	4.7
Oxytetracycline	Base	3.3, 7.3, 9.1
Papaverine	Base	6.4
Penicillamine	Base	1.8, 7.9, 10.5
Pentobarbital	acid	8.1
Perphenazine	Base	7.8
Pethidine	Base	8.7
Phenobarbital	Acid	7.2
Phenoxymethy l-penicillin	Acid	2.7
Phenylbutazone	Acid	4.5
Phenytoin	Acid	8.3
Physostigmine	Base	8.5
Piperazine	Base	5.7, 9.8
Practolol	Base	9.5
Prilocaine	Base	7.9
Probenecid	Acid	3.4
Procainamide	Base	9.2
Procaine	Base	8.8
Prochlorperazine	Base	8.1
Promazine	Base	9.4
Promethazine	Base	9.1
Propanolol	Base	9.45
Pyrazinamide	Base	0.5
Pyrimethamine	Base	7.2
Quinacrine	Base	7.7, 10.3
Quinalbarbital	Acid	7.9
Quinidine	Base	4.3, 8.4
Quinine	Base	4.3, 8.4
Reserpine	Base	6.1
Salbutamol	Base	9.3, 10.3
Salicylazosulfa-Pyridine	Acid	0.6, 2.4, 9.7, 11.8
Salicylic acid	Acid	3.0
Secobarbital	Acid	7.9
Succinylsulfa-thiazole	Acid	4.5
Sulfadiazine	Acid	6.3
Sulfadimethoxine	Acid	6.3
Sulfafurazole	Acid	4.9
Sulfamethiazole	Acid	5.4
Sulfamethoxy-pyridazine	Acid	6.7
Sulfamethoxazole	Acid	6.0
Sulfasalazine	Acid	0.6, 2.4, 9.7, 11.8
Sulfathiazole	Acid	7.1
Sultinpyrazole	Acid	7.1

Drug	Nature	pKa
Terbutaline	Base	10.1
Tetracycline	Base	3.3, 7.8, 9.7
Theophylline	Base	0.7
Thiopental	Acid	7.6
Tolazoline	Base	10.3
Tolbutamide	Acid	5.4
Tranexamic acid	Ampholyte	4.3, 10.6
Trifluoperazine	Base	8.1
Trimethorpim	Base	6.4
Vinblastine	Base	5.4, 7.4
Vincristine	Base	5.0, 7.4

Partition Coefficient (log p)

The partition coefficient, P, of a drug is a measure of its ability to distribute between a lipid and an aqueous phase when the drug is in its completely unionized state. The movement of a drug through biological membrane depends on the partition coefficient. Partition coefficient may be expressed as lipid/water partition coefficient (as the main component of the biological membrane is the lipid and water in the extra and intracellular space), chloroform/water partition coefficient, or blood/gas partition coefficient (considering the movement of drug from lung to blood and vice versa).

Phenobarbitone has a high lipid/water partition coefficient of 5.9. thiopentone sodium has chloroform/water partition coefficient of about 100, so is highly soluble in lipid. The relatively high solubility of thiopentone mainly reflects the presence of C = S moiety. Hexamethonium has chloroform/water partition coefficient of zero. This drug is used for the treatment of hypertension and is administered only by injection as because it is not absorbed from the gut.

Lipid/water partition coefficient of a drug can be changed when the polarity of a drug is increased either by its degree of ionization or by adding a carboxyl (– COOH), amino (– NH_2) or hydroxyl (–OH) group to the drug molecule, then the lipid/water partition coefficient will be decreased. And when the polarity of a drug is decreased either by decreasing its degree of ionization or by adding phenyl or butyle group, the lipid/water partition coefficient will be increased. The adding if 2-hydroxyl groups in estrone results in a 45- fold decrease in lipid/water partition coefficient, so there is decrease in coefficient.

Protein Binding

After absorption, drugs will enter into the systemic circulation where most of the drugs bind to plasma protein, mainly albumin. Each albumin molecules has more than one site to which a drug may bind. At pH 7.4, albumin has a negative charge and has high capacity but low affinity for binding cationic drugs. Many basic drugs like felodipine bind to α-1-acid glycoprotein and some drug even bind to enzyme (e.g., acetazolamide binds to carbonic anhydrase enzyme). The unbound fraction of a drug will cross the membranes and acts on receptors. There is equilibrium between bound and free drug however, protein binding is competitive and concomitant administration of other drugs may lead to a displacement of the equilibrium and alter the steady state. Different disease states can also change the amount of albumin (e.g., renal or hepatic failure) α-1-acid glycoprotein (e.g., myocardial infarction) and this can also effect steady state concentration of drug.

It has been found that 99% warfarin is bound to protein, while for ampicillins, the bound fractions account for only about 18%. Lithium is one drug, which remains totally free. [Table-2.2]

Bioavailability

Bioavailability measures the actual amount that reaches the systemic circulation following oral dosing, and expressed in the tables as a percentage of the administered dose.

Extent of absorption and first-pass biotransformation are the important factors on which bioavailability depends. Extent of absorption is the total amount of drug that undergoes and it is directly proportional to bioavailability. First-pass biotransformation is inversely proportional to the bioavailability.

The bioavailability factor (F) can be calculated by dividing the bioavailability by 100. For example, the F is estimated to be 0.62 for an orally administered digoxin tablet (bioavailability is 62%). This means that if 250 microgram of digoxin is given orally the absorbed amount can be calculated by,

$$F \times dose = 0.62 \times 250 = 155 \text{ microgram.}$$

Table 2.2 Protein Binding(%) of Drugs

Drug	Percent Bound	Drug	Percent Bound
Acetaminophen	25	Heparin	0
Acetazolamide	90	Imipramine	85
Ailopurinol	0	Indomethacin	90
Aminopyrine	18	Isoniazid	0
Aminosalicylic acid	65	Kanamycin	10
Amitriptyline	96	Lincomycin	85
Ampicillin	25	Mepacrine	90
Antipyrine	4	Meperidine	40
Atropine	50	Methadone	40
Barbital	10	Methicillin	45
Bishydroxycoumarin	97	Methotrexate	5
Carbamazepine	72	Nitrofurantoin	70
Carbenicillin	47	Nortriptyline	94
Cephalexin	22	Novobiocin	96
Chloramphenicol	25	Oxacillin	94
Chloroquine	55	Oxyphenbutazone	90
Chlorpheniramine	70	Oxytetracycline	28
Chlorpromazine	95	Phenacetin	30
Chlorpropamide	80	Phenylbutazone	95
Chlortetracycline	47	Phenytoin	87
Desipramine	80	Prednisolone	90
Diazepam	96	Probenecid	80
Diazoxide	99	Procainamide	15
Dicoumarol	97	Promethazine	8
Digitoxin	95	Quinidine	70
Digoxin	23	Rifampicin	85
Doxycycline	93	Streptomycin	34
Erythromycin	18	Sulfadimethoxine	95
Ethambutol	8	Sulfamethizole	90
Fenfluramine	32	Sulfathiazole	70
Furesamide	75	Theophylline	15
Glutethimide	54	Thiopental	75

The bioavailability can vary among different formulations and dosage formation of drug. Drugs such as glyceryltrinitrate, which are completely inactive following oral dosing, exhibit zero bioavailability and must be given by another route.

Tmax

It is a measurement of time in which maximum blood or plasma concentration of drugs reaches after oral administrations. For many drugs this is usually of the order of 2-4 hours but can vary largely between individuals and different factors like food, other drugs and different formulation can also affect the Tmax.

Volume of distribution (Vd)

After absorption, a drug distributes itself in the body. The extent to which a drug distributes in body is known as apparent volume distribution. Highly protein bound drugs have a low Vd value. On the other hand, drugs with very high volume distribution are usually taken up and retained by some tissue from which they are released only slowly. Vd is sensitive to the effects of other drugs. The Vd can also be changed in physiological and pathological changes of the body. Knowledge of Vd enables one to calculate the dose to be administered initially and subsequently to achieve these ends. The apparent volume distribution is an artificial but convenient mathematical concept related to the amount of drug administered and its apparent dilution in the body fluids as evidenced by its concentration in the body.

Fluid compartment	Mean volume Vd (kg^{-1})	Average value for 70 kg adult (L)	Approximate time for equilibration(t)	Type of substance with example
Blood, plasma	0.05	3.5	10 minutes	High plasma protein bound (e.g., warfarin) or molecular weight > 15000 (e.g., heparin, dextran)
Extracellular fluid	0.17	12	30 minutes	Highly ionized [e.g., (+) – tubocurarine, gentamicine]
Total body water	0.60	42	1 hour	Lipid soluble (e.g. ethanol)

Oral Absorption

Most of the drugs are given in oral route and absorption of drugs may vary due to nature of drugs. Absorption through oral route mean, absorption of drug via buccal cavity or via stomach or via intestine. The blood flow through buccal mucosa is high and drugs are absorbed in the systemic circulation by simple diffusion. Only a limited amount of drug is absorbed by the stomach. However a significant amount of aspirin and alcohol are absorbed from the stomach. Most drugs in nonionized form are absorbed from upper part of the small intestine by simple diffusion. Ionized drugs are incompletely and slowly absorbed by filtration. Some drugs such asmethyldopa, flurouracil, levodopa are absorbed from intestine by an active transport mechanism. Several factors related to drugs are molecular weight, size, lipid/water partition coefficient, pKa, formulation, disintegration, dissolution, inactivation and drug interaction. The factors related to patients are pH of GI tract, rate of gastric emptying presence of food in gut, bowel transit time, mucosal surface area available for absorption, regional blood flow and GI disease.

Active Metabolite

Some time some drugs may undergo metabolism to change to metabolite for quite different effects. Phenacetin after metabolism changes to active drug paracetamol. In aged person renal functions may decline with reduced renal clearance. So in this case the dose of the drugs should be adjusted which can produce active metabolite(s).

Clearance

In a particular time the blood or plasma is cleared of drug. Cl denotes that the volume [usually bold or plasma] cleared of drug in a particular time. t^{o} is depends on ratio between Vd and clearance. [Table 2.3 and 2.4]

Urine Excretion (AU)

The percentage of administered dose that is excreted unchanged via urine.

Table 2.3 Drugs which are Extensively (> 90%) Cleared Intact from the Kidneys and Which are Little Cleared (<5%).

Extensive Clearance	Little clearance	
Acetazolamide	Acetaminophen	Hydrallazine
Amantadine	Acetohexamide	Imipramine
Amiloride	Acetophenetidin	Indomethacin
Amphetamine	Aminopyrine	Levodopa
Barbital	Antipyrine	Lorazepam
Disodium cromoglycate	Aspirin	Nalidixic acid
Gentamicin	Bupivacaine	Novobiocin
Lithium	Carbenoxolone	Pentazocine
Methotrexate	Chlormethiazole	Phenacetin
Penicillins	Chlorpromazine	Phenytoin
Pentolinium	Desipramine	Prednisolone
Practolol	Diamorphine	Succinylcholine
Tranexamic acid	Diazepam	Suxamethonium
Vancomycin	Diazoxide	Thiopental
	Diphenoxylate	Thyroxine
	Griseofulvin	Vinblastine
	Heroin	Vincristine

Table 2.4 Clearance of Drugs in Different pH

Clearance Greater in Acidic Urine	Clearance Greater in Alkaline Urine
Amphetamine	Acetazolamide
Chloroquine	Amino acids
Codeine	Barbiturates
Imipramine	Nalidixic acid
Levorphanol	Nitrofurantoin
Mecamylamine	Phenylbutazone
Mepacrine	Probenecid
Meperidine	Salicyclic acid
Nicotine	Sulfonamides
Procaine	
Quinine	

PHARMACOKINETIC DATA

Drugs	Ionization constant (pKa)	Partition Coefficient (log p)	Oral Absorption (%)	Bio Availability (%)	Tmax	Volume Distribution (l/kg)	Protein Binding (%)	Half Life (hours)	Clearance (ml/min)	Urinary Excretion (%)
Abacavir (Anti retrovirus)			80					1-1.5 T1/2 of active metabolit e >12		
Acebutolol Beta-adrenoreceptor antagonist)	9.4	-0.4	90	40	2-4	1.2	20	3-6	500	10-55
Acetaminophen (Analgesic & antipyretic)			88	±0.3	Oat< 60 mg /ml		2		5	3
Acetohexamide (Anti diabetic)		2.4	Good		2	0.2	75-95	1-2	5	Low
Acetonide (Corticosteroid)				23 (oral) 22 (inhal^n)		1.3	40	2.0	7.7	1.0
Acetylprocainamide (Local anaesthetic)			83	1.4	10	0.6	3.1	81		
Acetylsaficylic acid (Analgesic)			68	6.15	49	0.25	9.3	1.4		
Acetylcysteine (Respiratory agent)	9.5	-0.6	Good	.1-3	0.4	64-78		6	Slow	81
Acrosoxacin (Quinolone antibiotic)	8.1	0,7		3-4		70	3-11			<5
Acetazolamide (Antiepileptic)	7.2	-0.3	Good		1-3	0.2	90-95	2-13	45	70-100
Actinomycin (Antiviral)			iv					36		
Acyclovir (Antiviral)	3.2	-1.7	20			0.7	9-33	3	200	40-70
Adrenaline (Sympathomimetis)	8.7	-1.4	Poor	0			50			<1
Ajmaline (Antiarrythmic)	8.2	1.3					80			
Albendazole (Anthelmintics)		3.5								

Drugs	Ionization constant (pKa)	Partition Coeffi-cient (log p)	Oral Absor-ption (%)	Bio Availa-bility (%)	Tmax	Volume Distribution (l/kg)	Protein Binding (%)	Half Life (hours)	Clearance (ml/min)	Urinary Excretion (%)
Alclofenac (Anti gout)	4.6	2.5				0.1	>99	3		
Aldesleukin (Anti Cancer)						0.08		1.2	1.44	
Alfentanil (Anti aesthetic)	6.5	2.2	iv			0.7	90	1-2	330	
Allopurinol (Antigout)	9.4	-0.6	Good	90	1-2	0.6	<5	0.5-2	800	Low
Alphaxalone (Anti aesthetic)			iv			0.8	46	0.5	1400	
Amiloride (Diuretic)	8.7									
Amlodipine (Antihypertensive)		2.8		52-88		21	97	30-40	450	
Aminocaproic acid (Antifibrinolytic)	4.4, 10.7									
Aminopyrine (Analgesic)	5.0									
Aminosalicylic acid (Antimycobacterial)	3.2									
Amitriptyline (Antidepressant)	9.4									
Amodiaquine (Antimalarial)		3	Good	4						
Amoxicillin (Antibiotic)	2.4	0.3	Good		1-2	0.2-0.4	20	1	200400	50-70
Amphetamine (CNS Stimulant)	9.8									
Amphoteracin (Antifungal)	5.5, 10.0		Poor			4	>90	360	28	<10
Ampicillin (Antibiotic)	*2.5, 7.2	0.6	Fair		2	0.2-0.5	20	1-2	200-280	30-90
Amrinone (Inotropic agent)		-0.6			<3		Low	3-12		
Amsacrine (Antineoplastic)		2.9	Poor					7		

Drugs	Ionization constant (pKa)	Partition Coefficient (log p)	Oral Absorption (%)	Bio Availability (%)	Tmax	Volume Distribution (l/kg)	Protein Binding (%)	Half Life (hours)	Clearance (ml/min)	Urinary Excretion (%)
Amylobarbitone (Sedative)	7.7	1.6	100	95	1-3	1	40-60	8-40	35	1
Anistreplase (Thrombolytic drug)						0.084		1.2	0.92	
Antipyrine (NSAID)	1.4	0.4			0.5	Low	8-12	50		
Apomorphine (Antispycotic)	7.2, 8.9									
Aspirin (Analgesic & antipyretic)	3.5	-1.1	Good	Low	0.25	0.15	70	0.3	650	<1
Astemizole (Antihistamin)		4.1	Good			250	>95	20 days		
Atenolol (AntihypertenSive)	9.6	-1.5	50	50	2-3	1.1	<5	5-9	100-180	40-50
Atracurium (Neuromuscular blocker)		Iv		0.1-0.2	82	0.3	375-450			
Atropine (Analgesic & antipyretic)	9.8	1.8	Good		0.5	2-3	50	2-4	1000	50
Auranofin (Antiimflarnmatory)				15-25		0.045	60	* 17-25	0.025	15
Aurothiomalate (Anti gout)			im				95	550		60-90
Azapropazone (Antiinflammatory)		1	Good	4-5	0.2	99	8-24	7-14	60	
Azathioprine(Immuno sup-pressant)	8.2	0.1	Good	1		30	0.5			10
Azelastin (Tropical Nasopha-ryngal Medication)		3.9	90	>80	4-5		78-88	25		
Azlocillin (Antibiotic)	2.8		Poor			0.2	30	1	1 50	50-60
Aztreonam (Antibacterial)	2.8		iv,im			.16-0.2	50-60	1.5-2	100-130	68-75

Drugs	Ionization constant (pKa)	Partition Coefficient (log p)	Oral Absorption (%)	Bio Availability (%)	Tmax	Volume Distribution (l/kg)	Protein Binding (%)	Half Life (hours)	Clearance (ml/min)	Urinary Excretion (%)
Azithromycin (Antibacterial)				37		31	7-50	40	9	12
Bacampicillin (Antibiotic)	6.8	2	65		0.5-1					Low
Bacitracin (Antibacterial)			Poor					1-2		9-31
Baclofen (Muscle Relaxant)		-1.4	var		2			2-5	260	High
Bacmecillinam (Antibiotic)						1			1	41 b
Bamethan (Calcium antagonist)	9	1.5			0.5-1					30
Barbital (Hypnotic)	7.8									
Beclomethasone (Cortico Steroid)		4.2	Good					15		
Benazepril (Anti hypertensive)				37		0.12	97	0.7 (parent)	0.3-0.4	<1
Bendrofluazide (Cardiovascular agent)	8.5		>90		2-3	1-2	95	4-9	520	30
Benorylate (Analgesic)		2.2	Good	Low			+	1		<!
Benoxaprofen (Anti inflammatory)		3.2						27		<10
Benperidol (Anti psychotic)	8									
Benzafibrate (Lipid lowering agent)			Good		2		94-96		2	
Benzylpenicillin (Antibiotic)	2.8	1.8	30		1	0.4	45-65	0.5-1	500	20-85
Bepridil (Calcium Chanel Blocker)				60		8	>99	12	5.3	<1
Betahistine (Antileutic)	3.5, 9.7	-0.1	Good		3-5					

Drugs	Ionization constant (pKa)	Partition Coefficient (log p)	Oral Absorption (%)	Bio Availability (%)	Tmax	Volume Distribution (l/kg)	Protein Binding (%)	Half Life (hours)	Clearance (ml/min)	Urinary Excretion (%)
Betamethasone (Corticosteroid)		1.8	Good			1.8	64	6-7	180	'
Betaxolol (Drug for Glucoma)		2.2	100	88	1-4	6	50	15	320	16
Bethanidine (Antirhypertensive)	12		Poor		2		<10		2-6	50-85
Bevantolol ($\beta_1$adrenoreceptor Blocker)	8.1	2.6	100	60		1.5	95		2	<10
Bishydroxycoumarin (Anticoagulant)	5.7									
Bupivacaine (Local Anesthetic)	8.1									
Buprenorphme (Analgesic & antipyretic)	8.5	3.2			3	2.5	96	2-6	1200	
Bupropion (Anti depressant)						7.2	84	12	35	<1
Burimamide (Anti ulcer Drug)	7.5									
Buserelin (Hormone)			Nasal	2-3				1-2		67
Busulphan (Antineoplastic)		-0.5	Good					2-3		1
Butobarbitone (Sedative)	, 7.9	1.7	Good		1-2	0.8	26	34-42	15	5-9
Butriptyline (Antidepressant)		5.1	Good		3		>90	20		<2
Cadralazine (Anti hypertensive)		0				0.7		3	180	
Caffeine (CNS Stimulant)	, 0.8	,0.1	Good					3-5		
Capreomycin (Antitubercular)	3.3		Poor		1-2					50
Captopril (Anti hypertensive)	9.8	1	75	65	0.5-1	0.7	30	1-2	900	50-70
Carbamazepine (Anticonvulsant)		2.5	100	>70	9	1	75	16-65	16-64	<10

Drugs	Ionization constant (pKa)	Partition Coefficient (log p)	Oral Absorption (%)	Bio Availability (%)	Tmax	Volume Distribution (l/kg)	Protein Binding (%)	Half Life (hours)	Clearance (ml/min)	Urinary Excretion (%)
Carbimazole (Antithyroid)			100	Low	1-3		Low			
Carbenicillin (Antibacterial)	2.6, 2.7	1.1	Poor			0.2	50	1.2	130	80-85
Carbenoxolone (Antiulcer)	7.1	13	>95		1-2	0.1	>99	8-20	s	<5
Carbocisteine (Respiratory agent)		-2.6			2-4			1	530	
Carboplatin (Antineoplastic)								120		
Carisoprodol (Muscle Relaxant)		1.7	Fair							
Carmustine (Antineoplastic)		VS.	Good			3.3		0.2	4000	
Carprofen (Antiinflammatory)		3.9						13-26		<5
Carteolol (β Blocker)		-0.5	100	>95	1-2		16	5-7		70-90
Carvedilol (Antihypertensive)			25		1.5	95		2.2	8.7	<2
Cefacetrile (Antibiotic)		-0.5	95			0.27	25	0.7		75
Cefaclor (Antibacterial)		-2.7	90-95	90	1-2	0.3-0.5	25	0.6	500	90-95
Cefadroxil (Antibacterial)		-2.7	85		1-3	0.2-0.4	20	1-2	200-300	70-90
Cephamandole (Antibiotic)						0.16	74	0.78	2.8	96
Cefapirin (Antibacterial)			Poor			0.2	50	0.5-1	730	75
Cefathiamidine (Antibacterial)								0.5		90
Cefatrizine (Antibacterial)			40			0.33	60	V-4	230	75
Cefazaflur (Antibacterial)		-0.3				0.35	65	0.4		90
Cefazedone (Antibacterial)		-1.5				0.13	95	1-2		80

Drugs	Ionization constant (pKa)	Partition Coeffi-cient (log p)	Oral Absor-ption (%)	Bio Availa-bility (%)	Tmax	Volume Distribution (l/kg)	Protein Binding (%)	Half Life (hours)	Clearance (ml/min)	Urinary Excretion (%)
Cefazolin (Antibacterial)						0.14	89	1.8	0.95	80
Cefbuperazone (Antibacterial)								1.6		75
Cefixime (Antibacterial)		0.2		40	3-5	0.2	70	3-4	150-320	
Cefmenoxime (Antibacterial)			im		1		77		1	
Cefmetazole (Antibacterial)		-0.6	im		0.7	0.13	85	1	90-165	75
Cefonicid (Antibacterial)		-1.7	im		1-2	0.13	98	4.4	27	95
Cefoperazone (Antibacterial)		-0.7	im		1-2	0.19	90	2	80	30
Ceforanide (Antibacterial)		-1.7	im		1	0.2	45-85	3	40-50	85
Cefotaxime (Antibacterial)		-0.2				0.4	30-40	1-1.5	250	50-60
Cefotetan (Antibacterial)		-1.2	im		2-3	0.13	90	3.5	35	80
Cefotiam (Antibiotic)		-4				0.36	40	0.8	390	70
Cefoxitin (Antibacterial)	3.5	0				0.2	75	1-2	250-330	77-90
Cefpimizole (Antibiotic)						0.27		2	119	80
Cefpiramide (Antibiotic)		0.5				0.1	96	5		25
Cefpodoxime (Antibacterial)		0.6		50		0.3		2-3	200	40
Cefprozil (Antibiotic)				90		0.22	40	1.5	3	73
Cefroxadinec (Antibacterial)		-0.2		90		0.2	10	1	340	80-96

Drugs	Ionization constant (pKa)	Partition Coefficient (log p)	Oral Absorption (%)	Bio Availability (%)	Tmax	Volume Distribution (l/kg)	Protein Binding (%)	Half Life (hours)	Clearance (ml/min)	Urinary Excretion (%)
Cefsulodin (Antibacterial)			85			0.2-0.4	30	1.5	80-145	60-70
Cefsumide (Antibacterial)		-1	90				13	2-4		90
Ceftazidime (Antibacterial)						0.2-0.3	15	2	110	60-90
Ceftezole (Antibiotic)		-2.2	3				85	0.9-3		90
Ceftizoxime (Antibacterial)						0.2-0.3	30	1.7	130-160	70-100
Ceftriaxone (Antibacterial)	3.2					0.1-0.2	83-96	8.5	20	65
Cefuroxime (Antibacterial)	2.5	-0.2	Low			0.2-0.3	40	1.3	130	>90
Celiprolol (Anti hypertensive)	9.7	1.7	80	55	2-4	2-3	26	4-6	130-180	11-28
Cephalexin (Antibiotic)	5.2, 7.3									
Cephalexm (Antibacterial)	2.5	0.7	90		1-2	0.2-0.3	10-25	0.8-1	250-380	50-90
Cephaloglycm (Antibiotic)	4.6	-1.3	25				25	1-2		15
Cephaloridine (Antibacterial)	3.4					0.21	20	1.4	1 70	70
Cephalothin (Antibacterial)	, 2.5	0.5				0.2-0.3	65-70	0.5	330-470	60-90
Cepnamandole (Antibacterial)		0.5				0.2	75	0.8	220-260	80-100
Cephapirm (Antibiotic)						0.21	62	0.72	6.9	48
Cephazolin (Antibacterial)	2.1	-0.2	Low			0.13	80-85	1 .8-2	50-65	65-95
Cephradine (Antibacterial)	2.5	-1.2	95			0.25	10	0.8	280-580	100
Chloralhydrate (Hypnotic)	10	0.6		Low		0.6		0.06		<-

Drugs	Ionization constant (pKa)	Partition Coefficient (log p)	Oral Absorption (%)	Bio Availability (%)	Tmax	Volume Distribution (l/kg)	Protein Binding (%)	Half Life (hours)	Clearance (ml/min)	Urinary Excretion (%)
Chlorambucil (Antineoplastic)	8.0	1.7	100	Rapid				1.5		<>
Chloramphenicol (Antibacterial)	5.5	1.1	Good		1-2	0.5-1	40-60	2-5	200-300	5-10
Chlorazepate (Amiolytic)	3.5	2.3			1-3	>95		2	7-21	
Chlordiazepoxide (Anxiolytic)	4.6	2.4	100	100	2-6	0.3-0.6	90-97	5-30	15-35	<1
Chlormethiazole (Cardiovascular agent)	3.2		Good		0.6	3-12	60-70	3-7	700-1 700	<5
Chlormezanone (Muscle Relaxant)		1.6	Good		4		50	20-30		<5
Chloroquine (Antimalarial)	8.4, 10.8	4.6	Good	85	1-6	820	50-70	40d	1080	40
Chlorothiazide (Cardiovascular agent)	9.5	-2	Poor	<30	1		95	2-13		
Cniorpheniramine (Antiallergic)	, 9.2	3.4	100	35	2-3	3	70	18040	100	3-10
Chlorpromazine (Anti psychotic)	9.3	3.4	Good	25	3	21	95-98	7-120	630	<5
Chlorpropamide (Antidiabetic)	4.8,	2.3	100		1-7	0.1-0.3	60-95	20-45	2	10-60
Chlorprothixine (Antipsychotic)	8.8	2.7		40	4	10-20		8-12	1000-1400	
Chlortetracycline (Antibacterial)	7.4, 9.3,	-0.9	Good			1.2	47-55	6		15
Chlorthalidone (Antihypertensive)	9.4	0.2	<90	65	1-3	4	75	35-70	70-140	25-50
Cisapride (Prokinetic)		3.7							-	
Ciclacillin (Antibiotic)			Good		0.5-1		20-25	0.5		60-70
Cilazapril (Antihypertensive)		0.6	Good	60	1-3	0.4		50-90	250	<!

Drugs	Ionization constant (pKa)	Partition Coefficient (log p)	Oral Absorption (%)	Bio Availability (%)	Tmax	Volume Distribution (l/kg)	Protein Binding (%)	Half Life (hours)	Clearance (ml/min)	Urinary Excretion (%)
Cimetidme (H$_2$ antagonistic)	6.8	0.4	>95	70	1-2	1-2	13-26	1-3	600	40-80
Cinnarizine (Anti vertigo)		6.1G			2			5		
Cinoxacin (Antibiotic)	4.7	-2	100		6	0.25	16-60	2-4	210	50-60
Ciprofloxacin (Antibacterial)	6	-1.6	100	70	1	3	20-40	3-6	500	30-50
Cisplatin (Antineoplastic)			iv				90	200	5	25-75
Clarithromycin (Antibacterial)				55		2.6	42-50	3.3	73	36
Clavulanic acid (Antibacterial)		-1.6			1	0.2	27	1	220	30-40
Clemastine (Antiallergic)		5.1			3-5					
Clindamycin (Antibacterial)	6.9,	2.2	90		1	0.8	93	3	200	5-15
Clioquinol (Antibiotic)	8.1	3.4	var		4			11-14	>	<T
Clobazam (Anticonvuisant)		1	>90	87	1	1-2	85-90	10-60	35	
Clofazimine (Antileprotics)	8.4		<90		4			70d		<!
Clofibrate (Lipid lowening agent)	3	3.7	c100	95	2-8	0.1-0.2	>95	12-25	10-20	15-30
Clomipramine (Antidepressant)	9.4	5.2	c100		2-4	12-17	90-98	20-80	400-750	1-3
Clomocycline (Antibiotic)		-1.9			2-3			6		30
Clonazepam (Anticonvuisant)	1.5	2.4	Good	>80	1-4	2-4	85	18-45	70-100	<!
Clomdine (Antihypertensive)	8.2	1.6	Good	100	1.5	2-4	20-40	6-25	3-12	30-50
Clorazepate (Anti anxiety)						0.33		2	1.8	<1

Drugs	Ionization constant (pKa)	Partition Coeffi-cient (log p)	Oral Absor-ption (%)	Bio Availa-bility (%)	Tmax	Volume Distribution (l/kg)	Protein Binding (%)	Half Life (hours)	Clearance (ml/min)	Urinary Excretion (%)
Cloxacillin (Antibacterial)	2.7,	2.4	var			0.1	94	0.3-2	200	35-65
Clozapine (Antipsychotic)	8	4.3	Good	50	1-4	5	Low	6-33		Low
Cocain (Anaesthetic)	8.7	2.3			1-2			<1	2000	10
Codeine (Antiillusive)	6.0,	1.1	Good	50	1-2	4-5	7-25	2-4	700-1600	6-16
Colaspase (Antineoplastic)			iv					8-48		<5
Colchicine (Antigout)	1,7	1	Good		1-2	0.7-2	30-50	1	600	5-17
Colistin (Antidiarrhoeals)			Poor		2-3			2-5		80
Cortisone (Corticosteroid)		2.1						0.5		
Cyclandelate (Peripheral Vasodilator)		4.6								
Cyclizine (Antihausea/ antivertigo)	8.2,	4			2			24		
Cyclobarbital (Barbiturates)	7.3,	1,8	Good		1-3	0.5	70	8-17	35	<10
Cydophosphamide (Neoplastic disorders)		0.6	Good	75	1	0.7	20	2-16	70	<10
Cyclosertne (Antitubercular)	4.5		100		2-4		<20	4-30		65
Cyclosporin (Immuno depressant)			var	40	3-4	3.5	98	9-27	280	<2
Cyproheptadine (Antiallergic)	8.9	4.7			6-9					5
Cyproterone (Hormone)		3.4	Poor		5-10					
Cytarabine (Neoplastic disorders)	4.3	-2.1	<20			2.5	13	2-3	920	
Dacarbazine (Antineoplastic)	4.4	-0.2	Poor				5	5		50

Drugs	Ionization constant (pKa)	Partition Coefficient (log p)	Oral Absorption (%)	Bio Availability (%)	Tmax	Volume Distribution (l/kg)	Protein Binding (%)	Half Life (hours)	Clearance (ml/min)	Urinary Excretion (%)
Danazol (Gouadal Hormone)		4.2						4-5		
Dantrolen (Muscle Relaxant)	7.5		Poor	4-6					9	Low
Dapsone (Antileprotic)	1.2-2.5	1							22	
Daunorubicin (Antineoplastic)	8.4	1.8	iv					19		
Debrisoquine (Anti Hypertensive)	11.9	0.8			2-4		25	3-30		8-80
Demeclocycline (Antibacterial)	3.3	-0.6	Good			1.8	40-90	10-15		
Demethylchlortetracycline (Antibiotic)	7.2, 9.4									
Desipramme (Antidepressant)	9.5,	4.9	Good		3-6	22	70-90	10-35	2200	<5
Desmethyldiazepam (Anxiolytic)				99		0.78	97.5	73	0.14	<1
Dexamethasone(Corticosteroid)		1.8	Good			1	67-77	2-5	245	
Dexamphetamine (CNS stimulant)	9.9	1.8	Good			3-4	15-40	4-12		1-75
Dextromethorphan (Steroid)	8.3	4	Good			2				<10
Dextromoramide (Opioid Analgesic)	7.0									
Dextropropoxyphene (Analgesic & antipyretic)	6.3	4	ioo	40	2	3-16	70-80	3-24	1000	<20
Dezocine (Analgesic)		3.6	*	iv		9-12		2-3	3500	

Drugs	Ionization constant (pKa)	Partition Coefficient (log p)	Oral Absorption (%)	Bio Availability (%)	Tmax	Volume Distribution (l/kg)	Protein Binding (%)	Half Life (hours)	Clearance (ml/min)	Urinary Excretion (%)
Diamorphine (Analgesic)	7.6	1	Good			3-5	20-35	0.05	1000-1400	<1
Diazepam (Anxiolytic)	3.3	2.8	100	75	1-2	0.5-2.5	>98	20-95	20-35	<1
Diazoxide (Antihypertensive)	8.5	1.2	iv			0.2-0.3	90	20-70	7	6-50
Diclofenac (NSAID agent)	4.2	1.5	Good	55	2-5	0.15	>99	1-2	240	<5
Dicloxacillin (Antibacterial)	2.7	2.9	Good			0.2	98	0.8	130	35-70
Dicoumarol (Anticoagulant)	5.7									
Dicyclomine (GI Sedative)		5.8	95	90	1.5			5		
Didanosine (Antiviral)				38		1	<5	1.4	16	36
Diethylpropion (Monoamine oxidase inhibitor)		2.5	Good					1.5-3		<1
Diflunisal (Analgesic)	3	4.4	Good		2	0.1	99	5-20	6-8	<5
Digitoxin (Cardiac glycoside)		1.8	Good	>90	2-3	0.4-0.8	95	200	3	20-50
Digoxin (Cardiac glycoside)		1.3	var	70	1	5-10	20-40	20-50	70-240	60-80
Dihydrocodeine (Analgesic)	8.8	-1.5	Good	20	1-2	1		4	280	
Dihydroergotamine (Antimigrairi)	6.9	4.9	Poor	<5	0.5	6-23		2-4	500-1000	<
Dilevalol (β Blocker)	9.5	1.2		30	2	17		12	2100	
Diltiazem (Antihypertensive)	7.7	2.7	100	40	3	4.5	>95	3-5	1000	<5
Diphenhydramine (Antiallergic)	8.3,	3.3	Good	50	2-4	4-8	80-98	5-9	700	<5
Diphenoxylate (Antidiarrhoeal)	7.1	5			2	4-5		2-3		<1

Drugs	Ionization constant (pKa)	Partition Coeffi-cient (log p)	Oral Absor-ption (%)	Bio Availa-bility (%)	Tmax	Volume Distribution (l/kg)	Protein Binding (%)	Half Life (hours)	Clearance (ml/min)	Urinary Excretion (%)
Diphenylhydantoin (AntiConvulsion Drug)	8.3									
Diphenylpyraline AntiHistamine	9.1	3.4	Good					20-40		<10
Dipyridamole (Antianginal)	6.4	2.1	Good	50	1	2.5	>90	12	140	<1
Disodium Cromoglycate (Anti Asthmatic Drug)	2.0									
Disopyramide (Antiarrhythmic)	8.4	1.4	100	85	1-3	2-3	35-80	3-11	600	50-60
Distigmine ((Parasym-pathomimetic)			Poor							
Disulfiram (Alcohol antagonist)		3.9			6-9		96		7	
Dobutamine (Inotropic agent)	9.5	2.2	inact	0		0.2		0.05	4000	
Domperidone (Antileutic)	7.9	4.1		20	0.5					<1
Dopamine (Inotropic agent)	8.8	0.4	inact	0				0.05	4000-6000	
Dopexamine (Vasodilator)	8.6	3						0.1		Low
Dothiepin (Anti depressant)		2.8	Good		3	70			2400	
Doxapram (Respiratory Stimulant)		3.1	Good	60		3		7	350	
Doxazosin (Antihypertensive)		3.8						11		
Doxepin (Antidepressant)	9	2.4	Good	30		20	80		1000	<1
Doxycycline (Antibiotic)	3.4, 7.7, 9.7									
Diflunisal (NSAID)	8.2	1.3	iv			43	71	30	400-1 200	5
Doxycycline (Antibacterial)	3.5	-0.2	100		2	0.7	82-90	16-22	28	30-40

Drugs	Ionization constant (pKa)	Partition Coefficient (log p)	Oral Absorption (%)	Bio Availability (%)	Tmax	Volume Distribution (l/kg)	Protein Binding (%)	Half Life (hours)	Clearance (ml/min)	Urinary Excretion (%)
Droperidol (Antidopaminergic)	7.6	3.5					85-90			<10
Dihydrogesterone (Gonadal Hormone)		3.5			Fast					
Edrophonium (Acetylcholinesterase inhibitor)						1.1			750	
Entosuximide (Anti Epilepsy)	9.5	-0.3	Good			0.7	<10	40-60	12	20
Emetine (Anti amoebic Drug)	5.8, 6.6									
Enalapril (Antihypertensive)	3	-0.1	Good	50-60		0.7	50	35	600	17
Encainide (Antiarrythmic)		3.8	>95	55			70-80		700	<10
Enoxacin (Antibiotic)	6	-2	Good	80	3	2.3	20-60		350	30-50
Enxaparin (Anti Coagulant)			93 (s.c)		0.12			3.8	0.3	
Enoximone (Phosphodiesterase inhibitor)		1 .6					70			<5
Epanolol (β-adrenoreceptor antagonist)		1		8		4	50	19	2000	<2
Ephedrine (Respiratory agent)	9.6	1	Good							50-75
Epirubicin (Antineoplastic)	8.3		iv					40		
Ergometrine (Obstetrics Drug)	7.3									
Ergonovine (Uterine Stimulant)	7.3									
Ergotamine (Antimigrain)	6.4	4.2	Poor	Low		2		2	350-1000	<1
Erythromycin (Antibiotic)	8.8,	2.5	var		2	0.7	70-80		400-500	1
Eserine (AntiCholinesterase inhibitor)	8.5									

Drugs	Ionization constant (pKa)	Partition Coefficient (log p)	Oral Absorption (%)	Bio Availability (%)	Tmax	Volume Distribution (l/kg)	Protein Binding (%)	Half Life (hours)	Clearance (ml/min)	Urinary Excretion (%)
Esmolol (Antiarrhythmic)	9.5	1.5	iv			3	55	0.2	230000	<2
Estramustine (Antineoplastic)		4.9	75	75						
Ethacrynic acid(Cardiovascular agent)	3.5	3.2	Good					0.5-1		20
Ethambutol (Antitubercuiar drug)	6.5, 9.0	0.1C	80			2.5		t	50-600	50-90
Ethanol (Alcohol)		-0.2	Good	80	0.5-1	0.5				<5
Ethinyloestradiol (Gonadal Hormone)		4	Good			2.9	97	13	380	
Ethosuximide (Anticonvulsant)	9.3					0.72	0	45	0.19	25
Etidocaine (Antiaesthetic)	7.7	3.2				2	94		1100	
Etintidine (Antispasmodic)					1					37
Ethyl biscoumacetate (Anticoagulant)	3.1									
Etodolac (NSAID)		3.6					99	7		
Etomidate (Anaesthetic Agent)	4.2	3				4.5	75		730	
Etoposide (Antineoplastic agent)	-1.1	c60	45			98-99			30-40	-1.1
Famciclovir (Antiviral)			77		0.9	<20	2.3	8	74	77
Famotidine (H$_2$ antagonist)	-0.6	<100	43		1	16		240-1000	72	-0.6
Felbamate (Antiseizure agent)			*	>80		0.76	22-25	21	0.5	40-50
Felodipine (Anti hypertensive)	7.1	100	15	0.5-2		>99	25	800	<1	7.1
Fenbufen (Antiinflammatory)	4.5	2.6	Good		2	3	>99	10		

Drugs	Ionization constant (pKa)	Partition Coeffi-cient (log p)	Oral Absor-ption (%)	Bio Availa-bility (%)	Tmax	Volume Distribution (l/kg)	Protein Binding (%)	Half Life (hours)	Clearance (ml/min)	Urinary Excretion (%)
Fenfluramine (Monoamine)	9.9,	3.4	Good				30-35			
Fenoprofen (Antiinflammatory)	4.5	0.8	Good		0.5-2	0.1	99		65	3
Fenoterol (Respiratory agent)	8.5	0.8	60	Low	2					<2
Fentanyl (Neuromuscular blocker)	8.4	4.1	iv			3	83	3	780	
Finasteride (Antiprostate)				63		1.1	90	7.9	2.3	<1
Flecamide (Antiarrythemic)	4.5			8	52	15	700			4.5
Floxuridine (Antineoplastic)	7.4	-1.2	Poor							Low
Flucloxacillin (Antibiotic)	2.7		Good		1	0.15	93	1.5	83	
Fluconazole (Antifungal)										
Flucytosine (Antiinflammatory)	2.9	-1 7	c100			0.7	Low	4	13	>90
Fludrocortisone (Corticosteroid)		2.2	Good				75	0.5		
Flufenamic acid (Antiinflammatory)	3.9	2					>90			
Flumazenil (Benzodiazepine Antagonist)		1.6	Good	16	0.5-1	1		<1	700-1 200	<ai
Flunitrazepam (Anxiolytic)	1.8	2.1	100	80-90		3.7	77-80	19-36	260	<5
5-Fluorouracil (Antineoplastic)	8.1	-1	var			0.25		0.25	1000	<20
Fluoxetine (Antidepressant)				>60		* 35	94	53	9.6	<2.5
Flupenthixol (Antipsychotic)	7.8	4.5	Good	55				14-36	500	
Fluphenazine (Antipsychotic)	8.1	3.5	Good				99	33		

Drugs	Ionization constant (pKa)	Partition Coeffi-cient (log p)	Oral Absor-ption (%)	Bio Availa-bility (%)	Tmax	Volume Distribution (l/kg)	Protein Binding (%)	Half Life (hours)	Clearance (ml/min)	Urinary Excretion (%)
Flurazepam (Hypnotic)	1.9	4.5	Good		1	3.4	>95	2		<!
Flurbiprofen (NSAID)	4.3	1.2	Good			0.1	99		20	25
Fluspirilene (Antipsychotic)	8.7	6.2								
Flutamide (Antineoplastic agent)		3.5					94-96			
Foscarnet (Antiviral)						0.6-2			150	
Fosfomycin (Antibiotic)								3	63	
Fosinopril (ACE inhibitor)				36		0.13	*9s	11.3	0.51	43
Frusemide (Diuretics)	3.7,	2.3	<90	65	1	0.1-0.2	95		70-210	70-90
Fusidic acid (Antibacterial)	5.4	5.6					95			<10
Gabapentin (Anticonvulsant)				60		0.8	0	6.5	1.6	100
Gallopamil (Calcium antagonist)		3.1C	100	15						
Ganciclovir (Antiviral)		-2.8		6		0.4-0.6	<5		200	>95iv
Gemfibrozil (Lipid lowering agent)		3.9	100				97-99			50
Gentamicin (Antibacterial/ Antifungal)	8.2		Poor			0.2	<30		75	80-98
Glibenclamide (Oral Antidiabetic)	5.3		Good		3	0.15	99		91	50
Glibornuride (Antidiabetic)		3				0.25	95	8		
Gliclazide (Oral Antidiabetic)	5.8	1.5	Good		4	0.3	85-95		13	<5
Glipizide (Oral Antidiabetic)		1.9	100	100		0.2	98		40	1

Drugs	Ionization constant (pKa)	Partition Coefficient (log p)	Oral Absorption (%)	Bio Availability (%)	Tmax	Volume Distribution (l/kg)	Protein Binding (%)	Half Life (hours)	Clearance (ml/min)	Urinary Excretion (%)
Gliquidone (Antidiabetic)		3.6	Good				99			<[1]
Glutethimide (Hypnotic Agent)	9.2	1.9								
Glyburide (Antidiabetic)	5.3	3.9	Good					10		<10
Glycerin (Antianginal/ coronary vasodilator)		1	Good	Low		3		<0.1	30000	<1
Glycopyrronium (Antisparmodic)			Poor					<0.1		
Glymidine (Antidiabetic)		1.3	>95				80			<1
Goserelin (Hormone)					0.2	Low		130		
Gold sodium (Thiomalate)						0.26	95	25days	7	70
Granisetron (antiemetic)				-60		3	65	5.3	11	16
Griseofulvin (Antifungal)		2.2	irreg			1.5		22		
Guanabenz (Antihypertensive)		3	Good				90	14-Dec	8000-17000	<-1
Guanadrel (Antihypertensive)		-2.2					20	10	*	50
Guanethidine (Antihypertensive)	11	-1 .7	Poor	<50	3		<10	4-8D		25
Guanfecine (Antihypertensive)		100	>95				20-30	15-17		30
Guanoxan (Antihypertensiv)	12.3	1.6								
Haloperidol (Antipsychotic)	8.3	3.4	Good	65			90		600-1300	<5
Heparin (Anticoagulant, Antithrombosis)						0.058	extensive	3.7	1	negligible
Heroin (Opioid Analgesic)	7.6									

Drugs	Ionization constant (pKa)	Partition Coefficient (log p)	Oral Absorption (%)	Bio Availability (%)	Tmax	Volume Distribution (l/kg)	Protein Binding (%)	Half Life (hours)	Clearance (ml/min)	Urinary Excretion (%)
Hexobarbital (Sedative)	8.2			>90		1.2	42	3.9		<i
Homatropine (Anticholinergic Drug)	9.7									
Hydrochlorothiazide (Diuretic)	9.2, 7.9	-0.1	<90	70		3	40		350	65-70
Hexobarbital (Sedative)				>90		1.2	42	3.9		<i
Hydralazine (Antihypertensive)	7.1	1			0.5		90	2	3000	<!
Hydrochlorothiazide (Diuretic)	9.2	-0.1	<90	70		3	40		350	65-70
Hexobarbital (Sedative)				>90		1.2	42	3.9		<i
Hydrocortisone (Corticosteroid)	5.1	1.6	Good		1	0.3-0,5	75-95		350-400	<1
Hydroxizine (Anxiolytic, Sedatives)	7.1	4.2						3		
Hydroxychloroquine (Antiprotozoal)		3.7	100		3			3d		8
Hydroxyprogesterone (Gonadal Hormone)										
Hydroxyurea (Antineoplastic)		-1.8	Good		2					<80
Hydroyzine (Antihistamin)	7.1	4.2						3		

Drugs	Ionization constant (pKa)	Partition Coefficient (log p)	Oral Absorption (%)	Bio Availability (%)	Tmax	Volume Distribution (l/kg)	Protein Binding (%)	Half Life (hours)	Clearance (ml/min)	Urinary Excretion (%)
Hyoscine (Antinausea)	8.1,	1.2	Good	Low	0.5	2			750	5
Ibuprofen (NSAID agent)	4.4	1	100			0.1	99	2	60	<10
Idoxuridine (Antinausea)							Low			Low
Ifosfamide (Antineoplastic)			Good		1					
Imipenem (Antibiotic)					0.23		<20	0.9	2.9	69
Imipramine (Antidepressant)	9.5	2.5	Good	50		20-Oct	85-95		1000	<10
Indapamide (Antihypertensive)	8,3		100		2-3		80	15	20	5-10
Indomethacin (NSAID agent)	4.5	-1.0	Good		1-4	0.2-1	90-99	3-15	70-140	5-20
Indoramin (AntiHypertensive Drug)	7.8	2.3			3-4	7	70-90	2-8	140	<10
Interferon(alfa) (Antiviral)				100(im)		0.4		0.67	2.8	
Interferon (beta) (Antiviral)				47		2.9		4.3	13	
Indoramin (antiadrenergic)	7.7	2.3			3-4	7	70-90	2-8	140	<10
Insulin (Pancreatic Hormone)			Inact				5		150-600	
Ipratropium (Antiasthamatic)			inhal	<1						Low
Iprindole (AntiDepressant)	8.2									
Iproniazid (Monoamine oxidase inhibitor)		0.2	Good					10		15
Isocarboxazid (Monoamine oxidase inhibitor)	10.4	1.5	Good					36		2
Isoniazid (Antituberculars)	3.5	-0.7	100	80	1-4	0.6-0.8	<5	1-5	200-500	5-30

Drugs	Ionization constant (pKa)	Partition Coeffi-cient (log p)	Oral Absor-ption (%)	Bio Availa-bility (%)	Tmax	Volume Distribution (l/kg)	Protein Binding (%)	Half Life (hours)	Clearance (ml/min)	Urinary Excretion (%)
Isoprenaline (Antiasthamatic)	8.6	0.1	irreg		1-2	0.5	68	0.05		<5
Isosorbide dinitrate (Antianginal)		0	Good	25	0.5	1.5	30-70	0.3-1	2500-4000	<1
Isosorbide mononitrate (Antianginal)		-0.4	100	90	1	0.6	<5	2-7	70-350	2
Isoxsuprine (Peripheral Vasodilator)	8.0, 9.8	2.6	Good		1			1.5		
Isotretinoin (Anti Acne Agent)				-25		7	99.9	14	5.5	<1
Isradipine (Calcium antagonist)		4.3	100	17	1	69-161	>90	9-16	750	<5
Itraconazole (Antifungal)			100	<90						<1
Kanamycin (Antibacterial)	7.2		Poor			0.3	<5	2-4	100	50-95
Ketamine (Anaesthetics)	7.5	2.2	iv			2	12	3	1000	3-20
Ketanserin (Antihypertensive)		3	Good	50	1		95	14		<1
Ketazolam (anticonvulsant)		3.7	Good					1.5		<1
Ketoconazole (Antifungal)	2.9	4.3			2-3		99	6-10		<5
Ketoprofen (NSAIDs)	4.6	1	Good		1-3	0.1-0.2	95	1-4	70-140	
Ketorolac (Analgesic & antipyretic)	3.5	1.9	100	90	0.5-1	0.2-0.3	>99	4-6	26-46	58
Labetalol (Antihypertensive)	8.7	1.2	90	30	1	10	50	2-6	1500	<5
Lanatoside C (Cardiovascular agent)		0.1	Poor		1	4	25	40		70

Drugs	Ionization constant (pKa)	Partition Coefficient (log p)	Oral Absorption (%)	Bio Availability (%)	Tmax	Volume Distribution (l/kg)	Protein Binding (%)	Half Life (hours)	Clearance (ml/min)	Urinary Excretion (%)
Latamoxef (Antibiotic)					0.2	50		2.5	70-115	75
Leucovorin (Antineoplastics)		97		3.2	35-45	9.3	3.9	10		
Levallorphan (Opoid Antidote)	4.5									
Levamisole (Anthelmintic)	8									
Levobunolol (Antiglucoma)	9.3	2.3	Good	75		5 .		6	800	15
Levodopa (Antirigidity/antitremor)	2.3, 8.7, 9.9,	-2.9	Good	33	1-2			1-2	1700	<1
Levorphanol (Analgesic)	9.2	3.4			1-2	10	40	15-30		
Levonorgestre (progestin Agent)				94		1.7	37	15	1.5	52
Lidoflazine (Antianginal)		5.8	High		1			24		
Lignocain (Anaesthetics)	7.9	2	Good	35		3	60-70	1-4	350-1400	3^20
Lincornycm (Antibacterial)	7.6	0.6	20-35			0.5	72	5		10-15
Liothyroine (Thiroid agent)	8.5	3	c100			0.5	99	2Drugs	17	
Lisinopril (Antihypertensive)	1.7	-2.9	50	25-50	6-8			30		
Lisuride (Antiparkinson agent)		2.7		20				2	750-1500	
Lithium (Antidepressant)			100	100	2	0.8		27	25	
Lodoqumol (Agent of STD)	8	4	var							
Lofepramine (antidepressant)		6.5	Good	Low	1		99			
Lomefloxacin (Antibacterial)		c100	c100	1				7-8	200-300	10-20
Loperamide (Antidiarrhoeal)	8.7	3.9	Poor	Low			97	7-15		1-2

Drugs	Ionization constant (pKa)	Partition Coeffi- cient (log p)	Oral Absor- ption (%)	Bio Availa- bility (%)	Tmax	Volume Distribution (l/kg)	Protein Binding (%)	Half Life (hours)	Clearance (ml/min)	Urinary Excretion (%)
Loracarbef (Antibiotic)				94		0.32	25	1.2	1.73	94
Loratidine (Antiallergic)		5.2			1-2			8-11		
Lorazepam (Sedative)	1.3, 11.5	2.5	Good	95	1-2	1-2	90	4-24	70	<1
Lorcainide (Antiarrythmic)		4.5				10	85	9	1000	<3
Lormustine (Antineoplastic)		2.8	Good							Low
Lornoxicam (Antiinflammatory)			2-3					3-5		<1
Lovastatin (Lipid lowering agent)			<5				95	1.1-1.7	4-18	negligible
Lymecycline (Antiinflammatory)										
Lysergide (Recreational Drug)	3.3, 7.8									
Maprotiline (Antidepressants)	10.5	4.2	Good	70	3-8	23-70	90	20-70	400-1400	<10
Mazindol (Monoarnine oxidase inhibitor)	8.6							36		12-24
Mebendazole (Anthelmintics)		3.1	Poor		3-7	2	95	2-9		<10
Mecamyramine (Anti Hypertention)	11.2									
Mecillinam (Antibiotic)	3.4		Poor					5-15	1	50-70
Meclizine (Antihistamine, H1 antagonist)	3.1	7								
Medazepam (Anxiolytic)	6.2	4.4	Good		1		>95	1-2		
Medifoxamine (Antidepressant)					1	8-12		1-2	5000	
Medigoxin (Cardiac glycoxide)			>90		1	6-10	10-30	40-70	140	30-50

Drugs	Ionization constant (pKa)	Partition Coefficient (log p)	Oral Absorption (%)	Bio Availability (%)	Tmax	Volume Distribution (l/kg)	Protein Binding (%)	Half Life (hours)	Clearance (ml/min)	Urinary Excretion (%)
Medroxy-progesterone (Gonadai Hormone)						0.6	94	36	1260	
Mefenamic acid (Analgesic, antipyretic)	4.2	5.3	Good		2-4		99	3-4		<50
Mefloquin (Antimalanal)		3.4	Good		2-14	19	98	21d	30	5
Mefruside (Diuretic)		1.4	90			6		3-12	350-2100	<1
Mepacrine (Anti Protozoal Drug)	7.7, 10.3									
Meperidine (narcotic analgesics)	8.7			52		44	58	3.2	17	1-25
Melphalan (Antineoplastic)		-0.5	var	var		0.5	50-60	1-2	520	13
Mepacrine (Antimalarial)	7.7	6.2	Good				90	120		
Mepenzolate (Antispasmodic)		Poor					10	7-14		
Mepivacaine (Anaesthetic)	7.7	1.8				1	77	1-2	780	
Meprobamate (Hypnotic)		0.7	Good		3.5	0.7	20		50	10-20
Meptazinol (Analgesic)	8.7	3.8	100		2-19	5	27	2	2100	<5
Mepyramine (Antihistamine)	8.9	0.5								
Mercaptopurine (Antineoplastic)	7.7	-1 .8	50	16	0.5-4		20	1-1.5		<10
Mesalazine (Antiinflammatory)	2.7	1.1	90			0.2-0.3	43	1		<10
Metaraminol (Cardiovascular agent)	8.6	-0.3						<0.1		
Metformin (Oral antidiabeticl)	2.8	-1.4	Good	55	2	1-4	<5	2-5	500-700	30-50
Methadone (Respiratory agent)	, 8.6	2.1	Good		4	5	80-90	10-25	140	33

Drugs	Ionization constant (pKa)	Partition Coeffi-cient (log p)	Oral Absor-ption (%)	Bio Availa-bility (%)	Tmax	Volume Distribution (l/kg)	Protein Binding (%)	Half Life (hours)	Clearance (ml/min)	Urinary Excretion (%)
Methaqualone (Hypnotic)	2.5	2.5	Good		2-3		High	10-40		<5
Methicillin (Antibiotic)	2.8	1 .2	Poor			0.4	40	0.6	500	25-80
Methimazole (Antithyroid drug)		0.1				0.5	Low	3-5	170	7-12
Methocarbamol (Muscle Relaxant)		-0.1								
Methohexitone (Anaesthetic)	7.9, 8.3	1.7				1	73		830	
Methotrexate (Antineoplastic)	4.8, 5.5	-0.5	Good			0.8	50-95		200	50-95
Methoxamine (Anti Hypotensive Drug)	4.8									
Methotrimeprazine (Antipsychotic)	9.2	4.7	Good			30		15-77		<1
Methylamphetamine (CNS Stimulation)	10.0									
Methyldopa (Antihypertensive)	1.2	-2.6	Poor		3	0.6	<20	1-2	200-400	20-60
Methylpheno-barbitone (Barbiturates)	7,8	2	<90	70	3-6		40-60	50-60	35	<2
Methylprednisolone (Corticosteroid)	4.6	2.2				0.7		3	250	
Metbyltestosterone (Hormone)		3.9							2	
Methyprylone (Barbiturates)	12	0.8		2			+	4		3
Methysergide (Analgesic)	6.6	2.1						10		56
Metoclopramide (Prokinetic)	7.3	2.6	>95	40	1-2	3	60-70	3-6	500-1200	10-25
Metocurine (Muscle Relaxant)						0.35	35	4.7	1.3	50
Metolazone (Diuretic)	9.7	2.6C	40-65		5	2	95	18	100	70-80

Drugs	Ionization constant (pKa)	Partition Coefficient (log p)	Oral Absorption (%)	Bio Availability (%)	Tmax	Volume Distribution (l/kg)	Protein Binding (%)	Half Life (hours)	Clearance (ml/min)	Urinary Excretion (%)
Metoprolol (Antihypertensive)	9.7	-0.1	>95	50	1-2	6	12	2-5	1000	<5
Metronidazole (Antibacterial/ antifungal)	2.5	0								
Mexiletine (Antiarrythmatic)	9	2,6	>90	90	5-8		70	7-25	500	10-20
Mezlocillin (Antibiotic)			Poor			0.25	35	1	200	60-70
Mianserin (Antidepressant)	7.1	4.3	Good	30	2	6-45	90-95	6-39	320	5
Miconazole (Antibacterial/ antifungal)	6.7	6D				20	92-99	24	760-	<1
Midazolam (Anxiolytic)	6.2	3.7	iv			1.3-2.2	>94	2-5	700-1700	<1
Midodrine (Antihypertensive)		-0.4								
Milrinone (Inotropic Agent)				380		0.32	70	0.8	6.1	85
Mifepristone (Anti progesterone)		4.9								
Minocycline (Antibacterials)	2.8	-1.4				1.5	70	15	120	<10
Minoxidil (Hair growth)		1.4				3	<5	3-4	600	<20
Misonidazole (Radiosensitizer)		-0.4								
Misopristol (Prostaglandin E1 (PGE1) analog)		2.9								
Mitomycin (Antineoplastic)	10.9	-0.4	iv							10
Mitotane (Antineoplastic)		5.6	<50							<10
Mitoxantrone (Antineoplastic)		Iv						43		Low
Moclobemide (Monoamine oxidase inhibitor)		2A		60						

Drugs	Ionization constant (pKa)	Partition Coeffi-cient (log p)	Oral Absor-ption (%)	Bio Availa-bility (%)	Tmax	Volume Distribution (l/kg)	Protein Binding (%)	Half Life (hours)	Clearance (ml/min)	Urinary Excretion (%)
Molindone (Antipsychotic)	6.9	2.6	Good							<5
Monosialog-anglioside						0.05-0.09			<3	
Moricizine (Antiarrythemic)		3.3	100	36	1-2		80-95	2-4	1300-2700	<10
Morphine (Analgesic, antipyretic)	7.9, 8.1, 9.9	0.2	60			3.5	35	2.5	1200	10-15
Moxalactam (Antibiotic)				3(oral) 70-100 (1.m)		0.25		2.1	1	76
Mustine (Antineoplastic)	6.4		iv					<0.05		^
Nabilone (Antinauseatic)		6.5	Good					2		
Nabumetone (NSAIDs)		2.8		Low			>99			
Nadolol (β-adrenoreceptor antagonist)	9.7	-1.3	25	25	2-5	2	20-30	15	150	25
Nafcillin **(Antibiotic)**				36	0.35	89.4		1.0	7.5	27
Naftidrofuryl (Cerebral vasodialator)	8.2			0.5-1						
Nalbuphine (Analgesic)		1.1	Good	50	1				3.5-5	
Nalidixic acid (Antibacterial)	6.7	-2	c100		1-2	1	93-95	2-9	160	<20
Nalorphine (Opioid Antidote)	7.8									
Naloxone (Antipoisoning)				~2		2.1		1.1	22	Negligible
Naltrexone (Opioid Antagonist)				5-40		19	20	2.7	48	<1

Drugs	Ionization constant (pKa)	Partition Coefficient (log p)	Oral Absorption (%)	Bio Availability (%)	Tmax	Volume Distribution (l/kg)	Protein Binding (%)	Half Life (hours)	Clearance (ml/min)	Urinary Excretion (%)
Naproxen (NSAIDs)	4.2	1.5	100		2-4	0.1	>99	10-20	5	<10
Natamycin (Antiinfective)		-2.9	Poor							
Nefopam (Analgesic, antipyretic)	9.2	3.7			1-3		71-76	3-8		<5
Neomycin (Antibacterial)			<5					2-3		
Neostigmine (Neuromuscular agent)	12					0.7		1.3	630	67
Netilmicin (Antibacterial)						0.25	<25	3	67	90-95
Nicardipine (Calcium antagonist)		4.3	100	35	0.3-2	0.8	>90	7-12	580	<5
Nicitinic acid (Anticoagulant)	4.8		100		1			0.3-1		35
Nicotine (Para-sympathomimetic)				30(oral) 90 (Smoking 80-90 (trans dertmal)		2.6	4.9		18.5	16.7
Nicoumalone (Anticoagulant)	*4.7*		Good			0.3	>95	8	35	<1
Nifedipine (Antihypertensive)		3.3	dOO	50		1-1.5	>90		100-700	<1
Nilvadipine (Calcium antagonist)		2.1		14			98	11	1250	<1
Nimodipine (Cardiovascular agent)		6	c100	13	2	1-2.5	>95	1	1000-13000	<10
Nisoldipine (Calcium channel blocke**)**		*7.1*	100				>90		1250	<5
Nitrazepam (Hypnotic)	3.2, 10.8	2.3	Good			2.5	85	30	60	<10

Drugs	Ionization constant (pKa)	Partition Coefficient (log p)	Oral Absorption (%)	Bio Availability (%)	Tmax	Volume Distribution (l/kg)	Protein Binding (%)	Half Life (hours)	Clearance (ml/min)	Urinary Excretion (%)
Nitrendipine (Antihypertensive)		6	80	Low			>99		1300	<5
Nitrofurantoin (Antibacterial)	7.2					0.8	40	1	680	
Nitroglycerine (Anti Anginal)			<1 (oral)		3.3			2.3	230	<1
Nizatidine (Antiulcer)		-0.6	>95	95		1.2	15-30	1.3	840	65
Noradrenaline (Sympathom imetic)	8.6	-1.1								16
Northiondrone (Hormone)				64		3.6	91-97	8.5	5.9	<4
Norethisterone (Gonadal Hormone)						4	80	10	450	
Norfloxacin (Antibacterial)	6.3	-1.4		40		2	15			30
Nortriptyline (Antidepressant)	9.7	1.7	Good	60		14-40	90-95	15-90	660	<5
Noscapine (Antitussive, Expectorant)	6.2	2.5	Good	30	0.5-2			1.5-3	1400	<1
Novobiocin (Antibiotic)	4.3, 9.1									
Nystatin (Antifungal)			Poor							
Octretide (Growth Hormone inhibitor)				<2(oral) 100(s.c) 25 (intra-nasai)		0.35	65	1.5	2.7	11-20
Oestradiol (Hormone)		4					50			<5
Ofloxacin (Antibacterial)		-2	100	90		1.2	20-30		560	85-95
Omeprazole (Proton Pump inhibitor)	2.2		Good	70	<0.5	0.17	94-96	0.5-1	560	<!
Ondansetron (Antieuetic, antinauseant)		3.2								

Drugs	Ionization constant (pKa)	Partition Coefficient (log p)	Oral Absorption (%)	Bio Availability (%)	Tmax	Volume Distribution (l/kg)	Protein Binding (%)	Half Life (hours)	Clearance (ml/min)	Urinary Excretion (%)
Orciprenaline (Antiasthamatic)	8.9, 11.8		Good	40				2		
Ornidazole (Antibacterial)	2.3	0.6				0.9	<15	14		
Orphenadrine (Antirigidity, antitremor)	8.4	1.5	Good				20	14-18		<5
Ouabain (Cardiac glycoside)		6,0	var							40-50
Oxacillin (Antibiotic)				33		0.33	92.2	0.4-0.7	6.1	46
Oxamniquine (Anthelmintic)	3.3	2.2								
Oxaprozin (NSAID)				95-100		0.14-0.24	>99.5	21-25	0.028-.042	negligible
Oxazepam (Anxiolytic, sedative)	1.7, 11.6	2.2	Good			0.5-2	95		70-140	<5
Oxprenolol (β-adrenoreceptor antagonist)	9.5	0.3	90	50		1.2	80-95		200	<5
Oxybutynin (Anticholinergic)		3.7								
Oxypentifylline (Anti Ulcer Agent)	0.3		High	Low	1-1.5	5		0.4-1	4900	<1
Oxyphenbutazone (NSAIDs)	4.7	2.7					99	45		
Oxytetracycline (Antibacterial)	3.3, 7.3, 9.1	-1.4				1.5	20-35	9		70
Paclitaxel (Antineoplastic)			Low			2	95-98	3	5.5	5
Pafenolol (Anti Hypertensive)		1.7	iv			1.1		3-4	300	50
Pamidronate (Nutritional supplement)			Low					2-3	300	iv30
Pancuronium (Neuromuscular blocker)					0.26	7	2.3	1.8	67	

Drugs	Ionization constant (pKa)	Partition Coeffi-cient (log p)	Oral Absor-ption (%)	Bio Availa-bility (%)	Tmax	Volume Distribution (l/kg)	Protein Binding (%)	Half Life (hours)	Clearance (ml/min)	Urinary Excretion (%)
Papaverine (Antispasmodic)	6.4	3	100	54	1-2		80	1-2		<!
Paracetamol (Analgesic, antipyretic)	9.5	0.5	Good	80	1-3	2	Low	1.5-3	350	<5
Paraldehyde (Antiepileptic)		0.7	Good		0.5	1		4-10	140	
Pargyline (MAO inhibitor)	6.9	2								
Paroxetine (Antidepressant)		3.4	Good	50	1-11		95			2
PAS (Antituberculosis)	3.3	0.9	Poor		1-2			58-73	1	50
Pefloxacin (Antibacterial)		-1.5	100	95	1-3	1.8	20-30	8-15	150	<10
Pelrinone (PDE inhibitor)							moderate	1-2		High
Pemoline (Monoamine oxidase inhibitor)	10.5				2-3		30-50	10-18		50
Penbutolol (β-adrenoreceptor antagonist)	9.3	1.9	>95	50	1-2		98	5-27		<5
Penicillamine (Antigout)	1.8, 7.9, 10.5	-2.5	Poor		2-3		90	2-6	1000	3-25
Pentamidine (Antimicrobial)		2	Poor			16		6.2	8500	<5
Pentazocine (Analgesic, antipyretic)	8.5	2	Good	20	1	5-6	60-70	2-4	1250	10
Pentobarbitone (Sedative)	8.1	2.1	Good		1-2		50	35-50		
Pentoxifylline (Peripheral vasodilator)			>90	31	2-3	2.2	Low	1		<1

Drugs	Ionization constant (pKa)	Partition Coefficient (log p)	Oral Absorption (%)	Bio Availability (%)	Tmax	Volume Distribution (l/kg)	Protein Binding (%)	Half Life (hours)	Clearance (ml/min)	Urinary Excretion (%)
Pergolide (Dopamine agonist)		3.8			1-2		90			
Pencyazine (Antipsychotic)		3.5								
Permdopril (Anti hypertensive)		1.3			1			3	500	
Perphenazine (Antipsychotic)	7.8	3.1	Good				10-35	8-12	840-2600	1-2
Pethidine (Analgesic)	8.7	1.6	Good	56	2	4	40-70	3-10	600-1000	5-10
Phenathicillin (Antibiotic)	2.7	2.2	var	86	2	0.3	75		295	50
Phenelzine (MAO inhibitor)		0.9	Good					7		<5
Phenformin (Oral antidiabetic)	3.1	-0.8				5	20	5	750	
Phenindamine (Respiratory agent)	8.3	0.7								
Phenindione (Anticoagulant)	4.1	3.7	Good				70	6		
Pheniramine (Antiallergics)	9.3	2			1-3			8-17		
Phenobarbitone (Anticonvulsant)	7.2	1.5	100	100	0.5-4	0.5-0.7	50	100	5	25
Phenoxy-Mepenicillin (Antibiotic)	2.7		Good	50	2	0.5	80	0.5	480	20-35
Phentermine (Monoamine oxidase inhibitor)	10.1	1.9	Good		4	3-4		19-24		70-80
Phenylbutazone (Antiinflammatory)	4.5	3.2				0.17	99	70	2	
Phenylethyl-malonamide (Anticonvulsant)				91	0.69		8	16	0.52	79

Drugs	Ionization constant (pKa)	Partition Coefficient (log p)	Oral Absorption (%)	Bio Availability (%)	Tmax	Volume Distribution (l/kg)	Protein Binding (%)	Half Life (hours)	Clearance (ml/min)	Urinary Excretion (%)
Phenylephrine (Mydriatic / cycloplegic)	8.9	-0.3	irreg	38	1-2	5		2-3	2100	<1
Phenylpro-panolamine (Psychoactive)				>70		4.1		4.7	10	65
Phenytoin (Antiepileptic)	8.3	2.5	100		2-4	0,7-0.8	90	7-60		<5
Pholcodine (Respiratory agent)	8	0.8			5			37		
Physostigmine (AChE inhibitor)	8.5	2.2			0.5	1-2	4-18	<0.3		
Pimozide (Antipsychotic)	7.3	6.3			4-8			18-48		<1
Pinacidil (Antihypertensive)		1.9	100	95	0.5-1		60-65	4		<10
Pindolof (b-adrenoreceptor antagonist)	8.8	0	>95	90	1-3	1	60	3-4	530	40
Pipecuronium (Neuromuscular Blocker)						0.35		2.5	2.1	37-41
Piperacillin (Antibiotic)			Poor			0.2	22	1	166	75-90
Piperazine (Anthelmintic)	5.7, 9.8	-1.2	Good							
Pipothiazine (Antipsychotic)		>12								1
Piracetam (cognitive enhancer)		-1.5								1
Pipothiazine (antipsychotic)		>12								1
Piracetam (Cognitive enhance)		-1.5								
Pirbuterol (Cerebral activator)	7	-0.5			2			2-3		10
Pirenzepine (Antimuscarinic agen)	8.1	1.2	Poor	25	2		10	11	240	20

Drugs	Ionization constant (pKa)	Partition Coefficient (log p)	Oral Absorption (%)	Bio Availability (%)	Tmax	Volume Distribution (l/kg)	Protein Binding (%)	Half Life (hours)	Clearance (ml/min)	Urinary Excretion (%)
Piretanide (Diuretic)		3.9	100		1	0.3	>90	1-2	200	51
Piroxicam (NSAIDs)	4.6	0.3	Good			0.1-0.2	99	30-60	2	10
Pirprofen (Antiinflammatory)		1	100		1-2	0.18	>95	6-7	20-25	1
Pivampicillin (Antibiotic)	7	2.4	Good		1					Low
Pivmecillinam (Antibiotic)	8.9		Good		1-2			0.7		30b
Pizotifen (Analgesic)	7				5-7			26		
Polymixin B (Antibacterial)	8.9		0		2			6		*60*
Polythiazide (Diuretic)	9.8	2.5	Good		5-12		80-85		25	20
Practolol (β-adrenoreceptor \ antagonist)	9.5	-1.7	>95	*95*	1-3		**7**	10	140	85
Pravastain (Hypolipidemic Agent)			18		0.46		43	1.8	305	47
Prazepam (Hypnotic)	2,7	3.7	var		2-8	0.5-3		70	5-20	<1
Praziquantel (Anthelmintic)		3.4	80		1-3			1-2		
Prazosin (Antihypertensive)	6.5	2.2		60	1-3	0.6	95	3	210	<5
Prednisolone (Corticosteroid)		1.6	>95	80	1-2	0.5-1.3	65-90	3-4	100-200	
Prednisone (Corticosteroid)				80		0.97	75	3.6	3.6	3
Prenalterol (Cerebral vasodialator)	9.5	1.1				2.4	Low	2-3	800	
Prenyleamine (Calcium channel blocker)		5.5	High				>95	7		

Drugs	Ionization constant (pKa)	Partition Coefficient (log p)	Oral Absorption (%)	Bio Availability (%)	Tmax	Volume Distribution (l/kg)	Protein Binding (%)	Half Life (hours)	Clearance (ml/min)	Urinary Excretion (%)
Primaquine (Antimalarial)		2.2	100		2-3	3-4		4-10		<5
Primidone (Anticonvulsant)		0.9	Good			0.6	<20	3-20	35-50	15-65
Prilocaine (Local Anesthetic)	7.9									
Probenecid (Antigout drug)	3.4	3.2	Good		3-4	0.1-0.2	90	4-17	23	1-10
Probucol (Anticoagulant)		>10	var							Low
Procainamide (Antiarrythmic)	9.2	0.9	>95	85	1-2	2	15	3	300-1000	45-60
Procaine (Local Anaesthetic)	8.8	1.9	Good							
Procarbazine (Antincoplastic)	6.6	-0.1	Good		0.5-1			0.2		5
Prochlorperazine (Antiemetic, antinauseants)	8.1	2.4		<20	2-6		High	7		
Procyclidine (Antirigidity, antitremor)		1:7	Good	75	1-8	1		8-16	75	
Progabide (Antiepileptic)	3.4	3								
Progesterone (Gonadal Hormone)		3.9		Low	1-3			0.05		
Proguanil (Antimalarial)	2.3		Good		3	2.9	75-90	82		30
Promazine (Antipsychotic)	9.4	2.5								
Promethazine (Anti emetic, antinauseants)	9.1	2.9	Good	25	2-3	13	75-93	10-15	1100	2
Propafenone (Antiarrythmatic)		3.2C	90	50	2.5-4		95	2-32	1200	<1
Propantheline (Prokinetics)			Poor	Low				2	1300	<5

Drugs	Ionization constant (pKa)	Partition Coeffi-cient (log p)	Oral Absor-ption (%)	Bio Availa-bility (%)	Tmax	Volume Distribution (l/kg)	Protein Binding (%)	Half Life (hours)	Clearance (ml/min)	Urinary Excretion (%)
Propofol (Anaesthetics)		3.8	Iv			5-25		3-10	1300-2000	<1
Propranolol (**Anti Hypertensive**)	9.5	1 .3	100	35	1-4	3	85-95	3-4	1000	<5
Propylthiouracil (Thyroid agent)	8.3		100		1	0.4	80	1-2	120-280	
Protriptyline (Antidepressant)		1.2	Good	90	6-12	22	95	140	140-350	<5
Pyrantel (Anthelmintic)	11	Poor							5	
Pyrazinamide (Antituberculers)	, 0.5	-0.6	Good		1-2		50	4-10		4-14
Pyridostigmine(AChE Inhibitor)			Poor	14		1.1		2-4	640	
Pyrimethamine (Antiprotozoal)	7.2	2.7	Good		2-4		80-94	3-4d	28	16-30
Quazepam (Hypnotic)		4.0	Good		1.5			39		
Quinacrine (**Anthelmintic**)	7.7, 10.3									
Quinalbarbitone (Barbiturate)	7.9	2	90		3	1.5	50-70	19-34	56	10-20
Quinapril (Antihypertensive)						0.4	97	2.2	2	28
Quindine (Antiarrythmic)	4.3, 8.4	3.2	90	75	1	2-3	75-90	4-12	300	10-50
Quinine (Antimalarial)	4.3, 8.4	3.4	100			2	70-90		90	
Quinapril (Antihypertensive)		1.8						3		
Ramipril (Antihypertensive)		1.6	Good	55-65	<1		73	1-5		<5
Ranitidine (H2 receptor antagonist)	8.2	0.3	Good	55	1-4	1-2	15	2-3	700	25-50
Reproterol (Respiratory agent)		-0.9								
Reserpine (Antihypertensive)	6.1	3.5	Poor				40-95	200	250	<5

Drugs	Ionization constant (pKa)	Partition Coefficient (log p)	Oral Absorption (%)	Bio Availability (%)	Tmax	Volume Distribution (l/kg)	Protein Binding (%)	Half Life (hours)	Clearance (ml/min)	Urinary Excretion (%)
Ribavirin (Antiviral)				45		9.3	0	28	5	35
Rifabutin (Antibiotic)				20		40	85	47	12	7
Rifampicin (Antftuberculers)	1.7	2.4	Good			1	80		170	15-30
Rimantadine (Anti Viral)						25	40	30	10	9
Rimiterol (Respiratory agent)	8.7	0.2	Good	Low				<0.1		10
Risperidone (Antipsychotic)			66(oral) 103(im)			1.1	89	3.2	5.4	3
Roxatidine (Antiulcer)	2.7				1					55
Roxithromycin (Antibacterial)					1		86-91	13	23	<5
Salbutamol (Antiasthamic)	9.3, 10.3	0.1	90		1-3		Low	2-7		50
Salicylate (Analgesic)	3	0.1				0.17	85	2-30	10-60	
Salsalate (Antiinflammatory)	3.5	3.6C	Good		1-2					<1
Salicylazo-sulfapyridine (Anti inflammatory Drug)	0.6, 2.4,9.7,11.8									
Scopolamine (Anti-acetylcholine)	7.8	1.2								
Secobarbital (Hypnotic)	7.9									
Selegiline (Antirigidity& antitremor)		2.2						39		
Semustine (Antincoplastic)		3.3	Good							Low
Sertraline (Antidepressant)				<5		76	99	23	38	<1
Simvastatin (Lipid lowering agent)							94	1.9	7.6	Negligible

Drugs	Ionization constant (pKa)	Partition Coeffi-cient (log p)	Oral Absor-ption (%)	Bio Availa-bility (%)	Tmax	Volume Distribution (l/kg)	Protein Binding (%)	Half Life (hours)	Clearance (ml/min)	Urinary Excretion (%)
Succinylsulfathiazole (Anti Microbial)	4.5									
Sodium cromoglycate (Antiasthmatic)	0.5	1.9	poor		0.25		60-70	1-2	560	<5
Sotalol (Antihypertensive)	9.8	-1.3	1oo	100	2-3	1	<5	15	150	60-70
Spectinomycin (Antibacterial)	8.7	-2.5			1	0.2	Low	2	100	35-90
Spironolactone (Antidiuretic)		2.3	<90		2-3		>95	18		Low
Streptokinase (Anticoagulant)					0.08			0.61	1.7	0
Streptomycin (Antibacterial)					1-2	0.3	50	3		30-90
Streptozocin (Antineoplastic)		-1.5	iv					0.5		
Sufentanil (Anaesthetic)	8.0	4.0	iv			2.0	93	2-3	730	
Sulfadiazine (Anti Microbial)	6.3			~100		0.29	54	9.9	0.55	57
Sulfadimethoxine (Anti Microbial)	6.3									
Sulfafurazole (Anti Microbial)	4.9									
Sulfamethiazole (Anti Microbial)	5.4									
Sulfamethox-ypyridazine (Anti MIcrobial)	6.7									
Sulfamethoxazole (Anti Microbial)	6.0			~100		0.21	62	10.1	0.32	14
Sulfametopyrazine (Antibacterial)			Good				60-80	C50		<20
Sulfasalazine (Anti Microbial)	0.6, 2.4, 9.7, 11.8									
Sulfathiazole (Anti Microbial)	7.1									

Drugs	Ionization constant (pKa)	Partition Coefficient (log p)	Oral Absorption (%)	Bio Availability (%)	Tmax	Volume Distribution (l/kg)	Protein Binding (%)	Half Life (hours)	Clearance (ml/min)	Urinary Excretion (%)
Sulfaurea (Antibacterial)			Good					2-3		
Sulfinopyrazone (Antigout)				100		0.74	98.3	4.0	2.4	39
Sulfisoxazole (Antimicrobial)				96		0.15	91.4	6.6	0.33	49
Sulindac (Antiinflammatory)	4.5	3.4	Good		1		95	7		<20
Sulipride (Antipsychotic)	8.9				3-4	2-3		6-41	420	20
Sulphadiamidine (Antibacterial)	7.4	2.0	Good		3-4	0.2-o.6	60-90	1-11	30	<15
Sulphadiazine (Antibacterial)	6.5	-0.1	Good		4	0.3	20-50	6-17	25	<50
Sulphadoxine (Antiprotozole)		0,7	Good		3-6		85-90	3-8d		<50
Sulphaguanidine (Antibacterial)	2.8	-1.2	var				<10			
Sulphamethoxazole (Antibacterial)	5.6	0.9	Good		2-4	0.2	60-70	9-12	15-25	60-80
Sulphasazine (antigout)	0.6	4.3	irreg		3	<1	>95	6-17		2-10
Sulphinpyrazone (Antigout)	2.8	2.3	Good		1-4	0.06	98	3-5	23	<50
Sultinpyrazole (Anti MIcrobial)	7.1									
Sumatriptan (Antimigrain)		0.8								
Sutamicillin (Antibiotic)		1.7	Good							
Tacrine AChE Inhibitor		3.3		<5	2			2-3	600	<3
Tacrolimus (AChE Inhibitor)				16		0.88	75-99	15	0.70	<1
Talampicillin (Antibiotic)		1.2C	Good		0.5-1					
Tamoxifen (Antineoplastic)		6.6			4-7			160		<1

Drugs	Ionization constant (pKa)	Partition Coefficient (log p)	Oral Absorption (%)	Bio Availability (%)	Tmax	Volume Distribution (l/kg)	Protein Binding (%)	Half Life (hours)	Clearance (ml/min)	Urinary Excretion (%)
Temazepam (Anxiolytic)	1.3	2.2	50-80		2	1	>95	15-20	65	<1
Teniposide (Anticancer)						0.22	>99	9	0.37	8
Tenoxicam (NSAIDs)					1			37		
Terazocin (Antihypertensive)				90		0.80	90-94	12	1.1	12
Terbutaline (Bronchodilator)	10.1	0.5		15	2-4	1	15-25	3-15	200-300	10
Terconazole (Anti-protozoal)		5.6								
Terfenadine (Antiallergic)							97	12	8.8	25
Testosterone (Gonadal Hormone)		3.3					98	0.25		Low
Tetrabenazine (Antirigidity & Antitremor)						1-2				
Tetracycline (Antibiotic)	3.3, 7.8, 9.7	-2.6				1.3-6	25-65	6-9	150-250	20-50
Tetrayhdrocannabinol (Hallucinogen)			Poor	10-20		10	97	>20	760-1190	0
Thalidomide (Immunomodulator/ anticancer		0.3								
Theobromine (Bronchodilator)	0.1	-0.8								
Theophylline (Bronchodilator)	0.7	-0.0			0.5-2	0.5	40-50	3-13	35-140	7-13
Thiabendazole (Anthelmintic)		2.3	Good		1-2			1		<1
Thiamphenicol (Antibiotic)		-0.3						2		
Thioguanine (Antineoplastic)	8.2	-0.1	Poor					0.5-4		<1
Thiopental (Sedative)	7.8	2.6	iv			3.0	80	10	130	

Drugs	Ionization constant (pKa)	Partition Coefficient (log p)	Oral Absorption (%)	Bio Availability (%)	Tmax	Volume Distribution (l/kg)	Protein Binding (%)	Half Life (hours)	Clearance (ml/min)	Urinary Excretion (%)
Thioridazine (Antipsychotic)	9.5	5.9	Good		1-4		>99	10-36		<1
Thiotepa (Antineoplastic)		0.5	Poor							<1
Thymoxamine (Calcium antagonist)			Poor		0.5-1					
Thyroxine (Thyroidal Hormone)	2.2		var			0.2	99.9	6-7 D	2	
Tiapamil (Calcium antagonist)		0.6		15-70		2	78	1-3	670-750	
Tiaprofenic acid (Antiinflammatory)	3.0	2.5	Good		1-2		98	1-2	75-100	
Ticarcillin (Antibiotic)	2.5	1.2	Poor			0.2	60	1.2	140	80-90
Ticlopidine (Anticoagulant)		4.0	90		1.2					<5
Timolol (Antiglucoma)	8.8	-0.1	72	60	1-2	2	60	3-6	500	20
Tinidazole (Antibacterial)	1.8	-0.3								
Tobramycin (Antibacterial)	6.7		Poor			0.3	<10	2-3	60-100	90-98
Tocainide (Antiarrythmic)	7.8	-0.1	High		1-2	1-3	10-50	8-25	140-210	20-50
Tolazoline (Vasodilator)	10.3									
Tolazamide (Antidiabetic)	3.5	1.8	Good		3		95	5-7		7-15
Tolbutamide (Hypoglycemic Drug)	5.4	2.3	Good		4	0.1-0.2	90-95	4-12	20	<5
Tolfenamic acid (Anti-inflammatory)		5.7				0.16	>99	2-3	155	
Tolmetin (Antiinflammatory)	3.5	1.0	Good		0.2-1	0.1	>99	1-6	70-140	<15
Tolrestat (Antidiabetic)			Good		2		99.5	10-12		High
Torasemide (Antihypertensive)			80		1	0.1-0.3		1-6	70	22-34

Drugs	Ionization constant (pKa)	Partition Coeffi-cient (log p)	Oral Absor-ption (%)	Bio Availa-bility (%)	Tmax	Volume Distribution (l/kg)	Protein Binding (%)	Half Life (hours)	Clearance (ml/min)	Urinary Excretion (%)
Tranexamic acid (Anti Fibinolic)	4.3, 10.6	-1.9	Good	40				10	120	
Tranylcypromine (Anti depressant)	8.2	1.5	Good					2		<2
Trazodone (Antidepressant)			100		1-3		90-95	4-7		<1T
Triamcinolone (Corticosteroid)										
Triamterene (Cardiovascular agent)	6.2	1.1	<90	50	1-2		45-70	2-4	1600	5-10
Triancinolone (Corticosteroid)		1.2				1.4-2.1		1.4	750-1100	
Triazolam (Anxiolytic)		3.2	100		1	1	80	3	330	
Trichloroethanol (sedative)					2.9	0.6	35	7-10		
Trifluoperazine (Anti Psychotic)	8.1	3.9			3-6			2-18		1
Trimeprazine (Respiratory agent)	9.0	4.6	Good		4-7					
Trimethoprim (Anti Bacterial)	6.4	0.9	100		1-4	1.4	40-70	8-17	75-150	40-70
Trimipramine (Antidepressant)		4.7	Good	40	3-6	20-50	95	10-40	700-1750	
Tripolidine (Respiratory agent)	6.9	3.9			2			1.5-2		
Tubocurarine (neuromuscular blocking agent))	8.0					0.4	50	2	140	63
Urapidil (Antihypertensive)		2.7	100	78	0.5-1	0.4-0.8	75-80	2-3	120-240	10-15
Valproate (Antiepileptic)	5.0	2.8	100	100	1-5	0.1-0.2	90	6-20	7-21	<5
Vancomycin (Antibacterial)			Poor			0.4-1	10-55	4-10	75	90-100
Vecuronium (Neuromuscular blocker)			iv			0.2-0.3	30-90	0.5-1	225-480	25

Drugs	Ionization constant (pKa)	Partition Coefficient (log p)	Oral Absorption (%)	Bio Availability (%)	Tmax	Volume Distribution (l/kg)	Protein Binding (%)	Half Life (hours)	Clearance (ml/min)	Urinary Excretion (%)
Venlafaxine (AntiDepressant)				~10		7.5	27	4.9	22	4.6
Verapamil (Antihypertensive)	8.9	3.8	100	20	2-3	4-5	90	2-7	700-1400	<5
Vidarabine (Antiviral)	3.5	-1.2						3-4		1-3
Vigabartrin (Antiepileptic)		3.1	100	2			Low	5-7		90
Viloxazine (Antidepressant)		1.3	100	1.5		0.5-1.5	85-90	2-5		12-15
Vinblastin (Anti Cancer)	5.4, 7.4	4.2	Poor				99.7			
Vincristine (Anti Cancer)	5.0, 7.4	2.8	Poor			8.4	75	23-85	128	<30
Vindesine (Antiepileptic)	5.4	2.4	Poor			8.8		24	300	
Warfarin (Anticoagulant)	5.0	2.5	Good	0.3-3		0.1-0.2	97-99	15-85	1.5-6.0	<1
Xamoterol (Cardiac stimulant) (β, adrenergic receptor Agonist)		0.5	9					7.7	224	62% unchanged in urine
Xipamide (Antidiuretic)	10	1.5	100	1			>95	5-8	19	30-50
Xylometazoline (Alpha agonist) (nasal decongestant)				poor				12		
Zalcitabine (Reverse transcriptase inhibitor)			80	0.53		<4		2	65	
Zidovudine (Antiviral)			100	60	0.5-2	14	<25	1-2	1600	57-72
Zimeldine (ssri antidepressant)	3.8	2.7						8.4		
Zolpidem (Anxiolytic)				67		0.54	92	2.2	4.3	<1
Zopiclone (Hypnotic)		1.0	Good	80	<1		45	2-3		<5
Zuclopenthixol (Antipsychotic)	6.7	5.7								

CHAPTER III

DRUG INTERACTIONS

DRUG INTERACTIONS

The drug interaction is a observable fact, which occurs when the effects of one drug are changed by the existence of other drug, food, drink or by some environmental chemical substances. The drug interaction may be beneficial or harmful effects. However, adverse or harmful effects are predominated. The mechanism of both types of interactions (beneficial or harmful) is very similar. I have discussed here only the adverse interactions. Drugs can interact with each other at any point from their being mixed during pharmaceutical formulation up to their final stage of excretion from the body. A patient takes more drugs, the greater will be the chances of adverse reactions. Many drugs are known to interact in some patients simply fail to do so in others. The dosage of the interacting drug may be important factor. The small dose of H_2 antagonist cimetidine may fail to inhibit the metabolism of the anticoagulant drug warfarin. However, a large dose may have great clinical effects. Sometime, the interactions can be avoided using another member of the same group of drugs. Doxycycline level in serum can fall below therapeutic concentration in phenytoin, barbiturates or carbamazepine are given concurrently, but member of tetracyclins do not affected in the same manner. Some doctors are over-anxious about drug interaction and other clinicians virtually disregard the existance of drug interactions. The responsible position lies between these two extremes. Very good number of interacting drugs can be given together safely if proper precaution can be taken.

Today, polypharmacy is the norm rather than an exception and there is enormous potential for drug interactions in these patients. Estimates of the incidence of Drug-Drug interactions have been reported as high as 20% of patients, who are on more than 5 medications at a time. Awareness of potential of drug interaction is essential for a practicing physician to enable the patient to receive the best medical care that he is entitled to.

A drug interaction refers to the possibility that one drug may alter the pharmacological effect of another drug given concurrently. The net result may be enhanced or diminished effect of one or both of the drug or a new effect that is not seen with either drug alone. Drug interaction is particularly important for those drugs with narrow therapeutic index, where even small elevations in plasma concentration can cause potentially serious adverse reaction.

There are two main type of drug interaction.

Pharmacokinetic interactions occur when one drug affects the plasma concentration, half-fife or both of another by altering its absorption, distribution, metabolism, or elimination. Example includes competition for protein binding in the plasma and alteration of hepatic cytocrome P450.

Pharmacodynamic interactions occur when one drug affects the ability of another to bring about its effects. This might occur with drugs that bind to multiple receptor type. Or it may even occur with the inadvertent concomitant use of mutually antagonistic agents such as β-agonists for bronchial asthma.

Drug interaction can be largely predicted on the pharmacological properties of the drugs being co-administered. A large number of drugs are metabolized (inactivated) by the hepatic microsomal cytochrome P450 enzymes. Some examples of drugs (with narrow therapeutic indices) being metabolized by these enzymes includes:

- Non-sedating antihistamines
- Long acting opiate analgesics
- Antiarrythmics
- Long acting benzodiazepines
- Ergotamines and dihydroergotamine
- Illicit drugs
- Coumarin anticoagulants

- Oral Contraceptives A number of drugs also alter the functioning of these enzymes. Some examples include:
- Cytochrome P450 inhibitors
    - HIV protease inhibitors
    - Non-nucleoside reverse transcriptase inhibitors
    - Macrolide antibiotics
    - Azole antifungal
    - Cimetidine
- Cytochrome P450 inducers
    - HIV protease inhibitors
    - Non-nucleoside reverse transcriptase inhibitors
    - Anticonvulsants (that are P450 inducers)

Co-administration of drugs having a narrow therapeutic index with either inducers or inhibitors of the cytochrome P450 enzymes could lead to either therapeutic failure or toxicity.

Similarly, drugs interactions are also particularly relevant for antibiotics, which are amongst commonest group of drugs prescribed. Many interactions take place at the absorption stage. Antacids and antidiarrhoeal preparations, in particular, can delay and reduce the absorption of anti-biotics such as tetracycline and clindamycin, by combining with them in the gastro-intestinal tract to form chelates or complexes. The potentiation of toxic side effects of one drug by another is a common type of interaction.Antibiotics, which are implicated in this type of interaction, are those, which themselves possesses some toxicity such as aminoglycosides, some cephalosporins, tetracyclines and colistin.Some of the most important adverse interactions with antibiotics are those which involve other drugs which have a low toxicity/efficacy ratio. These include warfarin; phenytoin and tolbutamide. Co-administartion of antibacterial drugs such as penicillin whose efficacy is dependent on bacterial cell division along with bacteriostatic drugs such as tetracycline would lead to significant reduced efficacy of the former.

This, one can easily appreciate the importance of awareness regarding drugs interactions to avoid iatrogenic adverse effects and therapeutic failure.

Outside the body interactions

Sometime, some drugs are added to infusion fluid to achieve better clinical effects. There is change for incompatibility between the drugs and the infusion fluid. Effect of soluble insulin can be reduced if it is drawn up with potassium zinc insulin in the same syringe or drip. If diazepum is added to infusion fluid, precipitation reaction will be caused.

Mechanism of drug interactions

The mechanism of drug interaction can be subdivided into two; (a) Pharmacokinetic interactions and (b) Pharmacodynamic interactions.

(a) Pharmacokinetic interactions:

In the interaction in which the process by which drugs are absorbed (A), distributed (D), metabolized (M) and excreted (E) [ADME interactions].

A. INTERACTION DURING ABSORPTION:

The majority of the drugs are orally given for absorption through the gastrointestinal tract. Resultantly, interaction within the gut will certainly alter the absorption pattern of the drugs. There are some drugs which are given chronically (e.g. oral anticoagulants) to the patients. In that case, total amount of drug absorption is important so, that should not be altered markedly. Besides this, there are drugs (e.g. hypnotics and analgesics) which are given as single doses. In this case absorption should be rapid, reduction of the absorption rate may cause failure to secure adequate serum levels.

A.1   Effect of the Gastrointestinal pH changes:

Absorption of a drug from gastrointestinal tract depends on the pKa value of the drug. Higher the non-ionized form (lipid soluble form) higher is the rate of drug absorption from the GI tract. The absorption of the salicylic acid from the stomach is much higher at low pH (more unionized form) than at high pH. So, alteration of gastric pH may alter the absorption of the drug.

A.2   Adsorption, chelation and other complex mechanisms:

Activated charcoal is used as an adsorbing agent which can adsorb drugs within the gut to hinder proper absorption of the drugs from GI tract. Antacids which can also adsorb a good number of drugs. Tetracyclin can chelate with di and tri-valent metallic ions such as aluminum, bismuth, calcium, iron etc., so, absorption of antibiotic will be reduced. Antacids and milk can also reduce the absorption of the tetracyclin from the gut. This type of interaction can be minimized by administering the two (tetracyclin + antacid or milk) at 2-3 hrs interval. Alteration of the gut flora by antibiotics may disrupt the enterohepatic cycling of oral contraceptives and digoxin. Cholestyramine (amonic exchange resin) binds to considerable number of drug if co-administered (e.g. digoxin, warfarin, thyroxine) and can reduce their absorption.

A.3   Altering gastrointestinal motility:

Alteration of gastrointestinal tract motility may influence the rate of drug absorption. Most of the drugs are absorbed from upper part of small intestine. There are some drugs, which can alter the rate of stomach emptying, and thereby absorption of drugs will alter. Anticholinergic drugs and metaclopramide decrease or increase gastrointestinal motility respectively and can alter the bio-availability of many drugs. Tricyclic antidepressants increase the absorption of dicumarol because they increase the time available for dissolution and absorption. On the other hand, in case of levodopa they reduce the absorption by increasing the intestinal mucosal metabolism of levodopa. Pethidine and diamorphine can reduce the absorption of other drug from gastrointestinal tract.

Malabsorption caused by drugs

The antibiotic neomycin may cause impairment of number of drugs like Digoxin, PenicillinV etc.

D.   INTERACTION DURING DISTRIBUTION

D.1   Displacement from plasma protein binding sites:

Some drugs during distribution in circulation can bind with plasma proteins, particularly albumins. There are drugs, which are extremely binding with plasma protein. The drug dico marol has only out of every 1000 molecules remain free at serum concentration of 0.5mg per 100 ml. Digoxin can bind to the muscle of heart to exert its pharmacological effects. The drug, which is greatly bound to albumin, can be displaced from its binding site by another drug which has greater affinity for the same binding site. The displaced (and now active) drug molecules come to the plasma water where its concentration rapidly rises. Drugs like aspirin competes with anticoagulant drug warfarin for same protein binding site thereby, the concentration of displaced warfarin will be high with increased adverse effects. Major metabolite of chloral hydrate is trichloroacetic acid which can displace warfarin, thereby increasing anticoagulant effects. Only drugs with low apparent volume of distribution (Vd) will be affected by this type of displacement phenomenon. Such drug includes tolbutamide (96% bound, Vd 101), oral anticoagulants such as warfarin (99% bound, Vd 91) and phenytoin (90% bound, Vd 351).

D.2. Displacement from other tissue binding sites:

Quinidine can displace digoxin from binding sites in the tissues. So, when a patient is given quinidine who is receiving digoxin, the concentration of digoxin will greatly increase pharmacological effects.

M. INTERACTIONS DURING BIOTRANSFORMATION

A large number of drugs are metabolized (biotransformed) inside the body to move water soluble forms for easy excretion from kidney. If this process (biotransformation) was not so, many drugs would remain in the body for a long period and pharmacological effects were also continued. Most of this biotransformation is carried out by this enzymes of liver cells. Some drugs are also metabolized in the serum, kidneys, the skin and the intestine.

M.1. Induction of enzymes:

Enzyme induction by drugs can enhance metabolism of drugs and therapeutic achievement will be less. Barbiturates increase the enzymes activities with increased metabolism and excretion. So, tolerance can develop with the repeated use of barbiturates.

If a drug D1 is biotransformed by the enzymes, then concurrent dosing of another drug D2 which can induce the same enzyme system, can enhance the metabolism of drug D1. Anticoagulant activity of the drug warfarin can be decreased with the concurrent administration of enzyme inducing agent, dichloralphenazone. Enzyme induction is very common mechanism of interaction. This type of interaction can also be caused by chlorinated hydrocarbon insecticides such as dichlophane and lindane. Tobacco smoking also act as enzyme inducer.

Phase1 oxidation is a metabolic pathway which is commonly affected by enzyme induction. Phase1 oxidation covers numbers of metabolic biotransformations, all of which require the presence of NADPH and P450. At the time of enzyme induction, endoplasmic reticulum amount of liver cells increases and cytochrome P450 level also rises.

M.2. Enzymes inhibition:

There are other drugs also which can act as enzyme inhibitors and potentiate of the other drugs whose pharmacological actions are limited by being metabolized. If a epileptic patient depends on phenytoin is given chloramphenicol (enzyme inhibitor) concurrently, the phenytoin level in blood may increase with possible toxicity. Metabolism of antocoagulant drug is increased by cimetidine. So, there is a change of excess warfarin accumulation with hemorrhage. Clinical significance of this type of enzyme inhibition depends on the increase of serum level of drugs. If this level remains within therapeutic concentration, the enzyme inhibition may be advantageous. If serum level of drug rises to the toxic range due to inhibitor drug, then interaction becomes adverse.

M.3. Alteration of blood flow through liver:

Orally absorbed drugs enter into the liver by portal circulation before they are distributed throughout the body for pharmacological effects. This phenomenon is called first pass. During this first pass a substantial number of fat soluble drugs undergo biotransformation. Some concurrently administered drugs can influence this first pass metabolism. For example, H_2 antagonist cimetidine, can reduce hepatic blood flow and thereby increase bioavailability of propranolol. A number of other drugs have opposite effect with increment of hepatic flow so that their biotransformation is increased.

E. INTERACTION DURING EXCRETION

Most of the drugs (axception : Inhalation anaesthetics) are excreted via bile or urine. The blood passes to the kidney tubules where drugs and its matabolites are removed from blood by active-energy transport system. This removed drugs along with metabolites deposited into the tubular filtrate. The tubular cells also possess active or passive transport system for reabsorption of drugs and metabolites. So, any action by drugs, with kidney tubules fluid pH, with active transport systems and with blood flow to kidney can alter the rate of excretion of other drugs and metabolites. For example, the drug probenecid interfere with penicillin for active transport process at the kidney and thereby prolongs the action of penicillins. This effect is pharmacologically beneficial.

E. 1.   Changes in urinary pH and drug interactions:

Any alteration of urinary pH influence ionization of drugs and its excretion. Only the un-ionized form of the drug is lipid soluble and can diffuse back through the lipid membrane of tubul cells. Hence, at high pH value (alkaline range) weakly acidic drugs with low pH value (3.0-7.5) will remain in ionized stage (lipid insoluble stage) and therefore pass through urine. Enhance excretion of absorption (acidic drug) occurs if sodium bicarbonate is given (alkaline pH). Similarly, weak organic bases (pKa value of 7.5-10.5) at low pH range (acidic) will excreted via urine rapidly. The basic drug amphetamine will rapidly excreted if ammonium chloride is given.

Clinically, significance of this phenomenon is largely metabolized in liver and a few drugs are excreted in urine in unchanged form. In case of overdosage, pH of urine is changed deliberately to increase the drug loss via urine. Example: phenobarbitone and salicylates.

E.2.   Interaction due to kidney blood flow:

Prostaglandins present in kidney act as vasodialator and blood flow through kidney partially depends on it. Indomethacin can inhibit the prostaglandin synthesis and serum excretion of lithium is reduced. Therefore, serum level of lithium will be high.

E.3.   Interactions due to biliary secretion and enterohepatic shunt:

Some drugs are excreted to bile in unchanged or conjugated form (as glucosonide to make them water soluble). Intestinal flora can change some conjugated drugs to parent drugs and these are then reabsorbed. The reabsorption process will help to prolong the stay of drugs inside the body. An antibiotic can effect this gut flora and recycling process of some drugs can be affected.

Possible sites of Drug Interaction

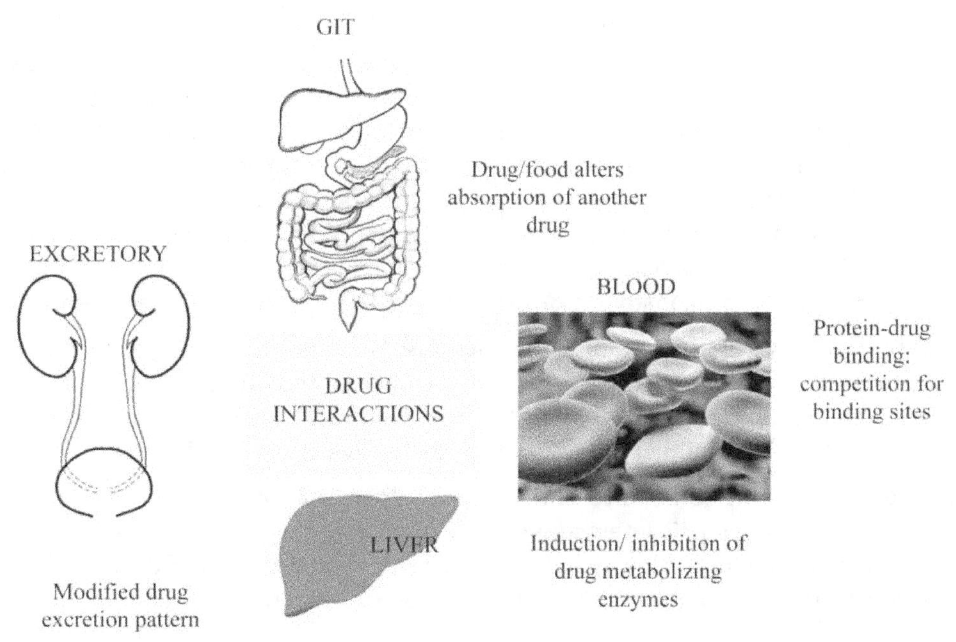

(b)   PHARMACODYNAMIC DRUG INTERACTIONS

Some times a patients can take two or more drugs at the same time. Pharmacodynamic interaction may happen in this case. The effects of one drug if changed by the presence of another drug at the site of action, this phenomenon is called pharmacodynamic drug interactions. The use of two or more drugs can induce either no effect, synergism or antagonism.

(b).1. Drug antagonism or opposing interaction:

When the effect of a drug is reduced or abolished by the presence of another drug, then the term can be said antagonism. Drug antagonism can be classified into three types (a) Chemical, (b) Physiological & (c) Pharmacological.

(a)   <u>Chemical antagonism:</u> When simple chemical reaction involves between two drugs, and effect of one drug is reduced or abolished, then it is called chemical antagonism. For example, non-absorbable antacids neutralized the gastric acid;

(b)   <u>Physiological antagonism:</u> Physiological antagonism is that when physiological effect of a drug is antagonized by another drug acting on two different types of receptors. Acetylcholin contracts smooth muscle of intestine through muscarinic cholinoceptors. But this action is antagonized by adrenaline via adrenoceptors;

(c)   <u>Pharmacological antagonism:</u> When a drug action is antagonized by other drug via same receptor, then it is called pharmacological antagonism. This is of two types: (i) competitive, (ii) non-competitive.

   (i)   **Competitive antagonism** – When two drugs compete for the same receptor and antagonism happens, then it can be said competitive antagonism. This type of antagonism is reversible. Acetylcholin can contract intestinal smooth muscle and this effect can be competitively antagonized by atropine.

   (ii) **Non-competitive antagonism** – When maximum response of an antagonist is reduced in presence of antagonist, then this is called non-competitive antagonism.

(b).2. Drug synergism:

The two drugs with same pharmacological effect are given together, the effect can be additive. This type of phenomenon is called drug synergism. It is of two types: (i) Additive, (ii) Potentiation.

   (i)   **Additive effect** – When two drugs are used together and effect is equal to the sum of individual effect, then it is called additive effect. For example, alcohol in moderate amounts with other hypnotics or tranquillizers may produce excessive depression of central nervous system. Additive effects can occur with therapeutic or toxic effects of two drugs. Sometimes the additive effects are solely toxic. (e.g. additive toxicity, nephrotoxicity or bone marrow depression)

   (ii) **Potentiation** – When the effect of two drugs concurrently used is greater than the sum of the individual drug effects, the effect is called potentiation. For example, combination of two antimicrobial like sulphamethoxazole and trimethoprim can produce potentiation.

Alteration of drug transport mechanism and drug interactions: There are some drugs which can prevent other drugs to reach adrenergic neurones for action. The drugs like tricyclic antidepressants prevent the re-up take of noradrenaline into peripheral adrenergic neurones so that its effects are increased. The tricyclic antidepressants are also able to prevent the up take of clonidine within CNS and therefore, its anyihypertensive effects are blocked.

Disturbances in fluid and electrolyte balance and cause of drug interaction: Some times, any change of fluid and electrolytes can cause pharmacodynamic interactions. For example, the antidiuretic drug frusemide depletes potassium in urine and plasma concentration may fall with increasing sensitivity and toxicity of digitalis glycoside. Thiazide diuretics can alter the sodium excretion via kidney which may cause decrease excretion of lithium and lithium concentration of plasma will rise.

DRUG INTERACTIONS TABLES

Alcohols

Drugs	Interaction with	Effects
Alcohol	Antihistamines (a) Promethazine, chlorpheniramine, dyphenylhydramines. (b) Astimizole, Loratidine terfenadine	(a) Additive CNS depression action. (b) Minimal or absence of additive effect.
	Aspirin	Prolongation of bleeding time can be increased.
	Atropine	Marked impairment of attention found.
	Barbiturates	Additive CNS depression.
	Benzodiazepines	CNS depressant action of benzodiazepines and alcohol are additive.
	Bromvaletone or Ethinamate	Additive CNS depressant action.
	Buspirone	Additive alcohol action.
	Butyraldoxime	Disulfiram action.
	Caffeine	No counteract effect found
	Calcium channel blockers	Blood alcohol level increased
	Cephalosporin antibiotics	Disulphiram like action.
	Chloral hydrate	Additive CNS depressant action.
	Cimetidine, Famotidine, Ranitidine	Additive CNS depressant action.
	CNS depressants	Additive action.
	Codeine	No interaction with small amount of codeine but additive reaction with higher doses.
	Dextropropoxyphene	Additive CNS depressant action.
	Dimethylformamide	Disulfiram like reaction.
	Disulfiram	Flushlessness and fullness of face and neck, tachycardia, breathlessness, giddiness and hypotension, nausea and vomiting.
	Fluoxetine, Femoxetine	No effects.
	Fluvoxamine	Additive effects.
	Clovaxamine	No effects.
	Glutethimide	Additive reaction, psychomotor skill is impaired.
	Glyceryl trintrate	Faint and dizziness may arise.
	Griseofulvin	The intoxicant effects of alcohol may increase.
	Hydromorphone	Additive CNS depressant action.
	Indomethacin or Phenylbutazone	Additive action of alcohol.
	Isomiazid	Additive action.
	Ketoconazole	Disulfiram like reaction may occur.
	Lithium carbonate	Additive action.
	Maprotiline	Additive action.
	Meprobamate	The intoxicant effects can be increased.
	Methaqualone or *Mandrax* (methaqualone + diphenhydramine)	Additive CNS depressant action.
	Metoclopramide	Sedative effects may increase.

Drugs	Interaction with	Effects
	Metronidazole	Disulfiram like reaction.
	Nitrofurantoin	No firm interaction found.
	Nitroimidazoles	Disulfiram like reaction.
	Paraldehyde	Additive CNS depressant action. (in the treatment of acute intoxication fatal effects results)
	Phenothiazines, Butyrophenones and other drugs	Additive effects
	Procarbazine	Flushing reaction.
	Sodium cromoglycate	No adverse interaction
	Tetracyclic antidepressant (a) Mianserin (b) Pirlindole	(a) additive action (b) no interaction
	Tolazoline	Disulfiram like reaction may appear.
	Trazodone	Additive action.
	Trichloroethylene	A flushing skin reaction similar to a mild disulfiram reaction.
	Tricyclic antidepressant (a) Amitriptylene (b) Doxepin (c) Nortriptylene, Clomipramine, Desipramine, amoxapine	(a) Impairment is increased. (b) Impairment is increased. (c) Only minimal interaction.
	Viqualine	No adverse interaction.
	Xylene	Dizziness and nausea, and a flushing skin reaction.
	Food: (a) Edible fungi *Coprinus atramentarius, Boletus luridus* and others. (b) Milk	(a) Disulfiram like reaction. (b) Blood level of alcohol and its intoxicant effects will be reduced.

Analgesic & Non - Steroidal Anti - inflammatory Drugs

Drugs	Interaction with	Effects
Alfentanil	Erythromycin	Prolonged and increased alfentanil effects.
Antirheumatic agents (indomethacin, salicylates etc.)	Mazindol	No adverse affects
Aspirin & Salicylates	Carbonic anhydrase	In high dose fatality may arise.
	Cimetidine or Ranitidine	Negligible clinical effect with cimetidine but no interaction with ranitidine.
	Corticosteroids	Gastrointestinal bleeding and ulceration may be increased.
	Levamisole	No effects confirmed yet.
	Methotrexate	Effect potentiate.
	Phenylbutazone	Reduces uricosuric effects by aspirin.
	Phenytoin	Level will increase.

Drugs	Interaction with	Effects
	Probenecid	Mutually antagonists
	Sulphinpyrazone	Mutually antagonists
	Spironolactone	Antagonistic action.
Azapropazone	Miscellaneous drugs	No significant effect
Buprenorphine	Amitriptyline	Potentiation with alcohol, other CNS depressant and MOIs Diazepam may produce respiratory and cardiac collaps.
Dextromoramide	Triacetyloleandomycin	An isolated report describes marked increase of dextromoramide and coma.
Dextropropoxyphene	Orphenadrine	Potentiation with alcohol, CNS depressant, decrease efficacy of heavy smokers.
	Tobacco smoking	Analgesic effect of the drug is less in those who smoke.
Diclofenac	Miscellaneous drugs	Increase blood level of lithium and digoxin, inhibit diuretics but potentiate sparing diuretics. Increase toxicity of methotrexate lowers serum level of salicylates.
Diflunisal	Non steroidal anti-inflammatory agents and analgesics (a) Aspirin (b) Indomethacin (c) Paracetamol & Naproxen	(a) Reduce the serum diflunisal levels (b) Serum Indomethacin level raises 2-3 folds (c) Paracetamol levels are increased but not those of naproxen.
Flufenamic, Mefenamic and Tolfenamic acids, Oxyphenbutazone or Phenylbutazone.	Antacids	Absorption of fenamates is accelerated by magnesium hydroxide but retarded by aluminum hydroxide. Sodium bicarbonate shows no effect.
Flufenamic or Mefenamic acid	Cholestyramine	Absorption of both are reduced.
Ibuprofen	Antacids	Aspirin displaces ibuprophen from serum binding sites hence should be avoided. Methotrexate and lithium toxicity may increase. Antagonises the effect of frusemide & thiazides. Anticoagulants may increase the risk of GI ulceration.
	Aspirin	
Ibuprofen or Flurbiprofen	Cimetidine, Nizatidine or Ranitidine.	Frusimide effects reduces, aspirin reduces serum level of Flurbiprofen. Digoxin absorption may be delayed. Anticoagulants effects may be interfered.
Indomethacin	Allopurinol	Alcohol and smoking associated with increased risk of peptic ulceration. Diflunisal may cause fatal GI haemorrhage in susceptible individuals. Anticoagulants may cause sever GI ulcers.
	Antacids	Irritation of the gut caused by indomethacin can be reduced by antacids.
	Aspirin and salicylates	No significant effect.

Drugs	Interaction with	Effects
	Cimetidine	Cause small reduction in the serum level of indomethacin without anti-inflammatory effects being altered.
	Probenecid	Serum indomethacin level can be doubled causing improvement in arthritis patients but toxicity may occur prominently in those whose kidney function is impaired.
	Vaccines	Limited evidence suggests more severe effect.
Isoxicam	Miscellaneous drugs	Blood loss is increased.
Vetoprofen	Probenecid	May reduce loss from the body and increase its serum level. Increased toxicity is a possibility.
Meclofenamic acid	Aspirin	Intestinal bleeding is increased by concurrent use.
Methadone	Anti –convulsants	Reduce methadone effect.
	Disulfiram	No adverse affect
	Rifampicin (rifampin)	Reduction in serum level.
	Urinary acidifers or alkalizers	If the urine is made acidic increment is observed from the body and if is made alkaline, reduction occurs.
Morphine	Cimetidine or Ranitidine	Isolated reports describe disorientation, confusion and agitation in a patient taking morphine and ranitidine. Other CNS depressants, alcohol, muscle relaxants, MAO inhibitor potentiate effect and cause respiratory depression. Diuretics antagonise morphine effect. Analgesic effects is potentiated with NSAID's.
	Contraceptives [oral]	The clearance of morphine is nearly doubled by concurrent use of the oral contraceptives.
	Metoclopramide	Increases the rate of absorption of oral morphine and enhance its sedative effects.
	Tricyclic antidepressants	The bioavailability and the degree of analgesia are increased by the concurrent use.
Nabumetone	Miscellaneous drugs	Does not interact.
	Antacids	Absorption can be altered using antacids with uncertain clinical importance.
	Aspirin and Salicylates	Serum naproxen levels may be increased or reduced without clinical effectiveness being disturbed.
Naproxen	Cholestyramine	Enhances the effect of oral anticoagulants, phenytoin, methotrexate, sulphonamides, sulphonylurea, hypoglycaemics. Diuretics increase risk of renal disorders. Absorption reduced by antacids and increased by bicarbonates.

Drugs	Interaction with	Effects
	Cimetidine	Does not effect.
	Probenacids	Serum levels are raised by 50% with probably minimum clinical importance.
Narcotic analgesics	Sulglycotide	Does not effect.
	Benzodiazepines	Having potent sedative effects of opiates appear to be opposed.
	Promethazone	Having potent sedative effects, would be expected to be additive with CNS depressant effects.
Nefopam	Miscellaneous drugs	Should avoid taking anticonvulsants or the MAOI. Side effects are somewhat increased. Concurrent use of tricyclic antidepressants may result in exaggerated antimuscarnic effects such as blurred vision, dry mouth, urinary retention.
	Antacids	No significant change in absorption rate except ketoprofen where a small reduction can occur.
	Sucralfate	Does not interact adversely and also possibly protect the gastric mucosa from damage.
Oxyphenylbutazone and phynylbutazone	Anabolic steroids	Serum oxyphenylbutazone levels are increased by 40%. Phenylbutazone appears to be unaffected.
Paracetamol(Acetaminophen)	Alcohol	Sever liver damage, fatal in some instances, who take moderate doses of paracetamol. Enhances anti-coagulant activities. Absorption of paracetamol is reduced by pethidine and propantheline.
	Anticholinergic agents	Delays gastric emptying
	Barbiturates	Hepatotoxicity developed in a woman.
	Cholestyramine	Absorption may be reduced if both taken at a time but if cholestyramine is given in a hour later, very little reduction in absorption.
	Cimetidine	No interaction of clinical importance.
Paracetamol and other drugs	Opioid analgesics	Morphine and diamorphine delay gastric emptying causing reduced rate of other drugs.
Paracetamol	Oral contraceptives	Cleared from the body move quickly in woman taking oral contraceptives. Paracetamol increases the absorption of ethinyloestradiol from the gut by about 20%.
D-Penicillamine	Antacids	Absorption can be reduced by 30-40% by antacids containing aluminum and magnesium hydroxides are taken concurrently.
	Iron Preparations	Can reduce as much as two thirds by the concurrent use.

Drugs	Interaction with	Effects
Pentazocine	Tobacco smoking and environmental pollution.	Those who smoke or urban dwellers require 50% or more for satisfactory analgesia than those who don't smoke or live where the air is clean. Respiratory depression effect with halothane, lidocaine.
Pethidine (Meperidine)	Acyclovir	CNS depression effect is potentiated by alcohol and other CNS depressants. Hydroxyzine enhances analgesic effects.
Pethidine	Chlopromazine and other phenothiazines.	An isolated report describes toxicity.
	Cimetidine or Ranitidine	Increased respiratory depression, sedation, CNS toxicity and hypotension can occur if used together.
Pethidine (Meperidine)	Furazolidine	Hyperpyrexic reaction may occur on concurrent use in man which is yet to be confirmed.
	Monoamine oxidase inhibitors (MAOI).	May result life threatening reaction in a few patients. Excitement, muscle rigidity, hyperpyrexia, flushing sweating occur rapidly. Respiratory depression, hypotension may occur.
	Phenytion	May reduce serum levels and increase toxic metabolite, clinical importance yet to be confirmed.
Phenazone (Antipyrine)	Miscellaneous drugs	Changes in the half life.
Phenoperidine	Antacids	An antacid showed the increase in the serum level.
	Beta-blockers	An isolated report describes a patient with tetanus showing fall in blood pressure.
Phenylbutazone	Allopurinol	No significant interaction.
	Barbiturates	No report having clinical importance.
	Indomethacin	An isolated report describes an insignificant deterioration in renal function.
	Methyl phenidate	May increase serum level.
	Pesticides	May increase the rate of metabolism.
	Tobacco smoking	The loss from the body is greater in smokers than in non-smokers.
Phenylbutazone or oxyphenylbutazone	Tricyclic antidepressants	Can delay the absorption from the gut.
Piroxicam and tenoxicam	Cholestyramine	May increase the loss of both from the body leading to loss by their therapeutic effects accordingly.
Piroxicam	Cimetidine	No significant interaction.
Sulindac	Dimethylsulfoxide (DMSO)	A single report describes serious peripheral neuropathy when applied on skin.

Antiarrythmic

Drugs	Interaction with	Effects
Ajmaline	Lignocaine(Lidocaine) or Quinidine	An isolated report describes cardiac failure in a patient administered concurrently.
Amiodarone	Anaesthetics	Risk of complication and death increased.
	Beta-blockers	Brabicardin, venticular fibrillation and asystole are reported on abdominal application.
	Calcium channel blockers	Sinus arrest and serious hypotension occurs.
	Cholestyramine	Reduce absorption.
	Cimetidine	Causes rise in the serum level.
	Disopyramide, propafenone or mexiletine	The risk of atypical ventricular tachycardia or seems to be increased.
Apridine	Amiodarone	Serum levels may be increased.
Disopyramide or procainamide	Antacids	Inconclusive evidence suggests that aluminum containing antacids may cause a small reduction in absorption.
Disopyramide	Anticholinergic	The effect may be expected to be additive.
	Beta-blockers	Adverse interactions between these drugs may be uncommon.
	Erythromycin	Cardiac arrythmias may occur.
	Phenobarbitone	Levels in the serum are reduced on concurrent use.
	Phenytion	Levels in the serum may be reduced on concurrent use and may fall below therapeutic concentration. Loss of arrythmic may occur.
	Quinidine	May be raised slightly.
Disopyramide	Rifampicin	May cause marked reduction in serum levels on concurrent use.
Encainide	Diltiazem	May cause sharp increase in serum levels with the slight increase of active metabolites
	Miscellaneous drugs	No interaction having clinical significance is reported except the effect of cimetidine which should be monitored.
	Quinidine	May cause a marked reduction in the clearance of encaidine in those who are extensive metaboliser of encaidine.
Flecainide	Amiodarone	Serum levels are increased.
	Cholestyramine	An isolated report describes reduced serum levels.
	Cimetidine	May increase serum levels.

Drugs	Interaction with	Effects
	Food or antacids	Absorption is not significantly altered in adults but may possibly be reduced by milk in infants.
	Quinine	Reduce the metabolism.
	Tobacco smoking	Tobacco smokers need larger doses.
Lignocaine (Lidocaine)	Beta blockers	Serum level may be increased.
	Cimetidine	Reduces the clearness of lignocaine and raises serum levels. Toxicity may occur if dosage is not reduced. Ranitidine appears to interact minimally.
	Disopyramide	No report having clinical justification is known.
	Morphine	No significant effect.
Lignocaine (Lidocaine)	Phenytoin	Central toxic side effects may be increased on concurrent intravenous infusion. Serum levels are slightly reduced but markedly reduced if given orally.
	Procainamide	An isolated case of delirium is reported.
	Tocainide	Toxic chronic Seizure in a man is reported.
Lorcainide	Rifampicin	Massed reduction in serum levels and failure to central ventricular tachycardia in a man is reported.
	Antacids, Urinary acidifiers and alkalinizers.	No remarkable effect.
	Antiarrythmic drugs	Concurrent use is reported to be beneficial with reduced side effects.
	Cimetidine or Ranitidine	No adverse interaction on concurrent administration.
Mexiletine	Diamorphine or Morphine	Absorption may be repressed in patients following a myocardial infraction and depression is marked and delayed if used concurrently.
	Phenytoin	Serum levels may be reduced on concurrent use.
	Rifampicin (Rifampin)	The clearness from the body is increased on concurrent use causing the need of increased dosage.
Moricizine (Ethomozine)	Cimetidine	Increases the serum levels.
Pirmental	Rifampicin (Rifampin)	Increases the loss from the body, then reduces the antirrythmic effect.
	Amiodarone	Serum levels are increased by about 60% and used concurrently. Reduction in dosage is required to avoid toxicity.
Procainamide	Beta blockers	Pharmacokinetics are wide changed.
	Cimetidine or Ranitidine	Serum level may be increased on concurrent application and toxicity may develop precisely to those having reduced renal clearance. Ranitidine appears not to interact significantly.

Drugs	Interaction with	Effects
	Para-aminobenzoic acid (PABA)	A single report describes the reduction in metabolism by increasing serum levels.
	Quinidine	A single report describes marked increase in serum levels on concurrent use.
	Trimethoprim	Causes marked increase in serum levels.
Propafenone	Cimetidine	No adverse interaction.
	Miscellaneous drugs	May oppose the effects of others. Shortness of breath and a worsening of the control of asthma is reported.
	Quinidine	It doubles the serum levels.
Quinidine	Amiodarone	Serum levels may be approximately doubled on concurrent administration. Reduction in dosage is advised to avoid toxicity and the risk of a typical ventricular tachycardia.
Quinidine	Anticonvulsants	Serum levels may be reduced on concurrent use. Loss of arrhythmia control is possible if quinidine dosage is not increased.
	Aspirin	A patient showed a two to three fold increase in bleeding times.
	Beta blockers	Normally an advantageous interaction.
	Calcium Channel Blockers	Depression in serum levels are reported on concurrent use of nifidipine and which doubled on being withdrawn. Diltiazem does not interact.
	Cimetidine and Ranitidine	Serum levels may rise and intoxication may develop on concurrent use. An isolated report describes ventricular bigenuiy when ranitidine was used.
	Kaolin-Pectin	Can reduce the absorption and reduce serum levels.
	Ketoconazol	Describes marked increase in serum levels in man.
	Laxatives	Serum level may reduce on concurrent use.
	Lignocaine (Lidocaine)	A single report describes sinoartrial arrest on concurrent use.
	Metoclopramide	May reduce the absorption from a sustained released formulation but may increase the absorption with other preparations.
	Rifampicine (Rifarnpin)	Serum levels and its therapeutic effects may be markedly reduced by the concurrent use.
Quinidine	Urinary alkalinizer and antacids	Large rise in the urinary pH due to concurrent use can cause the retention, which may lead to intoxication.
Tocainide	Urinary alkalinizer and antacids	Raising the pH of urine can reduce the loss of tocainide in urine.

Drugs	Interaction with	Effects
	Cimetidine	May reduce bioavailability and serum levels. Ranitidin appears not to interact.
	Rifampicine (Rifampin)	The loss from the body may be increased by the concurrent use.

Antibiotics and Antiinfectives

Drugs	Interaction with	Effects
Aminoglycoside antibiotics	Amphotericin	Nephrotoxicity attributed to the concurrent use.
	Cephalosporins	Nephrotoxic effects can be increased by concurrent use which may possibly be true for other aminoglycosides.
Aminoglycosides	Clindamycin	Three cases of acute renal failure have been attributed by concurrent use.
	Dimenhydrinate	The manufactures suggest that it may considerable mask the ototoxic effects of antibiotics.
	Ethacrynic acid	Concurrent use should be avoided because of their damaging action on the ear. Intravenous administration and renal impairment are additional causative factors. Sequential use is not safe.
	Extended spectrum penicillin	Gentamicin, netilmicin, tobramicin, and sisomicin are chemically inactivated if mixed in the fluids with carbenicillin, ticarcillin, piperacillins, mezlocillin.
	Frusemide (Furosemide) or Bumetanide	May develop nephrotoxicity and/or toxicity while taking both drugs.
	Indomethacin	No authentic report on effects.
	Magnesium salts	Respiratory arrest occurred in a baby.
	Miconazole	A report describes a reduction in serum level.
	Penicillin V	The serum levels can be halved by concurrent use when given orally.
Aminoglycosides	Vancomycin	Nephrotoxicity may be additive.
Aminoglycosidic acid (PAS)	Alcohol	Can nullify the blood-lipid-lowering effects of PAS.
	Aspirin and salicylates	Additive gastrointestinal irritation is possible. No report on other adverse effects.
	Diphenhydramine	May reduce the absorption to a little extent but clinial importance is uncertain.
	Probenecid	Serum levels may be increased by two to four folds by concurrent use.

Drugs	Interaction with	Effects
Amphotericin	Corticosteroids	May cause potassium loss as well as salt and water retention can have adverse effect on cardiac function.
	Low salt diet	Renal toxicity and sodium depletion.
Ampicillin or amoxycillin	Allopurinol	The incidence of skin rashes is increased by the concurrent use.
Antibiotics	Alcohol	Normally no adverse effect is reported.
Anti-infective agents	Cimetidine	No adverse effect is reported.
Anti-malarials	Antacids, antidiarrhoeals	Absorption may be reduced by 20% by the use of magnesium and about 30% by kaolin.
Cephalosporins	Cholestyramine	Absorption is delayed, importance of which is very small.
	Frusemide (Furosemide)	Nephrotoxoic effects may be increased by concurrent use of frusemide and levels in the brain are reduced as well.
Cephalosporins	Penicillins	Reduce the less from the body.
	Probenecid	Serum levels of many but not all are raised by the concurrent use.
Cephalothin	Colistin sulphomethate sodium	Renal failure is reported on concurrent use.
Chloramphenicol	Paracetamol (Acetaminophen)	May increase, decresae or to have no effect on serum levels.
	Penicillin, streptomycin or Cephalosporins	Antagonism has been described in a case.
	Phenobarbitone	Serum levels may be depressed supported by studies in children. A single report suggests increased serum levels.
	Rifampicin	Serum levels may be markedly lowered on additional treatment.
	Cimetidine or Ranitidine	Cimetidine reduces metabolism and loss of chlorquinine from the body. Ranitidine does not interact.
Cotrimoxazole	Folic acid	The effects of folic acid may be reduced.
	Kaolin-pectin	Very small action with no clinical importance.
	Prilocaine-lignocain (Lidocain) cream	Methaemoglobinamia may develop in a body.
Cycloserine	Alcohol, Isoniazid, Phynytoin	May increase the effects of alcohol and phenytoin CNS side-effects are increased by isoniazid.
Dapsone	Clofazimine	May reduce the anti-inflammatory effects.
	Probencid	The serum levels can be raised by concurrent use.
	Rifampicin (Rifampin)	Increases the excretion of dapsone and thus lowers its serum levels.
Erythromycin	Antacids	May prolong the absorption time without any clinical importance.

Drugs	Interaction with	Effects
	Other antibiotics	The effectiveness may be more and sometimes less effective than with only one antibiotic.
	Urinary acidifier or alkalinizers	Activity is maximal in alkaline urine and minimal in acid urine.
Ethambutol	Antacids	Aluminum hydroxide causes small reduction in the absorption with no clinical importance.
Ethinamide	Miscellaneous drugs	May cause mental depression, psychiatric disturbances, hypoglycemia, hypothyroidism and alcohol related psychotoxicity.
Flucytosine	Cytarabine	May oppose the activity.
	Miscellaneous drugs	No interaction of clinical importance.
Griseofulvin	Phenobarbitone	Anti-fungal activity may be reduced and even abolished by concurrent use.
Hexamine compounds	Urinary acidifier or alkalinizers and sulphonamides	Urinary alkalinizers and these antacids capable of raising pH above 5 should not be used. Older less soluble sulphonamides may cause the risk of kidney damage due to crystalluria as the low urinary pH values.
8-hydroxyquinoline	Zinc oxide	Inhibits the therapeutic effects in ointments.
Imipenem	Aminoglycosides	Nephrotoxic effects may be there.
Influenza vaccine	Paracetamol (Acetaminophen), Alprazolum and Lorazepam	Does not affect.
Interferon	Aspirin, Paracetamol, Prednosone	No evidence of interaction excepting that Prednisone may reduce the biological activities.
Isoniazide	Antacids	Absorption may be reduced by concurrent use. The Isoniazid may be given at least an hr. before the antacid to minimize the effects of interaction.
	Cheese or Fish	May experience a reaction with headachem, difficulty in breathing, nausea and trachycardia.
	Cimetidine or Ranitidine	No interaction reported.
	Disulfirum	Difficulties in co-ordination and changes in affects and behavior by concurrent use are reported.
	Ethambutol	Optic neuropathy may be increased by concurrent use.
	Food	Absorption is markedly reduced.
	Levodopa	Hypertension, tachycardia, flushing and tremor by concurrent use are reported.
	Pethidine (Meperidine)	An isolated report describes hypotension and lethargy following concurrent use.
Isoniazid	Propanolol	May cause reduction in the clearance from the body.

Drugs	Interaction with	Effects
	Rifampicin	Hepatotoxicity, acetylators in presence may be increased.
Ketoconazole	Antacids and/or cimetidine	Reduce the gastrointestinal absorption of ketoconazole.
Ketoconazole or Itraconazole	**Food**	Though the normal trends suggest the use with food, background evidence supporting this is confusing & contradictory.
	Phenytoin and phenobarbitone	Reduction in serum levels and relapse in the treatment of a fungal infection is reported.
	Rifampicin (Rifampin) and isonizid	50-90% reduction in serum levels is reported by concurrent use.
Lincomycin or Clindamycin	**Food or drinks**	Serum levels may be depressed by up to two-thirds if taken in presence of food but clindamycin is not significantly affected.
	Kaolin	Absorption may be reduced which may be avoided by giving lincomycin 2 hr. after kaolin.
Metronidazole	Antacid, kaolin-pectin and cholestyramine	Absorption is unaffected by Kaolin-pectin but small reduction occurs if aluminum hydroxide antacid is given.
	Barbiturates	Increases the loss from the body.
	Chloroquine	An isolated report describes acute dystonia.
	Cimetidine	May increase the loss to some extent with very small clinical importance.
Metronidazole	Corticosteroids	May increases the loss from the body suggesting the increased dosage of metronidazole.
	Disulfirum	Acute psychoses and confusion is reported by concurrent use.
Nalidixic acid	Nitrofurantoin	Uncertain in clinical practice.
	Probenecid	Serum levels is markedly increased by the concurrent use.
Nitrofurantoin	Antacids	Effectiveness in the treatment of urinary tract infections is reduced markedly by magnesium trisilicate, but aluminum hydroxide is reported not to interact.
	Anti-cholinergics and Diphenoxylate	May double the absorption in some patients.
Penicillins	Chloroquine	Absorption may be reduced by concurrent use but bacampicillin is not affected.
	Dietary fibre	May reduce the absorption.
	Miscellaneous drugs	Aspirin, Indomethacin, Probenecid, phenylbutazone, sulphaphenazole. Prolong the half life whereas chlorothiazide, sulphamethizole, sulphamethoxypyridazine do not.
	Tetracyclins	May reduce the effectiveness in scarlet fever.

Drugs	Interaction with	Effects
Piperazine	Phenothiazines	Convulsion in a child is reported.
Priziquantel	Corticosteroids	Continuous use can reduce serum levels by 50%.
Primaquine (Quinacrine)	Mepacrine	Does not affect adversely.
Prothionamide	Rifampicin (Rifampin) and/or Dapson	Hypertoxicity may appear.
Pyrantel	Piperazine	May opposes the anthelmintic action.
Pyrazinamide	Miscellaneous drugs	Pyrazinamide may cause hyperuricaemia which may be modestly reduced by aminosalicylic acid or probenecid but more extensively by aspirin. May have adverse effect on control of diabetes.
	Cotrimoxazole or Sulphonamide	Pancytopemia and megaloblastic anaemia is reported.
Quinine	Antacids or Urinary acidifier and alkalinizers	Alkalinizers may increase the retension time in man but reduce in animals.
	Cimetidine or Ranitidine	Loss may be reduced by concurrent use.
	Rifampicin (Rifampin)	Serum levels may reduce.
Quinolone antibiotics	Antacids	Serum levels may reduce by concurrent use of aluminum and magnesium antacids.
	Cimetidine or Ranitidine	Cimetidine reduces the clearance from the body whereas ranitidine reduces the absorption.
	Iron preparations	May reduce the absorption of ciprofloxacin and ofloxacin. Quinolone-iron complexes formed have reduced antibacterial effects.
	Rifampicin (Rifampin)	Serum levels may be reduced but no interaction is also reported.
Quinolone antibiotics	Sucralfate	Causes marked reduction in the absorption if taken together but a smaller reduction is reported if dosage are separated by 2hr.
	Zinc	May reduce absorption.
Rifampicin	Aminosalicylic acid (PAS)	Serum levels may be halved.
Rifampicin (Rifampin)	Antacids	Reduction up to 30% may be caused by concurrent use with uncertain clinical importance.
	Clofazimine	No interaction is reported.
	Dipyrone	No significant interaction.
	Food	May delays and reduce the absorption.
	Probenecid	Unpredictable.
	Triacetyloleandomycin	Cholestatic jaundice have been reported.
Rifampentine	Other drugs	Have ten times greater potency and a linger half-life. So far no clinical important interaction reported.
Sulphasalazine	Antibiotics	The release in the colon of the active drug is markedly reduced by concurrent use.

Drugs	Interaction with	Effects
Sulphasalazine or Sodium fusidate	Cholestyramine	Cholestyramine can bind with two drugs thereby reducing their activity.
Sulphasalazine	Iron salts	May bind but the therapeutic response is uncertain.
Suphasalazine	Metronidazole	Does not interact.
	Barbiturates	Anesthatic effects are increased but shortened.
	Local anaesthetics	May reduce the effects and allow the development of local and generalized infections.
	Para-aminobenzoic acid (PABA)	Antibacterial effects are reduced.
Tetracyclins	Alcohol	Serum levels may fall below minimal therapeutic concentration but tetracyclin itself is not affected.
	Antacids	Effectiveness may be reduced markedly and even abolished by concurrent use of antacids containing aluminum, bismuth, calcium or magnesium. Other antacids may raise the gastric pH.
	Anticonvulsants	The serum levels may be reduced and may fall below the accepted therapeutic minimum.
	Cimetidine	Does not interact.
	Colestipol	May markedly reduce the absorption.
	Diuretics	Concurrent use should be avoided because of their association with rises in blood urea nitrogen level.
	Iron preparations	Absorption from the gut of both is remarkably reduced by concurrent use which leads to depressed serum levels. Effectiveness may be reduced and even abolished.
	Milk and diary products	Absorption may be remarkably reduced if come in contact in gut leading to reduction and even abolishment of therapeutic effects. Doxycyclin is the least affected.
	Rifampicin (Rifampin)	Serum levels may be reduced up to 50%.
Tetracyclins	Thiomarsal	May experience on inflammatory ocular react ion.
	Zinc sulphate	Reduction as much as 50% is reported.
Tinidazole	Rifampicin (Rifampin)	Increases the loss from the body.
Trimethoprim	Antacids	Magnesium trisilicate and kaolin-pectin reduce the bioavailability of trimethoprine with uncertain clinical importance.
	Guar or food	May reduce the absorption.

Drugs	Interaction with	Effects
Vidarabine	Allopurinol	Toxicity of vidarabin may be increased by concurrent use.
Zidovudine (Azidothymidine)	Miscellaneous drugs	Paracetamol increases the haematological toxicity to considerable extent but acyclovir, aspirin, ketoconazole, and cotrimoxazole appear not to interact.

Anticoagulants

Drugs	Interaction with	Effects
Anticoagulants	ACE inhibitors	No interaction reported.
	Acitretin	Does not alter the effects.
	Alcohol	No alteration of effects who drinks small or moderate amount of alcohol but heavy drunker with liver disease shows fluctuation in prothrombin times.
	Allopurinol	No adverse interaction on oral administration in most patients but monitoring the initial anticoagulant response is necessary since excessive hypoprothrombinaemia and bleeding may occur.
	Aminoglutethinide	Concurrent use may reduce the effectiveness remarkably.
	Aminoglycoside antibiotics	If the intake of vitamin K is normal, either small or no interaction takes place.
	Aminosalicylic acid (PAS) and/or Isomiazid	A report describes anticoagulant response on concurrent use.
	Amiodarone	Effectiveness may be increased and bleeding may occur if dosage is not being reduced.
	Anabolic steroids and related sex hormones	Anticoagulant effects are markedly increased by concurrent use. Bleeding may occur if dosage is not changed/reduced appropriately.
	Antacids	Aluminum hydroxide does not interact with warfarin or dicoumarol and magnesium hydroxide does not interact with warfarin. Evidence supports that absorption may be increased by magnesium hydroxide with no clinical supports.
	Ascorbic acid (Vitamin C)	Isolated case describes that effectiveness may be reduced.
	Aspirin and other salicylates	Aspirin in doses of 500 mg/day increases the bleeding 3-5 times.
	Azapropazone	The effectiveness may be increased and bleeding may occur if dosage is not reduced.

Drugs	Interaction with	Effects
	Barbiturates	The effectiveness may be reduced. 30-60% increase in dosage is required to obtain full therapeutic effects.
	Benfluorex	Does not alter the effects.
	Benziodarone	The effectiveness is increased. The dosage should be reduced approximately.
	Benzodiazepines	The anticoagulant effects are not affected.
	Benzydamine hydrochloride	The effects are not altered.
	Beta-blockers	Oral anticoagulants are not affected by the concurrent use.
	5-bromo-2-deoxyuridine (BUDR)	The effectiveness is markedly increased.
	Calcium channel blockers	Does not interact adversely.
	Carbamazepine	The effectiveness may be markedly reduced. The dosage needs to be doubled.
	Carbon tetrachloride	Single report describes the increment in the effectiveness
	Cephalosporins	May increase the effectiveness.
	Chloral hydrate	The effectiveness may be increased but this is of little or no clinical importance.
	Chloramphenicol	Concurrent use may increase the effectiveness.
	Cholestyramine or colestipol	The effectiveness may be reduced.
	Cimetidine, Ranitidine or Nizatidine	The effectiveness may be increased by concurrent use of cimetidine. Ranitidine and nizatidine does not interact.
	Cinclophen	Concurrent use may increase the effectiveness. Bleeding occurs if the dosage is not reduced appropriately.
	Cisapride	May cause a small increase in the effectiveness.
	Clofibrate, Bezafibrate or Gemfibrozil	Bleeding may occur with the increment in the effectiveness so dosage should be reduced appropriately.
	Contraceptives (oral) and Related Sex hormones	The effects of dicoumarol can be increased but for nicoumalone, the effect may be decreased by the concurrent use.
	Corticosteroids or ACTH	Unpredictable but small change may occur.
	Cytotoxic (antineoplastic) agents	Concurrent use may increase the effectiveness supported by single report . A decrease in the effects is also reported with cyclophosphamide, reaptopurine and mitotane.
Anticoagulants	Dextropropoxyphene	Five patients showed a marked increase in the effects.

Drugs	Interaction with	Effects
	Dichloralphenazone	The effectiveness is reduced by the concurrent use.
	Diflunisal	Limited causes describes the increment of the effects with warfarin but phenprocoumon appear not to interact.
	Dipyridamol	Mild bleeding may occur on concurrent use.
	Dipyrone	One report describes no interaction while another claims a rapid but transient increase in the effectiveness.
	Disopyramide	Effectiveness may be reduced but reverse report is also there.
	Disulfiram	May increase the effectiveness. Bleeding may occur if dosage is not reduced appropriately.
	Ditazole	No alteration of effects reported.
	Diuretics	Does not affect the effectiveness. Rare occurrence in the increase in the effects is reported with ethacrynic acid. Bleeding may occur.
	Erythromycin	Increase in the effects associated with bleeding is reported.
	Ethchlorvynol	Effectiveness may be well reduced by concurrent use.
	Fenofibrate (procetofene)	Increase in the effectiveness with bleeding is reported unless the anticoagulant dose is reduced by one-third.
	Feprazone	Effectiveness may be increased.
	Flutamide	May increase the effects.
	Food	Rate of absorption is increased. Soy protein may reduce the absorption rate.
	Glucagon	Effectiveness is rapidly and markedly increased in large doses. Bleeding may occur if warfarin dosage is not reduced appropriately.
	Glutethimide	Concurrent use may reduce the effects.
	Griseofulvin	Effectiveness may be reduced by concurrent use.
	Halofenate	Increase in the effects by concurrent use is reported.
	Haloperidol	Concurrent use may reduce the effectiveness.
	Heparinoid	Bleeding is reported by a single report.
	Herbal remedies	Herbal remedies itself containing anticoagulating effects is expected to increase the effectiveness.
Anticoagulants	Hydrocodone	Effects may be increased.
	Indomethacin	No particular case is reported to have altered effectiveness. Caution is required to be taken because indomethacin may cause irritation and bleeding.

Drugs	Interaction with	Effects
	Influenza vaccines	Concurrent use is safe but report of bleeding is attributed to an interaction.
	Insecticides	An isolated report describes a patient having forted to respond after very heavy exposure to an insecticide.
	Isoxicam and Peroxicam	Effectiveness may be increased.
	Ketoconazole	Three elderly patients showed increase in the effects. But no interaction is also reported.
	Laxatives, Liquid Paraffin or Psyllium	No change either in the absorption rate or anticoagulant effects is reported.
	Meclofenamic acid or Mefenamic acid	Increase in the effectiveness is reported.
	Meprobamate	After the effectiveness in significant amounts.
	Meptazinol	No change in the effects is reported.
	Methaqualone	May cause small change but clinically unimportant.
	Methylphenidate	No change in the effects is reported.
	Methonidazole	May cause marked increase in the effects. Bleeding may occur if dosage is not altered appropriately.
	Miconazole	Effectiveness may be markedly increased on concurrent use. Bleeding may occur if dosage is not reduced appropriately.
	Monoamine oxidase inhibitors	No confirmed clinical report is attributed.
	Nalidixic acid	Two out of three, developed hypoprothrombinaemia and one bled.
	Nizatidine	Does not interact.
	Nomifensine	A single report supports the increase in effectiveness.
	Non-steroidal antiinflammatory drugs (NSAID's) Arylalkanoates	Effectiveness may be increased in a few patients and may bleed. No interaction takes place with normal & doses.
	Omeprazole	May cause very small change in the effectiveness.
	Oxametacin	Concurrent use may increase the effects.
Anticoagulants	Oxpentifylline	No significant change in effects by concurrent use.
	Paracetamol (Acetaminophen)	No significant change in the effects is reported.
	Penicillins	No change takes place on oral administration of anticoagulants but isolated report describes increased prothrombin times and bleeding also occur. Isolated case also supports the reduction in the effectiveness.

Drugs	Interaction with	Effects
	Phenazone (Antipyrine)	Effectiveness may be reduced.
	Phenothiazines	Does not interact.
	Phenylbutazone	Effect iveness is markedly increased by concurrent use. To avoid bleeding, concurrent use may be restricted.
	Phenyramidol	Increase in effects associated with bleeding may takes place. So, reduction in dosage is recommended.
	Piracetam	A single report describes who began to bleed within a month of starting to take piracetam.
	Prolintane	No alteration in the effectiveness is reported.
	Profagenone	Concurrent use may cause increase in the effectiveness. Reduction in the dosage is necessary.
	Proquatone	No change in the effects.
	Quinidine	Effectiveness may be increased with bleeding. A decrease in the effect is also reported.
	Quinine	No change in the effects is reported on oral administration.
	Quinolone antibiotics	Enoxacin does not interact, nor ciprofloxacin with nicoumalane or ethylbicoumacelate nor ofloxacin with phenprocoumon. Increase in the effect is also reported.
	Rifampicin (Rifampin)	Concurrent use may reduce the effectiveness which demands the dosage to be increased accordingly.
	Reoprostil	May reduce the effectivenees.
	Roxithromycin	Does not interact.
	Simvastatin	May cause small but clinically unimportant increase in the effectiveness.
	Sucralfate	Two cases describe marked reduction in the effects. Uncommon interaction is also reported.
	Sulindac	Occasional increase in the effectiveness is reported.
	Suloctidil or Zomepirac	Does not intertact significantly.
	Sulphinpyrazone	May increase the effects markedly associated with serious bleeding provided the dosage is not reduced appropriately.
	Sulphonamides	Concurrent use may increase the effects. Bleeding may occur if dosage is not changed appropriately.
	Tamoxifen	Concurrent use may increase the effects significantly. Reduction in dosage by a half and even more may be necessary to avoid bleeding.
	Terodiline	Does not alter the effects.
	Tetracycline, Tricylic and other antidepressants	Oral anticoagulants does not alter the effects. A single report describes increase in the effectiveness with mianserin and lofepramine.

Drugs	Interaction with	Effects
	Tetracycline	Generally no change in the effects is reported. Isolated case describes increase in the effects.
	Thyroid or Antithyroid compounds	Concurrent use may increase the effects. Bleeding may occur if dosage is not reduced appropriately. A reduction in the effectiveness is expected if antithyroid compounds are used.
	Ticlopidine	The concurrent use may cause liver damage.
	Trazodone	Concurrent use can be uneventful while an isolated case describes a woman who needed increased dosage.
	Vitamin E	Limited cases are reported that it may increase or decrease effectiveness.
	Vitamin K	Effectiveness may be reduced and even abolished by the concurrent use.
Heparin	Aspirin	May be effective in the prevention of post-operative thromboembolism but risk of bleeding occur.
	Dextran	Although successful and uneventful evidence is also there which suggests the increment of the effectiveness. Dosage may be reduced to a third or a half during concurrent use.
	Glyceryl trinitrate (Nitroglycerin)	The effectiveness may be reduced by concurrent use.
	Probenecid	May possibly increase the effectiveness associated with bleeding.

Anticonvulsants Drugs

Drugs	Interaction with	Effects
	Acetazolamide	Severe osteomalacia and rickets is reported by concurrent use. A marked reduction in serum level is also attributed.
	Aspartame	May cause convulsions.
Anticonvulsants	Calcium channel blockers	Verapamil may cause marked rise in serum level which is also similar with dilitiazem. Nifedipine does not interact, but may cause phenytoin intoxication. The serum level of felodipine may markedly deduced by carbamazepine, phenobarbitone and phenytoin.
	Cinromide	May depress the serum level.
	Cytotoxic drugs	Serum level may be reduced markedly by concurrent use with cytotoxic drugs.

Drugs	Interaction with	Effects
	Denzimol	Marked and rapid rise in serum level accompanied by acute toxicity is reported.
	Dextropropyphene	Concurrent use may rise the serum level associated with toxicity.
	Disulfiram	Serum levels are markedly and rapidly increased by concurrent use.
	Felbamate	May rise the serum level.
	Folic acid	Fall in the serum levels leading to adverse seizure control may occur by concurrent use.
	Influenza vaccines	May rise in the serum level.
	Nafimidone	May rise the serum level. Dosage reduction is needed to prevent toxicity.
	Progabide	Serum level can rise by concurrent use.
	Pyridoxine	Large dose (200mg daily) can cause reduction up to 40-50% in the serum level.
	Quinolone antibiotics	Ciprofloxacin and enoxacin may cause occational convulsions.
	Stiriprentol	May cause marked rise in serum levels, Dosage to be reduced to avoid toxicity.
	Tobacco smoking	No important interaction.
	Vigabatrin	May reduce in serum level.
	Viloxazine	Serum levels may rise up to 50% by concurrent use.
Barbiturates	Caffeine	The hypnotic effects may be reduced and even abolished by concurrent use.
	Cimetidine	May reduce the absorption of cimetidine.
	Miconazole	Serum levels may be increased.
	Rifampicin (Rifampin)	May markedly increase the clearance from the body. The effects of both are expected to be reduced.
	Sodium valproate	Concurrent use may cause the increase in serum levels. A reduction in the dosage by a third to a half can be safely carried out.
	Triacetylobandomycin	Concurrent use may cause marked reduction in the serum levels.
Carbamazepine or Phenobarbitone	Benzodiazepines	No effects reported but serum level may be reduced of limited clinical importance.

Drugs	Interaction with	Effects
	Cimetidine or Ranitidine	Transient increase in serum levels is reported. Cimetidine appears to produce some side effect, which disappears rapidly. Ranitidine does not interact.
	Danazol	Concurrent use may rise in the serum level. Dosage reduction in recommended to avoid toxicity.
	Diuretics	Hyponatraemia may be caused by concurrent use.
	Erythromycin	Serum levels may be raised rapidly to toxic concentration by concurrent use. Erythromycin does not interact with Phenytoin.
	Isoniazid	Concurrent use may rise the serum level rapidly. Reduced dosage is required to avoid intoxication.
	Macrolide antibiotics	Serum level may rise rapidly leading to intoxication within 1-3 days.
	Miconazole	A single report describes adverse response by concurrent use.
	Monoamine oxidase inhibition	No interaction is reported.
	Phenobarbitone	Reduction in serum levels is reported by concurrent use.
Carbamazepine	Primidone	Marked reduction in serum levels is reported.
	Sodium valproate	Serum levels of both may fall by 20-25% by concurrent use.
	Valpromide	Intoxication (carbamazepine) may occur if valpromide is not replaced by sodium valproate.
	Barbiturates, Phenytoin or Primidone	Fall in the serum levels may be caused by concurrent use. Phenytoin intoxication is also reported.
	Carbamazepine	Serum levels may be reduced.
Ethosuximide	Isoniazid	An isolated report describes psychotic behaviour and signs of ethosuximide intoxication by concurrent use.
	Sodium valproate	Significant rise in the serum levels is reported by concurrent use.
	Alcohol	Chronic heavy drinking reduces serum concentration. Excessive drinking also increases the frequency of seizures in epileptics.
Phenytoin	Allopurinol	A single report describes intoxication in a body by concurrent use.

Drugs	Interaction with	Effects
	Amiodarone	Serum levels may be raised. Phenytoin intoxication may occur if dosage is not reduced appropriately.
	Antacids	Some, but not all cases can reduce serum level.
	Anticoagulants	Serum level may be increased. Effectiveness may be reduced.
	Aspirin	Phenytoin toxicity is reported. Adverse interaction occurs in most patients.
	Azapropazone	Concurrent use may rise in the serum levels. Phenytoin intoxication is likely to develop.
	Barbiturates	Concurrent use is uneventful. Phenytoin intoxication has been reported.
	Benzodiazepines	May cause to rise, fall or remain unaltered in the serum levels.
	Carbamazepine	Rise or fall in the serum levels are reported by concurrent use.
	Chloramphenicol	Concurrent use may rise the serum levels. Phenytoin intoxication in two patients.
	Chlorpheniramine	Concurrent use reports phenytoin intoxication in two patients.
	Cholestyramine or colestipol	No change in absorption rate is reported.
	Cimetidine, famotidine and ranitidine	Serum levels may be raised by cimetidine with toxicity. Others two don't react.
	Cloxacillin	Concurrent use may cause marked reduction in serum levels.
	Diazoxide	Reports of four children who showed marked reduction in serum levels are attributed with reduced effectiveness.
	Dichloralphenazone	Concurrent use may lead to reduction in serum levels.
	Floconazole	Serum levels may rise rapidly. Toxicity may develop if dosage is not being reduced appropriately.
	Food	The absorption may be affected by some food.
	Carbapentin	Concurrent use shows no interaction of clinical importance.

Drugs	Interaction with	Effects
	Hypoglycaemic agents	Large and toxic doses may cause hyperglycaemia.
	Ibuprofen	No interaction of clinical importance is reported.
	Influenza vaccines	Reports to increase, decrease or to have no effects on the serum levels have been documented.
	Isoniazid	Serum levels may be raised by concurrent use.
	Loxapine	Depressed serum levels by concurrent use is reported.
	Methylphenidate	Serum levels may be raised associated with intoxication.
	Metronidazole	Small and clinically unimportant rise in the serum level is reported.
	Miconazole	Intoxication is reported in two cases.
	Omeprazole	The loss from the body is reduced.
	Pheneturide	Serum levels may be raised up to 50% by concurrent use.
	Phenothiazines	Serum levels may be raised or lowered.
	Phenylbutazone	Serum levels may be raised. Intoxication may appear if dosage is not reduced appropriately.
	Phenyramidol	Serum levels may be raised up to three folds by concurrent use. Phenytoin dosage is to be reduced to avoid intoxication.
	Rifampicin (Rifampin)	Clearance is doubled by the concurrent use.
	Sodium valproate	Uneventful.
	Sucralfate	The absorption may be reduced to 7-20% by concurrent use.
	Sulphinpyrazone	Concurrent use may rise the serum levels markedly. Dosage is to be reduced appropriately to avoid intoxication.
	Sulphonamides	Serum levels may be raised by co-trimoxazole, sulphamethizole, sulphamethoxazole,

Drugs	Interaction with	Effects
		trimethoprinete by concurrent use. Others like sulphadimethoxine etc. don't interact.
	Sulthiame	Concurrent use may raise the serum levels to double resulting intoxication if dosage is not being reduced appropriately.
	Theophyllin	Serum levels and effectiveness may be markedly reduced by concurrent use leading to need of increment in dosage to maintain concentration.
	Teinilic acid (Ticrynoden)	Intoxication is reported.
	Trazodone	Concurrent use may result intoxication.
	Tricyclic antidepressants	Very limited evidence supports that serum level may be raised by concurrent use.
Primidone	Barbiturates	Elevated serum phenobarbitone levels may develop by concurrent use.
	Carbamazepine, Clonazepam or Clorazepate	Carbamazepine may reduce but clonazepam may raise the serum level.
	Isoniazid	Serum level may be reduced by concurrent use.
	Phenytoin	Concurrent use may raise the serum level.
	Sodium valproate	Serum levels may be increased or decreased by concurrent use.
Sodium valproate	Antacids	Absorption is slightly accelerated by (aluminium-magnesium hydroxide) but no interaction with magnesium trisilicate or calcium carbonate.
	Aspirin	Large dose may develop toxicity by concurrent use. Blood levels increased by aspirin.
	Benzodiazepines	Side effects may be increased.
	Cimetidine or Ranitidine	Cimetidine interact minimally whereas ranitidine does not.
	CNS depressants and alcohol	Potentiate the activity of Sodium Valproate.

Antihypertensives

Drugs	Interaction with	Effects
ACE inhibitors	Allopurinol	Concurrent use may cause serious Stevens-Johnson syndrome and hypersensitivity.
	Antacids	May reduce the absorption by concurrent use.
	Azathiprine	Leucopenia in the occational case may be resulted by concurrent use.
	Diuretic	Generally safe and effective. But a few patients may have felt lightheaded within an hour of first dose resulting hypotension. Hyperkalaemia is also possible if potassium-sparing or potassium supplements are used.
	Non-steroidal antiinflammatory drugs	The effectiveness may be reduced or even abolished by indomethacin, ibuprofen and aspirin.
	Other antihypertensives	The effects may be delayed to occur. Dosage reduction is required to avoid hypotension.
Acetazolamide	Beta-blockers	Patients with chronic obstructive lung disease may witness acidosis.
Amlodipine + Linisopril	Diuretics	Fall in BP, hypokalemia with concommitant use of potassium sparing diuretics.
	Indomethacin	It may alternate antihypertensive effect of linisopril.
	Thiazides	Linisopril reduce the potassium loss.
Antihypertensives	Alcohol	Blood pressure may be raised by moderate to heavy drinking. Postural hypertensive, dizziness and fainting shortly after having a drink may also be experienced.
	Fenfluramine	May increase the blood pressure thus lowering the effectiveness.
	Food	Absorption may remain unaltered and if lowers, very little.
	Phenothiazine	Side effects of phenothizines may increase the side effects of others, the patients may fell faint if they stand up quickly.
	Pyrazolone compounds	Effectiveness may be reduced.
	Salbutamol	Severe hypotension is reported.
Atenolol	Indomethacin	Reduces antihypertensive effect of atenolol.
Benazepril	Diuretics	Increases the risk of hyperkalaemia.
	Thiazides	Excessive fall in blood pressure.
	Food	Rate of absorption delayed.
Bisoprolol	Anaesthetic agents, clonidine, calcium antagonists, digitalis, hypoglycaemic agents, NSAIDs.	The action of these Drugs are enhanced by Bisoprolol.
	Rifampicin	May cause reduction in plasma concentration and elimination half-life of the Bisoprolol.

Drugs	Interaction with	Effects
Captopril	Immunosuppressive Drugs	Risk of bone marrow depression increased.
	Probenecids	It delays the excretion of captopril and increases the blood level of captopril.
	Morphine	The analgesic and respiratory depression produced by morphine may be accentuated by captopril.
Carvedilol	Rifampicin	Pretreatment with rifampicin results in a decreased Cmax and AUC.
	Verapamil	Severe bradycardia and myocardial depression.
	Clonidine	Hypotensive and cardiodepressive actions are potentiated.
Clonidine	Beta-blockers	Concurrent use may cause a sharp and serious rise in blood pressure. The effectiveness may also be abolished which is reported.
Clonidine or apomorphine	Oral contraceptives	Concurrent use may reduce the sedative effects.
Clonidine	Prazosin	Effectiveness may be reduced by concurrent use.
	Tricyclic antidepressants	Reduction or even abolition of effectiveness may be reduced.
Diazoxide	Hypoglycaemic agents and hypotensive agents	Severe hypotension is reported. Excessive hypoglycaemia may also occur by concurrent use.
Diltiazem	Digoxin, Cyclosporine	Elevates serum digoxin and cyclosporin levels.
	Propanolol	Potentiate the action of propanolol.
	Cimetidine	It may increase the plasma concentration of diltiazem.
Diuretics (Potassium-sparing)	Potassium suppliments and salt subastitutes	Severe and life threatening hyperkalaemia may result if potassium level is not monitored.
Diuretics	Trimethoprim	Excessive low serum levels is reported by concurrent use.
Enalapril	Cyclophosphamide, azathioprine	Risk of bone marrow suppression increased with concomitant therapy with the immunosuppressive Drugs.
Enalapril	Diuretics/potassium supplements	Hyperkalaemia and potentiates the hypotensive action.
	Probenecids	It delays the excretion of the enalapril.
	Morphine	Potentiates the analgesia and respiratory depression produced by morphine.
Frusemide	Chloralhydrate	Intravenous injection of frusemide after being treated with chloral may cause sweating, hot flushes, a variable blood pressure.
	Clofibrate	Diuresis and muslcular symptoms is reported by concurrent use.
	Food	May reduce the bioavailability of frusemide and diuretic effects.

Drugs	Interaction with	Effects
Frusemide or Bumetanide	Indomethacins and others NSAID's	The antihypertension and diuretic effects may be reduced or even abolished by concurrent use.
	Phenytoin	The effectiveness may be reduced up to 50% by the concurrent use.
	Probenacid	May cause the reduction of urinary loss of sodium.
Guanethidine and related drugs	Haloperidol or Thiothixene	Concurrent use may reduce the effectiveness.
	Indirectly acting sympathomimetic amines and related drugs	Concurrent use reduces the effectiveness to even abolition. Blood pressure may be increased.
	Monoamine oxidase inhibitors	The effects may be reduced by the concurrent use.
	Phenothiazines	Large doses may cause reduction or even abolition of the effectiveness by the concurrent use.
	Pizotifen	The effectiveness may be even abolished.
	Tricyclic antidepressants	The effects may be reduced and even abolished by the concurrent use.
	Tyramine – rich foods	Serious hypertension is reported.
Hydralazine	Diclofenac	Diclofenac is reported to oppose the effectiveness of hydralazine. It is uncertain in the case of indomethacin.
Indapamide	Thiazide/Potassium losing diuretics	Hypokalaemia and hypercalcuria enhanced.
Indoramin	Alcohol	Concurrent use may raise the serum levels of both.
Ketanserin	Beta-blockers	Acute hypotension have been reported by the concurrent use.
	Diuretics	Sudden deaths, abnormal heart rhythym may be markedly increased by concurrent use.
Labetalol	Halothane	Hypotensive effect of halothane enhanced by labetalol.
	Anti-arrythmics & antagonists	Potentiates action of anti-arrythmics and Ca-antagonists.
	Cimetidine	Bio-availability of labetalol increases.
Lacidipine	Cimetidine	It increases the plasma lacidipine levels.
Linisopril	Indomethacin	It may reduces the hypotensive effect of linisopril.
	Hydrochlorthiazide	Hypotensive effect of linisopril is potentiated leading to severe hypotension and hyperkalaemia.
Linisopril	Alcohol	Hypotensive effect of linisopril is potentiated by alcohol.
	Cyclo-oxygenase inhibitors	Co-administration of cyclo-oxygenase inhibitors may cause sharp reduction in renal function.
	Diuretics	Hypotensive effect of losartan is potentiated by diuretics.

Drugs	Interaction with	Effects
Losartan potassium	NSAIDs	It may blunt anti-hypertensive response of losartan.
	Cimetidine	It may inc rease the AUC of losartan by about 18%.
	Phenobarbital	It may reduce the AUC of losartan and its active metabolite.
	Ketoconazol	It inhibits the conversion of losartan to its active metabolites.
	Barbiturates	Concurrent use does not alter the effects.
Methyldopa	Cephalosporin	Pustular eruptions may occur by concurrent use.
	Disulphiram	Abolition of effectiveness may be caused.
	General anaesthetics	It enhance the effect of methyldopa.
	Haloperidol	Concurrent use may result dementia but no serious problem is reported.
	Iron salts	Concurrent use may reduce the effectiveness.
	Phenoxybenzamine	Total urinary incontinence is reported by concurrent use.
Metoprolol	Tricyclic antidepressants	Concurrent use does not adversely alter the effects but hypertension, tachycardia, tumor are reported.
	Verapamil	Hypotension, bradycardia asystole with verapamil in the presence of AV nodal block and LVF.
	Antidiabetics	Masking of hypoglycaemic symptoms.
	Cimetidine	Metoprolol activity is potentiated.
	Nifedipine, nitrates, verapamil	Enhancement of anti-anginal activity.
	Diuretics and vasodialators	Enhancement of anti-hypertensive activity.
Nifedipine	Quinidine	Plasma quinidine levels may be reduced.
	Theophylline, phenytoin	Levels of plasma theophylline and phenytoin levels increased.
	Beta-blockers	Synergism and reduce depression of cardiac function.
	Cimetidine	Bio-availability of Nifedipine increases and hypotensive action is potentiated.
Nitrendipine	Theophylline, phenytoin	Levels of plasma theophylline and phenytoin levels increased.
	Beta-blockers	Synergism and reduce depression of cardiac function.
	Cimetidine	Bio-availability of Nitrendipine increases and hypotensive action is potentiated.
Perindopril	Diuretics	Diuretics that lead to salt depletion increase risk of hypotension with the drug, potassium sparing diuretics can cause hypokalaemia, increase in lithium level.
	NSAIDs	Reduction in anti-hypertensive effect.

Drugs	Interaction with	Effects
Prazosin	Beta-blockers	May cause some patients to faint.
Prazosin	Calcium channel blockers	Blood pressure may fall sharply. Close monitoring of the response is required.
	Diuretics	Diuretics aggravates Sodium depletion.
Propranolol	Adrenaline	Marked hypertension and bradycardia.
	Anaesthetic agents	Reduced heart rate and output.
	Digitalis & Calcium channel blockers	Severe bradycardia may occur (especially with impaired left ventricular function)
	Chlorpromazine	Blood levels of both the drug increases and additive hypotensive effect.
	Cimetidine	Blood levels of propranolol increases.
	Indomethacin	Hypotensive effect is reduced.
	Smoking	Reduced efficacy.
	Vasodilators	Tachycardia inhibited.
	Other antihypertensives and diuretics	Additive effect.
Ramipril	Diuretics	Concommitant administration may lead to serious hypotension and with potassium sparing diuretics dangerous hyperkalaemia may result. Serum lithium concentration may increase.
	NSAIDs	Effect of the drug may be reduced, and cause deterioration of renal function.
	Alcohol	Effect is exacerbated.
	Vasodilators	Inhibits tachycardia.
Rauwolfia alkaloids	Tricyclic antidepressants	May be successfully used in some resistant form of depression by concurrent use.
Sotalol	General anaesthetics	May impair myocardial contractility.
	Antidepressants & quinidine	Polymorphic ventricular trachycardia.
Spironolactone	Dextropropoxyphene	Gynaecomastia and rash is reported.
Terazocin	Beta-blockers, calcium channel blockers, diuretics	Orthostatic hypotension is potentiated.
Thiazides	Calcium carbonate	Hypercalaemia and metabolic alkalosis is reported by concurrent use.
	Cholestyramine or Colestipol	The absorption may be reduced by the concurrent use. The diuretic effect is likely to be reduced accordingly.
	Indomethacin and other NSAID's	Reductoin in the effectiveness by indomethacin of moderate clinical importance is reported. Ibuprofen has less impacts where as others interact resulting no adverse effects.

Drugs	Interaction with	Effects
	Propantheline	May increase the absorption by concurrent use.
Triamterene	Cimetidine or Ranitidine	Ranitidine may reduce the absorption and diuretic effects of uncertain clinical importance. Cimetidine does not interact.
	Indomethacin	Acute renal failure is reported by concurrent use.

Antiparkinsonian

Drugs	Interaction with	Effects
Amantadine	Miscellaneous drugs	Various problems are reported.
	Thiazides	Successful and unsuccessful concurrent uses are reported. Intoxication is also reported.
Anticholinergics	**Betel nuts**	Controls of side effects are reported by concurrent use.
Benzohexol	Tricyclic antidepressants, antiparkinsonian Drugs, antihistaminic and quinidines	Additive anticholinergic activity.
Bromocriptine	Alcohol	Alcohol reduces tolerance to the drug and vice-versa.
	Erythromycin	Bioavailability of the bromocriptin is increased.
	Griseofulvin	Effectiveness may be opposed.
	Macrolid antibiotics	Toxicity may occur with Josamycin. Marked serum level is reported with erythromycin.
Levodopa	Anticholinergics	Effectiveness may be reduced.
	Benzodiazepines	Concurrent use may reduce and even abolish the effects.
	Beta-blockers	Concurrent use may appear favorable but long time effects of the elevated growth hormones is uncertain.
	Clonidene	The effects may be opposed by the concurrent use.
	Ferrus sulphate	May reduce the bioavailability.
	Food	May reduce the effectiveness by concurrent use.
	Methionine	Concurrent use may reduce the effects.
	Methyldopa	May cause in the increment of effects there by reduction in dose is essential.
	Metoclopramide	Some of the effects may be increased and a few may be opposed.

Drugs	Interaction with	Effects
Levodopa	Monoamine oxidase inhibitors (MAOI)	Concurrent use may cause a rapid, serious and potentially life-threatening hypertension.
	Papaverine	May cause deterioration in the control of parkinsonism with no confirm trial report.
	Phenothiazines or butyrophenones	Concurrent use may oppose the effects by each other.
	Phenylbutazone	The effects may be antagonised by concurrent use.
	Phenytoin	Concurrent use may reduce and even abolish the effects.
	Piperidine	Concurrent use may oppose the effectiveness.
	Pyridoxine (Vit - B6)	The effectiveness may be reduced and even abolished by the concurrent use.
	Rauwolfia alkaloids	The effects may be opposed by the concurrent use.
		The concurrent use is uneventful although very small reduction in the effectiveness is reported. Hypertensive crisis is also reported.
Orphenadrine	Anticholinergics, alcohol, other CNS depressants, MAOIs and antidepressants	These drugs are potentiated by orphenadrine.
	Propoxyphene	May cause tremors and mental confusion.
	Chlorpromazine	Plasma chlorpromazine level decreased.
	Levodopa	Synergistic effects.
Selegiline	Reserpine, Tetrabenazine	Interfere with the effect of Selegiline.

Beta – blockers

Drugs	Interaction with	Effects
Beta – blockers	Antacids	A few antacids may cause small reduction in the absorption of proporanolol, atenolol, and others while absorption may be increased with metaprolol are reported by concurrent use.
	Anticholinesterases	Bradycardia and hypotension is reported by the concurrent use.
	Barbiturates	May cause reduction in the removal process from the body by liver.
	Calcium channel blockers	Concurrent use is reported to be useful. However some level may be raised of clinically unimportance.

Drugs	Interaction with	Effects
	Cholestyramine or colestipol	Serum level may be reduced.
	Cimetidine	The blood leves may be doubled by the concurrent use. Bradycardia (heart rate 36 beats/min) and hypotension is also reported.
	Cimetidine phenylephrine	Lowering of blood pressure by the concurrent use is reported. Bronchospasm may also occur.
	Contraceptives (Oral)	The blood levels may be increased with uncertain clinical importance.
	Dextromoramide	Bradycardia and severe hypotension is reported.
	Diltiazem	Although mainly safe and uneventful but bradycardia is also reported.
	Ergotamine or methylsergids	Although mainly very effective and useful but severe peripheral vasoconstriction is also described.
	Erythromycin or Neomycin	Serum levels may be increased.
	Etintidine	Serum levels may be increased.
	Food	Food may increase, decrease or have no effect on the bioavailability.
	Halofenate	Concurrent use may reduce the serum levels and the therapeutic effects.
	Haloperidol	Hypotension and cardiopulmonary assets in women may be occurred.
	Hydralozine	Serum levels may be increased with no adverse impact.
	Indomethacin and other NSAID's	Effectiveness may be reduced. Sulindac don't interact. Aspirin appears to be uncertain. Indomethacin may cause hypertension.
	Morphine	Serum levels may be increased.
	Nifedipine	Concurrent use is effective but excessive hypotension and heart failure is also reported.
	Phenothiazines	Serum levels may be increased the both. Excessive hypotension is reported.
	Propafenone	Serum levels may be raised by 2-5 folds by the concurrent use.
	Rifampicin (Rifampin)	May increase the serum levels.
	Sulphinpyrazone	Concurrent use may reduce and even abolish the effectiveness.
	Thallium scans	May provide false information of stress thallium scans, used for the diagnosis of coronary heart disease.

Drugs	Interaction with	Effects
	Tobacco smokings and/or coffee and tea drinking	Smoking may reduce the effectiveness considerably while drinking of tea or coffee may have same but smaller effects.
	Verapamil	Serious cardiodepression may occur by the concurrent use. Hence initial close supression and monitoring is recommended.
	x-ray contrast media	Hypotension is reported by the concurrent use.

Calcium-channel blockers

Drugs	Interaction with	Effects
Calcium-channel blockers	Aspirin	The antiplatelet effect of ca-channel blockers may be increased by the concurrent use. Bruising is reported.
	Calcium salts	The effectiveness may be antagonized by the concurrent use.
	Cimetidine or ranitidine	Serum levels may be increased by cimetidine. Ranitidine interact minimally but famotidine appears to be reduce the heart activity.
	Dantrolene	Hyperkalaemia and cardiovascular collapse is reported.
	Food	Don't interact with clinical importance.
	Clonidine	Clonidine may provide additional effects.
	Local anaesthetics	Bradycardia and hypotension may occur by the concurrent use.
	Magnesium salts	Muscle weakness paralysis is reported by the concurrent use.
	Miscellaneous drugs	Concurrent use should be avoided to escape from the risk of the development of the torsodes depointes.
	Rifampicin	Serum levels may be reduced to that level making therapeutically ineffective if the dosage is not increased appropriately.
	Sulphinpyrazone	The clearance may be markedly increased.
	Vancomycln	The effectiveness may be increased by the concurrent use.
	x-ray contrast media	The hypotensive effects is increased by the presence of calcium-channel blockers. Ventricular tachycardia is reported by the concurrent use.

Oral contraceptives and related sex hormone drugs

Drugs	Interaction with	Effects
Oral contraceptives	Alcohol	Although blood alcohol remains unaltered, the detrimental effects may be reduced by the concurrent use.
	Antacids	A few evidence suggest the concurrent to be safe, but magnesium ticitrate may reduce the effects and reliability is also reported.
Oral contraceptives	Anti-asthmatic preparations	No recorded interaction is available. But asthmatic condition may be worsened and sometimes may be improved as well.
	Antibiotics and anti-infective agents	Concurrent use may lead to the failure of oral contraceptives to prevent pregnancy.
	Anticonvulsants	Concurrent use reports uncertainty towards action of oral contraceptives. Intermediate breakthrough bleeding, spotting and even pregnancies may occur. Sodium valproate does not interact.
	Antihypertensive agents	Anti-hypertensive agents appear resistant towards the hypertension caused by oral contraceptives.
	Cimetidine	Cimetidine may raise the serum oestradiol levels.
	Fluconazole	May reduce the effectiveness and even pregnancies may occur.
	Griseofulvin	Concurrent use may reduce the effects by the effects of oral contraceptives.
	Ketoconazole	May reduce the effectiveness of oral contraceptives by the concurrent use associated with intestinal bleeding.
	Penicillins	May cause the oral contraceptives to fail.
	Rifampicin	Concurrent use may cause the reliability of oral contraceptives uncertain.
	Tobacco smoking	May increase the rise of thromboembolic disease.
	Triacetyloleandomycin	Concurrent use may produce severe pruritis and jaundice.
	Vitamins	Oral contraceptives may rise the serum levels of vitamin A and lower levels of ascorbic acid, cyanocobalamin, folic acid and pyridoxin.
	Anti-inflammatory agents	Concurrent use may produce oceatin failure to prevent pregnancy.
	Aminoglutethimide	May reduce the serum levels markedly.
Intrauterine contraceptive diuretics (IUD's)	Aspirin, Codein, Paracetamol	Concurrent use may produce failure to prevent pregnancy.
	Mefenamic acid	Concurrent use may produce failure to prevent pregnancy.
Medroxyprogesterone	Aminoglutethimide	Aminoglutethimide markedly reduces the serum level of medroxyprogesterone.

Cytotoxic drugs

Drugs	Interaction with	Effects
Cytotoxic drugs	Aclarubicin	The effectiveness of aclarubicin can be increased.
Aminoglutethimide	Bendroflumethiazide	Prolong treatment with drug may cause serious loss of sodium.
Azathioprine/Mereaptopurine	Allopurinol	Concurrent use may increase the effectiveness if cytotoxic agents is given orally. To avoid intoxication, dosage of cytotoxic drugs should be reduced to a third or a quarter. No interaction takes place on intravenous administration of cytotoxic drug.
	Cotrimoxazole or trimethoprin	Concurrent use may increase the risk of life-threatening haematological toxicity.
	Doxorubicin (Adriamylin)	Concurrent use may increase the effectiveness.
Bleomycin	Cisplatin	Pulmonary toxicity of bleomycin is reported.
	Oxygen	Serious and fatal pulmonary toxcity can develop.
	Radiotherapy	Toxicity enhanced.
	Various cytotoxic regimens	The effectiveness, the bleomycin-induced pulmonary reactions in particular is increased by the concurrent use.
	Vincristin	Debilitation syndrome is produced.
Busulphan	Vaccination	Immunisation will live viruses can acuse life threatening infection.
	Thioguanine	Combination may results in nodular regenerative hyperplasia, portal hypertension, varices.
	Cyclophosphamide	Enhances haemopoietic therapeutic recovery.
Carmofur	Alcohol	A disulfiram-like reaction may occur.
Carmustine (BCNU)	Cimetidine	Concurrent use may increase the effectiveness but the fall in neutrophil and thrombocyte counts may become serious.
Chlorambucil	Myelosuppressive agents	Potentiation.
	Phenylbutazone and Warfarin	Effect of chlorambucil is potentiated.

Drugs	Interaction with	Effects
Cisplatin	Aminoglycoside antibiotics	Potentiate neurotoxicity.
	Antihypertensive agents	Kidney failure by the concurrent use is reported.
Cisplatin	Ethacrynic acid	The effectiveness may be increased by the concurrent use.
	Methotrexate	Fetal methotrexate toxicity may develop by the concurrent use.
	Probenecid	No report is available with certain support.
Cyclophosphamide	Allopurinol	Increased risk of bone-marrow toxicity.
	Benzodiazepines	Toxicity of cyclophosphamide may be increased by the concurrent use.
	Myelotoxic drug or radiotherapy	Serious toxicity is reported.
	Chloramphenicol	Increased risk of bone marrow toxicity.
	Corticosteroids	The effects may be reduced by the concurrent use.
	Dapsone	The effects may be reduced.
	Doxorubicin (Adriamycin)	Increased risk of cardiotoxicity.
	Morphine or Pethidine	The toxicity may be increased by the concurrent use.
	Phenobarbital	Metabolism & leukopenic activity increases.
Cyclophosphamide or Mustine	Sulphaphenazole	May increase or decrease the effects of cyclophosphamide.
Cyclophosphamide	Calcium channel blockers	The efficiency may be increased but reduction in absorption is reported.
Cytotoxic drugs	Food	Absorption may be reduced while other effects remain unaltered.
	Gentamycin	Hypomagnesaemia is reported by the concurrent use.
	Vaccines	The immune response of the body is suppressed by cytotoxic drugs. The effectiveness of vaccine may be poor.
Cytarabin	Radiotherapy & other myelotoxic Drugs	Bone marrow depression is potentiated.
Daunorubicin	Vaccination	Not recommended.
	Radiation	Enhanced radiation reaction.
	Heparin, Aluminum dexamethasone	Incompatable.
Doxorubicin (Adriamycin)	Actinomycin, Plicamycin, Methranycin	Concurrent use may cause fatal cardiomyopathy.

Drugs	Interaction with	Effects
	Barbiturates	The current use may cause reduced effects.
	Mercaptopurine	Cholestasis induced by mercaptopurine may be potentiated by the drug.
	Beta-blockers	Cardiotoxicity is reported.
	Streptozotocin	Toxicity may be increased.
Etoposide	Cytotoxic Drugs	Synergism.
5-fluorouracil	Aminoglycosides	Gastrointestinal absorption may be delayed by the concurrent use.
	Cimetidine	Serum levels may be increased by 75%.
	Other bone marrow depressants and immuno-suppressive agents	Additive adverse effects.
	Vaccination	Simultaneous live viral vaccination may produce generalised and life threatening infection, killed virus vaccines are ineffective.
Hexamethylmelamine	Antidepressants	Severe orthoststic hypotension is reported.
Hydroxyurea	CNS depressants	Increased CNS depression is reported.
	Cytarabin	Risk of haematological toxicity increased.
Infosfamide	Barbiturates	Encephalopathy is reported by the concurrent use.
	Cisplastin	Intoxication of ifosfamide may be increased.
	Warfarin	Effect of warfarin increased.
L-asparaginase	Methotrexate or cytarabin	Striking synergistic effect.
Leukovorin	Methotraxate	Reduces methotrexate activity.
	Fluorouracil	Enhance cytotoxic effect of fluorouracil.
Lomustine (CCNU)	Theophylline	Thrombocytopenia and bleeding is reported by concurrent use.
Melphalan	Cimetidine	Bioavailability of melphalan be reduced by the concurrent use.
Mercaptopurine	Food	The absorption is reduced and delayed by the concurrent use.
	Allopurinol	Effect drug enhanced by allopurinol.
	Hepatotoxic Drugs	Toxicity of mercaptopurine is potentiated.
	Myelosuppressive Drugs	Antineoplastic effect is potentiated.
	Warfarin	Anticoagulant effect of warfarin may be inhibited.

Drugs	Interaction with	Effects
Methotrexate	Alcohol	Risk of hepatic cirrhosis and fibrosis may be increased.
	Amiodarone	Toxicity of methotrexate is reported by concurrent use.
	Aminoglycosides	Absorption may be reduced by the concurrent use of the paromomycin, neomycin and other oral aminoglycosides.
	Barbiturates	Alopecia caused by methotrexate may be increased by concurrent use.
	Chloramphenicol, PAS, Sodium Salicylate, sulphomethoxy pyridazine, Tetracycline, Tolbutamide.	Intoxication may be enhanced by the concurrent use.
	Cholestyramine	The serum level can be markedly reduced by the concurrent use.
	Corticosteroids	The intoxication may be increased with the reduction of efficacy of methotrexate.
	Co-trimoxazole or trimethoprine	Bone marrow depression and even fatal is reported.
	Diuretics	Concurrent use may reduce the bone-marrow supression.
	5-Flurouracil (5-FU)	The effectiveness may be reduced by the concurrent use.
	Nitrous oxide	Methotrexate induced stomatitis and other toxic effects may be enhanced by the concurrent use.
	Non-steroidal antiinflammatory drugs (NSAID's)	Concurrent use may cause rise in the serum levels and life threatening toxicity.
	Penicillins	The loss of methotrexate from the body may be reduced considerably by the concurrent use.
	Probenecids	Serum levels may be increased even by 3-4 folds by the concurrent use.
	Retinoids	Although concurrent use may be useful but toxic hepatitis is also reported.
	Teracyclins	Methotrexate intoxication may develop by the concurrent use.
	Urinary alkalinizers	May increase the solubility of methotrexate in urine but may increase its excretion.

Drugs	Interaction with	Effects
	Salicylate, sulphonamides, phenytoin, phenylbutazone, tetracyclines, chloramphenicol, para-amino-benzoic acid	Toxicity of methotrexate increases.
Misonidazole	Cimetidine	Does not interact.
	Miscellaneous drugs	Clearance from the body may be increased by phenytoin, phenobarbitone, dexamethazone. Metoclpramide does not interact.
Mitomycin	Chlorozofocin	Pneumonitis by the concurrent use is reported.
	Adiramycin	Adiramycin induced cardiotoxicity is potentiated.
	Nitrosourea, doxorubicine	Enhancement of pulmonary damage.
Mitozatrone	5-Flurouracil, vincristin, dacarbazine, methotrexate	Synergistic affect.
Mustin HCl	Other mytotoxic and bone marrow suppressive drugs	Severe myelosuppression.
Procarbazine	CNS depressants or antihypertensives	The effectiveness may be increased by the concurrent use.
	Mustiline (Mechlorethamine, Nitrogen mustard)	Neurological toxicity may develop by the concurrent use.
	Tyramine-containing food and sympathomimetic amines	Itching skin reaction is reported by the concurrent use.
Streptozocin	Phenytoin	Concurrent use may reduce and even abolish the effectiveness.
Tamoxifen	Warfarin	Warfarin enhanced fatal results.
	Aminoglutethimide	Plasma Tamoxifen concentration reduced.
Vinblastin	Bleomycin, Cisplatin	Cardiovascular toxicity is reported.
Vinca alkaloids	Mitomycin	Pulmonary toxicity of mitomycin may be increased.
Vincristine	Colaspase, Isaoniazid and Pyridoxine	Concurrent use may increase the vincristine neurotoxicity.
	Mytomycin C	Acute Bronchospasm.
	Other myelosuppressive Drugs	Potentiation.
	Digoxin	Serum digoxin level decreased.
	Methotrexate	Synergistic effect.

Digitalis glycosides

DRUGS	Interaction with	Effects
Digitalis glycosides	ACE inhibitors	Serum levels may be raised up to 20-25% by the concurrent use. Enalapril, lisinopril and ramipril appear not to interact.
	Amiloride	Amiloride may reduce the contractibility of heart by concurrent use.
	Aminoglutethimide	Concurrent use may increase the clearance of digitoxin.
	Aminosalicylic acid (PAS)	Concurrent use may reduce the blood levels of digitoxin.
	(Para)- Aminosalicylic acid (PAS)	No certain and important information is reported.
	Amiodarone	Concurrent use may make double the blood levels of digoxin. Dosage reduction is necessary to avoid digitalis intoxication.
	Amphotericin	Digitalis toxicity is reported.
	Antacids	Antacids may reduce the bioavailability of digoxin. A gap by 1-2 hr. may be advised to avoid admixture in the gut.
	Azapropazone	Very occational small rise in blood level is reported.
	Barbiturates	Effectiveness is expected to be reduced by the concurrent use.
	Benzodiazepines	Digoxin intoxication and reduction in the urinary clearance is reported by the concurrent use.
	Beta-blockers	Concurrent use may cause bradycardia by the concurrent use.
	Clacium channel blockers	May rise the serum levels so dosage reduction is required.
	Calcium preparations	The concurrent use may enhance the effectiveness of digitalis and life threatening heart-arrhythmias may occur if intravenous calcium is administered.
	Carbamazepine	Bradycardia is reported by the concurrent use.
	Carbenoxolone	Carbenoxolone may raise blood pressure, disturb sodium-potassium level which may leads to congestive heart-failure.
	Cholestyramine	Reduction in serum levels for both are reported.
	Cimetidine	Rise raise or fall in serum levels are reported.
	Cisapride	May cause very small and clinically unimportant change in absorption.
	Colestipol	No interference in the absorption is reported.
	Cylosporin (e)	Kidney dysfunction and increased serum levels are reported by concurrent use.

DRUGS	Interaction with	Effects
	Cytotoxic (Antineoplastic) agents	Concurrent use may increase the absorption if digoxin is provided in fatal form.
	Dietary fibre (Bran) and laxatives	Dietary fibre in large amount and bulk-forming laxatives containing isphagula may have a significant effects on the absorption from the gut.
	Diltiazam	20-85% increase in the serum levels is reported by the concurrent use.
	Diuretics, potassium depleting agent	May cause increased digitalis toxicity.
	Edrophonium	Bradycardin and AV-block may occur by concurrent use.
	Enoximone	No change in serum level reported.
	Erythromycin, Tetracycline or other antibiotics	10% patients treated with erythromycin may show increment in serum level to double leading to digitalis intoxication.
	Enoldopam	Very small and unimportant change in serum levels is reported.
	Guanethidine and related drugs	No change in the effects is reported.
	Hydroxychloroquine and chloroquine	70% increment in the serum levels is reported.
	Ibuprofen	Concurrent use may increase the serum levels by the concurrent use.
	Indomethacin	Serum levels may be increased up to 40% by the concurrent use. Dosage reduction is required to avoid intoxication.
	Kaolin-Pectin	Serum levels may be reduced. Taking dosage by 2 hr apart is advised to avoid interaction.
	Methyldopa	Bradycardia is reported by the concurrent use.
	Metoclopramide	Metoclopramide interferes with absorption of solid dosage forms of digitalis glycosides.

Hypoglycaemic agents

DRUGS	Interaction with	Effects
Hypoglycaemic agents	ACE inhibitor	Concurrent use is reported to be uneventful.
	Alcohol	Delayed hypoglycaemia may occur if one drinks beyond moderation and accompanied by food.
	Allopurinol	Increment in the half life of chlorpropamide and decrease of tolbutamide is reported by the concurrent use.
	Amiloride	Hyperkalaemia may occur by the concurrent use.
	Anabolic steroids	The effects of the insulin may be reduced by the concurrent use.

DRUGS	Interaction with	Effects
	Anaesthetics	Extreme adverse effects is not reported. However for extensive surgical procedure, a change from oral antidiabetic treatment is advisable.
	Anticoagulants	Increased hypoglycaemia and anticoagulants effects is reported by the concurrent use of dicoumarol and tolbutamide.
	Azapropazone	Severe hypoglycaemia is reported by the concurrent use.
	Beta-blockers	Hypoglycaemia may occur and increased sweating is reported by the concurrent use.
	Calcium channel blockers	Calcium channel blockers are reported to have effects on insulin secretion and glucose regulation.
	Chloramphenicol	Concurrent use is reported to have increased hypoglycaemia.
	Chlorpromazine	Blood sugar may be increased by chlorpromazine and hence the dose of hypoglycaemic agent is required to be increased.
	Cimetidine or Ranitidine	Cimetidine or ranitidine may increase the effects of glipizile, gliclazide.
	Clofibrate	The effectiveness may be increased by clofibrate.
	Clonidine	May suppress the sign of hypoglycaemia in patients.
	Contraceptives (oral)	Oral contraceptives are reported to cause the dose of hypoglycaemic agents to be increased or decreased.
	Corticosteroids	The effects are opposed by corticosteroids.
	Cytotoxics	Control of diabetics may be severely disturbed by the concurrent use.
	Ethacrynic acid	May oppose the effects of hypoglycaemic action.
	Fenfluramine	May increase the effects.
	Frusemide	Increment in blood sugar.
	Guanethidine and related drugs	Increment in hypoglycaemic action is reported.
	Halofenate	May cause enhance blood sugar and lowering effects of chlorpropramide, tolbutamide tolazamide and phenformin.
	Heparin	Hypoglycaemia is reported by the concurrent use.

DRUGS	Interaction with	Effects
	Isoniazid	Raise of blood sugar by concurrent use.
	Lithium carbonate	May rise blood sugar by concurrent use.
	Methylsergide	The effectiveness of tolbutamide may be increased by the concurrent use.
	Miconazole	Hypoglycaemia is reported by the concurrent use.
	Monoamine oxidase inhibitors (MAOI)	Concurrent use may enhance the effectiveness.
	Non-steroidal antiinflammatory drugs (NSAID's)	Severe hypoglycaemia is reported when fenclofenac is given with chlorpropamide and metformin. Ibuprofen may increase the effects of glipizide.
	Phenylbutazone	Phenylbutazone may increase the effectiveness.
	Phenylephrine	Elevated blood pressure is reported by the concurrent use.
	Phenyramidol	The effects may be increased.
	Probenecid	Clearance from the body may be prolonged.
	Quinine or Quinidine	Severe hypoglycaemia is reported by the concurrent use.
	Rifampicin	Rifampicin may reduce the serum levels by concurrent use.
Hypoglycaemic agents	Salicylates	Aspirin and other salicylates may reduce the blood sugar.
	Sugar-containing pharmaceuticals	Liquid antibiotics, cough linctuses, bulk laxatives may cause additional diabetic problems.
	Sulphin pyrazone	Severe hypoglycaemia may occur by concurrent use.
	Sulphonamides	Effects may be increased.
	Tetracyclines	Oxytetracycline may enhance the effects which is also similar with doxycycline.
	Thiazides, chlorthalidone or related diuretics	May reduce the effects of hypoglycaemic agents and hyponatraemia is also reported.
	Tobacco smoking	Smikers requires more insulin.
	Tricyclic antidepressants	Hypoglycaemia is reported.
	Urinary alkalinizers and acidifiers	The effects of chlorpropamide is decreased if urine is made alkaline and increased if urine is acidified but no adverse interaction is reported.

Immunosupressant agents

DRUGS	Interaction with	Effects
Corticosteroids	Aminoglutethimide	The effects of dexamethasone may be reduced and even abolished by the concurrent use.
	Antacids	The absorption may be reduced by large.
	Anti-infective agents	Corticosteroids generally suppress the normal potential of the body to attack by micro organism, it is required to make sure that anti-infective agent is capable to prevent the threat of potential infection.
	Barbiturates	Concurrent use may decrease the effects by concurrent use and hence corticosteroids dosage may require to be increased.
	Caffeine	Falsified information may be provided.
	Carbamazepine	The loss from the body may be increased by concurrent use.
	Carbimazole or Methimazole	The loss of prednisolone from the body may be increased. Hence its dosage is required to be increased.
	Cimetidine or Ranitidine	Cimetidine or Ranitidine appears not to interact.
	Contraceptives (Oral)	Oral contraceptives may increase the serum levels by concurrent use.
	Diuretics, Potassium losing	Concurrent use may cause excessive loss of potassium from the body which may lead to depletion. So, intake of potassium should be increased to balance the loss.
	Ephedrine	Dexamethasone loss from the body is enhanced by ephedrine while other does not interact.
	Ketoconazole	May reduce the absorption by concurrent use.
	Macrolide	May show higher toxic effects.
	Non-steroidal antiinflammatory drugs (NSAID's)	Gastrointestinal bleeding and ulceration may occur by concurrent use.
	Phenytoin	The effects may be reduced by concurrent use.
	Primidone	The effectiveness may be reduced by primidone by concurrent use.
	Rifampicin (Rifampin)	Rifampicin may reduce the effects by concurrent use.
	Live vaccines	Life threatening infections may occur by concurrent use.
Cyclosporins	Aminoglycosides antibiotics	Kidney toxicity may be enhanced by concurrent use.

DRUGS	Interaction with	Effects
	Amphotericine B	Kidney toxicity may be enhanced by concurrent use.
	Anticoagulants	May increase the need of higher dose of the both by concurrent use.
	Anticonvulsants	Serum levels may be reduced by concurrent use and 2-3 folds increase in the dosage may be needed.
	Calcium channel blockers	Cyclosporin serum levels may be enhanced.
Cyclosporin	Cholestyramin and food	Absorption may be affected by concurrent use.
	Corticosteroids	Convulsion is reported by the concurrent use.
	Diuretics	Concurrent use may cause nephrotoxicity.
	Etoposide	May be effective in the leukaemia treatment but severe side effect is reported.
	Fluconazole, Itraconazole, Ketoconazole	5-10 fold rise in serum level may occur if ketoconazole is used concurrently. A small rise is observed with other two.
	Macrolide and related antibiotics	Marked rise in serum levels is reported by the concurrent use leading to cyclosporin toxicity. Dosage reduction is required.
	Metoclopramide	May increase the absorption increasing the serum levels.
	Non-steroidal antiinflammatory drugs (NSAID's)	Nephrotoxicity is reported by the concurrent use.
	Octreolide	Sharp fall in serum levels is reported.
	Probucol	Serum level reduction is reported.
Cyclosporine	Rifampicin	Sharp and marked fall in serum level is reported if dosage is increased by 2-3 folds.
	Sex hormones and related drugs	Hepatotoxicity is reported when used with oral contraceptives.
Cyclosporin	Sulphonamides, trimethoprin or Cotrimoxazole	Renal disfunction is reported by concurrent use. Drastic fall in serum level may on when both given intravenously.
	Vaccines	May cause immunity deficiency when given with influenza vaccine.

Lithium Drug Interaction

Drugs	Interaction with	Effects
Lithium carbonate	ACE inhibitors	Lithium toxicity is reported by the concurrent use.
	Acetazolamide, Chlormerodrin, Spironolactone, Triamterene	Excretion of may be increased by triamterene and acetazolamide. Lithium intoxication is also reported.
	Baclofen	Huntington's chorea showed aggregation by the concurrent use.
	Calcium channel blockers	Increase in the effects, lithium intoxication and decrease in serum levels is reported. Bradycardia is also reported.
	Carbamazepine	Neurotoxicity is reported by the concurrent use.
	Cisplantin	Fall in serum levels with no clinical importance is reported.
	Co-trimoxazole	Lithium intoxication is reported by concurrent use.
	Diazepam	Hypothermis may develop by the concurrent use.
	Fluoxetine	Lithium toxicity is reported by concurrent use.
	Frusemide or Bumetamide	Although concurrent use is reported to be safe, but serious lithium intoxication is also reported.
	Haloperidol	Adverse reaction is reported by the concurrent use.
	Iodides	Additional hypothyroidic and goitrogenic effects is reported.
	Isphagula husk	Reduced serum level is reported by the concurrent use.
	Low sodium diet	Can increase tubular reabsorption of lithium and cause increased toxicity.
	Mazindol	Lithium intoxication is reported by the concurrent use.
	Methyldopa	Lithium intoxication is reported by the concurrent use.
	Metronidazole	Concurrent use reports rise in serum levels.
	Non-steroidal antiinflammatory drugs (NSAID's)	60% rise in serum levels is reported with clometacin and Indomethacin whereas around 15-34% rise with diclofenac and ibuprofen is reported.
	Phenytoin	Concurrent use may cause lithium intoxication.
	Sodium chloride or bicarbonate	May rise the serum levels and ingesion of sodium may prevent the maintenance of lithium serum levels.
	Spectinomycin	Concurrent use may cause intoxication.
	Tetracycline	Lithium intoxication is reported by concurrent use.
	Theophylline	Reduced serum level by 20-30% is reported by the concurrent use.
	Thiazides or related diuretics	Serum levels may be increased leading to lithium intoxication.

Monoamine oxidase inhibitor

Drugs	Interaction with	Effects
Monoamine oxidase inhibitor	Amantadine	An isolated report describes a rise in blood pressure in a patient on amantadine when given phenelzine.
	Barbiturates	Generally MAOI can enhance and prolong the activity of the barbiturates but a few isolated report describes an interaction in man.
	Benzodiazepines	Concurrent use may cause adverse effects like oedema, chorea.
	Chloral hydrate	Fatal hyperpyexia is reported by the concurrent use.
	Cyproheptadine	Hallucination is reported by the concurrent use.
	Dextropmethorphan	Hyperpyrexia may be occurred by the concurrent use.
	Dextropropoxyphene	Increament in the sedative effect is reported by the concurrent use.
	Fenfluramine	Concurrent use is effective.
	Ginseng	Adverse effects are reported by the concurrent use.
	Mazindol	Increase in the blood level is reported by the concurrent use.
	Methyldopa	Delayed development of hallucinosis is reported. The order of administration is reported to be important.
	Monoamine oxidase inhibitor	Stroke and hypertensive reaction is reported by the concurrent use.
	Morphine or Methadone	Hypotension is reported although very rare.
	Oxtriphylline	Tachycardia and apprehension may be occurred by concurrent administration.
	Phenothiazine	Fatal reaction with methotrimeprazine is reported.
	Rauwolfia alkaloids or tetrabenazine	Central association with hypertension may occur if MAOI is administered first.
	Sulphonamides	Weakness, ataxia and other adverse effects may occur by concurrent use.
	Tricyclic antidepressants	Concurrent use is contraindicacious. However extreme careful monitoring may bring advantageous result.
	L – tryptophan	Neurological sign of toxicity is reported by concurrent use.

Neuroleptic, Anxiolytic and Tranquilizing drugs

Drugs	Interaction with	Effects
Benzodiazepines	Antacids	The absorption may be delayed by concurrent use with antacids.
	Beta-blockers	Patients on diazepam may be more accident prone while taking beta-blockers.
	Cimetidine, Ranitidine, Famotidine, Nizatidine	Except cimetidine, no interaction is reported with others. Serum levels may be raised by cimetidine. Dose of alprazolam should be reduced to 1/3 rd when administered concurrently with cimetidine.
	Contraceptives, Oral	Oral contraceptives may raise the effectiveness of alprazolam, chlordiazepoxide diazepam, nitrazepam & triazolam but reduction in effects of oxazepam, lorazepam and temazepam are reported.
Benzodiazepines	Desipramide	Alprazolam enhances the activity of desipramide.
	Dextropropoxyphene	Serum levels may be raised by concurrent use.
	Disulfiram	Serum levels may be increased leading to drowsiness is reported.
	Ethambutol	No interaction is reported by the concurrent use.
	Imipramine	Alprazolam enhances the activity of imipramine.
	Indomethacin	No adverse effects is reported except increament in the filling of dizziness.
	Isoniazid	Reduces the loss from the body. Increase in the effect of diazepam & triazolam is expected. No interaction is reported with oxazepam or clotiazepam.
	Lithium	May produce hypothermia in case of diazepam.
	Macrolide antibiotics	Erythromycin, triacetyloleandomycin and Josamycin may alter the serum level to higher side. Hence dosage reduction may be necessary.
	MAOIs	Potentiate action of diazepam and lorazepam.
	Omeprazole	Clearance from the body may be delayed. Prolongation of clobazam action is reported.
	Probenecids	May reduce the loss from the body thus higher sedative effects may be expected.
	Rifampicin (Rifampin)	May cause marked increase in the loss from the body.

Drugs	Interaction with	Effects
	Theophylline and caffeine	Caffeine may reduce the sedative effects.
	Tobacco smoking	Smokers may require larger doses than the non-smokers.
	Valproate	May increase plasma clobazam concentration.
Buspirone	Fluoxetine	Concurrent use may reduce the effects of buspirone.
Droperidol/Hyoscine	Mnoamine oxidase inhibitors (MAOI)	Hypotension is reported by concurrent use.
Haloperidol	Alcohol	CNS depressant effects enhanced.
	Antituberculars	The serum levels of haloperidol may be reduced by concurrent use.
Haloperidol	Carbamazepine	Neurotoxicity is reported during concurrent use. Reduce plasma concentration.
	Fluoxetine	Development of extrapyramidal symptoms is reported by concurrent use.
	Guanethidine	Guanethidine effect may be decreased.
	Lithium	Increases lithium blood levels and may predispose to neuroleptic malignant syndrome.
	Metoclopramide	Adverse effect may be increased.
	Indomethacin	Confusion and drowsiness is reported by concurrent use.
	Rifampicin	Plasma concentration may be reduced by concurrent administration.
	Tobacco smoking	Smokers require more doses than nonsmokers.
	Tricyclic antidepressants	Increases adverse effects of tricyclic antidepressants.
Hydroxyzine	Alcohol	Potentiates CNS depression.
	Barbiturates	Potentiates CNS depression.
	Opoid analgesic	Potentiates CNS depression.
	Monoamine oxidase	Potentiates antimuscarinic effects.
	Atropine	Potentiates antimuscarinic effects.
	Tricyclic antidepressants	Potentiates antimuscarinic effects.
	Aminophylline	Incompatibility with hydroxyzine.
	Chloramphenicol	Incompatibility with hydroxyzine.
	Benzylpenicillin	Incompatibility with hydroxyzine.
	Miscellaneous drugs	High dose of hydroxyzine may cause ECG abnormalities.
Neuroleptics (Butyrophenones, Phenothiazines, Thioxanthenes)	Anticholinergics	Mainly uneventful but occasional life-threatening reaction may occur.
	Bromocriptine	Concurrent use though mainly successful but re-emergence of schizophrenic symptoms is also reported.

Drugs	Interaction with	Effects
Phenothiazines	Antacids	Antacids may reduce the serum levels.
	Antimalarials	Serum levels of phenothiazines may be enhanced.
	Ascorbic acid	Serum levels may be reduced is reported by concurrent use.
	Attapulgib	Fall in absorption is reported.
	Barbiturates	Presence of one reduces the other in serum levels.
	Cimetidine	Serum levels may be reduced by a third by concurrent use.
	Disulfiram	Re-emergence of psychotic symptoms is reported by concurrent use.
	Lithium carbonate	Extra-pyramidal side effects or neurotoxicity has been reported by the concurrent use.
	Naltrexone	Lethargy occurrence is reported by the concurrent use.
	Phebnylpropanolamine	Concurrent use may cause ventricular fibrillation.
	Tricyclic antidepressants	Mutual interaction is reported which causes rise in the serum levels of both drugs.
Sulpiride	Antacids or sucralfate	The absorption of sulpiride may be reduced by concurrent use.
Tetrabenazine	Chlorpromazine	Parkinson – like symptoms are reported by concurrent use.
	Haloperide	Can cause severe dopamine deficiency.
	Metoclopramide	Can cause severe dopamine deficiency.
Zolpidem	Alcohol	Enhances sedative action.
	Rifimpcin	Significantly reduces the plasma concentration and effect of zolpidem.
	Haloperidol	The effectiveness of haloperidol may be increased.
	Smoking	Heavy smoking may also reduces the effects.

Neuromuscular blocker & anaesthetic drugs

Drugs	Interaction with	Effects
Anaesthetics	Adrenaline, Noradrenaline and Terbutaline	Heart arrhythmias may develop by concurrent use unless control of dosage is not monitored.
	Alcohol	Who regularly drinks require higher dosage than those who don't drink.
	Anaesthetics	Myoclonic Seizures is reported by concurrent use.
	Antibiotics	The effectiveness may be increased by the concurrent use with aminoglycoside antibiotics.
	Antihypertensives	The normal homeostatic response of the cardiovascular system may be impaired.

Drugs	Interaction with	Effects
Anaesthetics	Beta – blockers	Concurrent use appears to be safe excepting methoxyflurane, cyclopropane, diethyl-ether, trichloroehylene.
	Calcium channel blockers	Impaired myocardial conduction is reported by concurrent use.
	Fenfluramine	Cardiac arrest of fatal nature is attributed by concurrent use.
	Monoamine oxidase inhibitors	MAOI should be withdrawn well before anaesthesia is generally advised. In most cases it seems unnecessary. Though hypo and hypertension is reported by the concurrent use.
	Neuromuscular blockers	Nitrous oxide is reported to be noninteractive. Others inhalation anaesthetics may increase neuromuscular blockers.
	Phyrnylephrine	Phenylephrine eye drops may cause cyanosis and brady cardia.
Anaethetics (Metroxyflurane)	Phenytoin or phenobarbitone	Phenytoin intoxication, hepatic necrosis are reported by concurrent use.
Anaesthetics and/or Neuromuscular blockers	Theophylline	Cardiac arrhythmias is reported by concurrent use.
	Tricyclic antidepressants	Tachyarrhythmias has been reported by concurrent use.
Anaesthetics (Local)	Alcohol and antirheumatics	Person who receives anti-rheumatic drugs and drinks may practice increased chances of failure rate of spinal anaesthesia.
	Anaesthetics (local)	Normally combined use is safe. However increased toxicity is supposed to be occured.
	Benzodiazepines	Conflicting evidence is reported about wheather diazepam can increase or decrease the concentration in the serum levels.
	Beta-blockers	Propanolol reduced the clearance of bupivacaine.
Neuromuscular blockers and/or anaesthetics	Cimetidine or Ranitidine	Both cimetidine and ranitidine are reported to raise bupivacaine levels.
	Aminoglycoside antibiotics	Having neuromuscular blocking activity, aminoglycoside antibiotics should be appropriately measured to accommodate the increased neuromuscular blockade and prolonged fatal respiratory depression.
Neuromuscular blockers	Aprotinin	Apnoea is reported by concurrent use.
	Benzodiazepines	The effectiveness of neuromuscular blockers may be enhanced.
	Beta-blockers	Bradycardia and hypotension is reported. May increase or decrease in the extent of neurovascular blockade.
	Calcium channel blocker	Increased and prolonged neurovascular blockade is reported by the concurrent use.

Drugs	Interaction with	Effects
	Carbamazepine	Carbamazepine reduces the time of recovery from neurovascular blockade.
	Cimetidine or Ranitidine	Ranitidine appears not to interact. Cimetidine however enhance the recovery time from neurovascular blockade.
	Cyclophosphamide	The effects may be enhanced and prolonged by concurrent use with cyclophosphamide.
	Cyclosporine	The effectiveness may be increased by concurrent use.
	Dantrolene	The muscle relaxant effects of dantrolene can be additive.
	Dexpanthenol	The effects may be increased by concurrent use.
	Ecothiopate iodide	The effects may be increased and prolonged.
	Fentanyl citrate-droperidol (innovar)	The effects may be prolonged by concurrent use.
	Frusemide	Lower doses of frusemide increases the effects, higher doses oppose the effectiveness.
	Immunosupresants	The effects may be reduced even by 2 - 4 folds by concurrent use.
	Insecticides	The neuromuscular blocking effects may be enhanced.
	Lignocaine, procaine or procainamide	The effectiveness may be enhanced and prolonged by concurrent use.
	Lithium carbonate	Normally safe. However prolonged blockade and respiratory difficulties are also reported.
	Magnesium salts	The effects may be increased and prolonged by concurrent use.
	Metoclopramide	Increament and prolongation in the effects is reported by concurrent use.
	Miscellaneous antibiotics	Antibiotics having neuromuscular blocking activity should be appropriately measured to accommodate increased blockade. Metronidazole, Chloramphenicol, Penicillin are reported not to interact.
	Monoamine oxidase inhibitor	Concurrent use may enhance the effectiveness.
Neuromuscular blockers & anaesthetics	Morphine	Hypertension and tachycardia are reported by concurrent use.
	Phenytoin	Phenytoin may reduce the effects of most drugs except tubocurarine where the effect is minimum and atracurium with no interaction.
	Promazine	Apnoea is reported by concurrent use.
Neuromuscular blockers	Quinidine	Quinidine may enhance the effects of both depolarizing and nondepolarizing type. Recurarization and apnoea are reported.
	Quinine	Recurarization and apnoea are reported by concurrent use.

Drugs	Interaction with	Effects
	Testosteron	Interference to the effects is reported.
	Thiotepa	Increament of effects are expected.
	Trimetaphan	The effects may be enhanced to prolonged apnoea.

Sympathomimetic Drug

Drugs	Interaction with	Effects
Amphetamines and related drugs	Chlorpromazine	The effects of both are opposed by one another.
Amphetamines	Lithium Carbonate	The effects are likely to be opposed by lithium carbonate.
	Nasal decongestants	Antagonism of l-amphetamine is reported.
	Urinary acidifiers or alkalinizers	Acidifiers increases the loss in the urine while it is reported being reduced by alkalinizers.
Directly acting sympathomimetics	Beta-blockers	Life-threatening hypertensive reaction resulting due to increament in the pressure effects of adrenalin may lead to bradycardia. Anaphylaxis is reported to be enhanced by concurrent use.
Directly or indirectly acting sympathomimetic amines	Furazolidone	Concurrent use may raise the blood pressure seriously.
Directly acting sympathomimetics	Guanethidine and related drugs	The pressure effects may be increased even by 2-4 folds by concurrent use.
	Mianserin or Trazodone	Generally no adverse effect is found. However toxicity on trazodone by pseudoephedrine is reported.
	Monoamine oxidase inhibitor (MAOI)	Moderate increment in the effects is reported.
Directly and indirectly acting sympathomimetics	Rauwolfia alkaloids	Slight increment in the effects is reported by rauwolfia alkaloids. The effects of indirectly acting or mixed activity may be even abolished.
Directly acting sympathomimetic amines	Tricyclic antidepressants	Hypertension, cardiac arrhythmias are reported to injection of noradrenalin and to a lesser extent to phenylephrine.
Dopamine	Ergometrine	Development of gangrene is reported by concurrent use.
	Phenytoin	Serious hypotension is reported by concurrent use.
Indirectly acting sympathomimetic amines	Methyldopa	No serious interaction is reported. Methyldopa however may depress the effects.
	Monoamine oxidase inhibitor (MAOI)	Hypertensive abnormalities and cricis is reported by concurrent use.

Drugs	Interaction with	Effects
3, 4, – methylene-dioxymethamphetamine (MDMA)	Monoamine oxidase inhibitor (MAOI)	Hypertoxicity, altered mental status are reported by concurrent use.
Phenylpropanolamine	Indomethacin	Concurrent use of a single dose of indomethacin reported to develop serious hypertension.
Phenylephrine	Monoamine oxidase inhibitor (MAOI)	Concurrent use may lead to even life-threatening crisis.

Theophylline and related xanthine drug interactions

DRUGS	Interaction with	Effects
Theophylline	Allopurinol	Concurrent use may enhance the effects of theophylline.
	Aminoglutethimide	Theophylline loss from the body may be increased.
	Barbiturates	Theophylline serum level can be reduced.
	BCG vaccine	The theophylline serum levels may be increased by small extent.
	Beta-antagonist bronchodilators	No adverse interaction is reported. Due to side effect, hypokalaemia may occur.
	Beta-blockers	Bronchospasm may occur by concurrent use.
	Ephedrine	Chronic concurrent treatment increases adverse effects.
	Sympathomimetics	Cardiac arrhythmias (especially with preexsisting cardiac disease) may develop with concurrent use.
	Pancuronium	Trachycardia may develop with concurrent use.
	Cimetidine	Inhibition of metabolism is found with concurrent use.
	Propanolol	Inhibition of metabolism is found with concurrent use.
	Halothan	Potentiate cardiac arrythmias.
	Erythromycin	Reduce clearance.
	Phenobarbitone	Induces metabolism & clearance.
	Phenytoin	Induces metabolism & clearance.
	Rifampicin	Induces metabolism & clearance.
	Sulphinpyrazone	Enhances clearance.
Caffeine	Cimetidine	The stimulant effects of caffeine is increased by concurrent use.
	Oral contraceptives	The effects of caffeine may be enhanced by concurrent use.
	Disulfirum	The caffeine loss from the body may be reduced complicating the withdrawal from alcohol is reported.
	Idrocilamide	Retention time of caffeine in the body may be increased, resulting intoxication which may leads to insomnia, nervousness, anxious agitation.

DRUGS	Interaction with	Effects
Theophylline	Methoxsalen	Loss of caffeine from the body may be reduced thus increases the possibility of caffeine intoxication.
	Mexiletine	30-60% reduction in caffeine clearence from the body is reported by concurrent use.
	Quinolone antibiotics	Enoxacin and pipemidic acid may increase the blood levels.
Theophylline	Erythromycin	Reduces clearance.
	Food	The bioavailability of theophylline from many preparation may be increased or decreased.
	Frusemide	Potentiate cardiac arrythmias.
	Halothane	Frusemide may increase, decrease or may be noninteractive.
	Idrocalamide	Theophylline levels may be increased.
	Influenza vaccine	Toxicity is reported in few patients by concurrent use.
	Interferon	Interferon reduces the clearance of theophylline from the body.
	Isoniazid	Concurrent use may increase the theophylline serum levels.
	Ketoconazole	May reduce theophylline levels in asthmatics.
	Macrolide antibiotics	Triacetylolcandomycin may raise theophylline serum levels.
	Mexilatine	Increased theophylline level and intoxication is reported.
Theophylline & related drugs	Probenecid	Serum theophylline level remain unaltered but diprophylline and enprofylline levels can be raised.
	Pyrantel	Increased serum theophylline level is reported.
	Quinolone antibiotics	Enoxacin or ciprofloxacin may raise serum theophylline level markedly. Nonfloxacin, lomefloxacin.
	Quinolone antibiotics	Ofloxacin and pefloxacin may cause to less extent.
	Rifampicin	Serum theophylline levels may be reduced.
	Sucralfate	Absorption of sustained release theophylline is reduced by sucralfate.
Theophylline	Sulphinpyrazone	Serum theophylline levels may be reduced to small extent.
	Tetracycline or cephalosporins	No adverse interaction of clinical importance is reported.
	Thiabendazole	Serum theophylline levels may be significantly increased by concurrent use leading to theophylline intoxication.
	Thyroid & antithyroid compounds	Serum theophylline levels may be increased leading to intoxication.
	Ticlopidine	Clearance of theophylline from the body may be reduced.
	Tobacco smoking	Smokers may require more theophylline dose to obtain the desired effects.

DRUGS	Interaction with	Effects
	Vidarabine	Concurrent use may cause increase in the serum theophylline levels.
	Viloxazine	The serum theophylline levels may be increased by concurrent use leading to theophylline intoxication.

Tricyclic antidepressants & related drug interactions

DRUGS	Interaction with	Effects
Femoxetine	Cimetidine	Concurrent use may raise the femoxetine serum levels by 140%.
	Miscellaneous drugs	No adverse reaction is reported by concurrent use.
	Monoamine oxidase inhibitors (MAOI)	Serious reaction occur with concurrent use.
	Antidepressants	Two-fold increase in plasma levels of other antidepressants when concurrently use with fluoxetine.
	Diazepam	Half life of diazepam is prolonged.
	Warfarin	May cause transient shift in plasma concentration of warfarin resulting in adverse effects.
	Digoxin	May cause transient shift in plasma concentration of digoxin resulting in adverse effects.
Fluoxetine	L – Tryptophan	Concurrent use may cause central & peripheral toxicity.
Mianserin or Nomifensine	Anticonvulsants	Serum levels of both may be reduced by concurrent use.
Tetracyclic antidepressants	Beta-blockers	Maprotiline toxicity is reported by concurrent use.
Trazodone	Phenothiazine	Hypotension is reported by concurrent use.
Tricyclic antidepressants	MAOIs	Dangerous combination. Trazodone should not be given within 2 weeks of discontinuing drug 76 Multiple sclerosis is reported.
	Baclofen	
	Barbiturates	
	Benzodiazepines	The serum levels may be reduced by the concurrent use of barbiturates.
	Cannabis	Drowsiness, forgetfulness are reported by concurrent use.
	Carbamazepine	Tachycardia is reported on smoking cannabis.
		Carbamazepine intoxication is reported by concurrent use.
Tricyclic antidepressants	Cholestyramine	Marked reduction in serum doxepine level is reported.
	Cimetidine or Ranitidine	Serum amitrittyline, desipramine, dexepin, imipramine, nortriptyline levels can be raised by concurrent use.
Tricyclic and related antidepressants	Co-trimoxazole	The symptoms may be relapsed by concurrent use.
Tricyclic antidepressants	Dextropropoxyphene	Increased lethargy and day time sedation is reported.
	Disulfirum	Disulfirum reduces the clearance from the body. The increament in the effects is reported.

DRUGS	Interaction with	Effects
Tricyclic and related antidepressants	Ethchlorvynol	Concurrent use may cause transient delerium.
	Fenfluramine	A confusing situation is reported.
	Fluoxetine	Serum desipramine, imipramine, nortriptyline and trazodone is increased by concurrent use.
Tricyclic antidepressants	Food	No effect in the absorption is reported.
	Furazolidone	Development of toxic psychosis, hyperactivity, sweating is reported by concurrent use.
	Haloperidol	Serum level of tricyclic antidepressants may be increased by concurrent use.
	Methadone	Serum levels may be doubled by methadone.
	Methylphenidate	Clinical improvement may be caused by concurrent use.
Tricyclic antidepressants	Oestrogens (estrogens)/oral contraceptives	The effects of imipramine may be reduced by oestrogens.
	Quinidine	Quinidine may reduce the losses of nortriptyline.
	Sucralfate	Absorption of amitriptyline is reduced by concurrent use.
	Thyroid preparations	Peroxysomal atrial tachycardia, thyrotoxicosis are reported by concurrent use.
	Tobacco smoking	Serum amitriptyline, clomipramine, desipramine, imipramine and nortriptyline levels may be reduced. However free and unbound antidepressants may offset the effects of interaction.

Miscellaneous drug interactions

Drugs	Interaction with	Effects
Acipimox	Cholestyramine	No significant interaction is reported.
Allopurinol	Antacids	Aluminum hydroxide antacid may reduce the effects.
	Iron	No adverse reaction is reported.
	Probenecid	No adverse interaction is reported.
	Tamoxifen	Concurrent use may cause marked enhancement in the effects of allopurinol.
	Thiazides	Renal failure and allergic reactions are attributed by concurrent use.
Anistreptase (APSAC)	Streptokinase	The effects of streptokinase may be reduced or even abolished.
Anticholinesterases	Miscellaneous drugs	Acetazolamide may oppose the actions. Dipuridamole, procainamide and quinidines also appear to oppose the action of drug used for myasthenia.
Antihistamines	Contraceptives, oral	No adverse reaction is reported.
Baclofen	Ibuprofen	Baclofen intoxication is reported by concurrent use.

Drugs	Interaction with	Effects
Benzbromarone	Miscellaneous drugs	No confirmed interaction is reported.
Bismuth sublitrate	Miscellaneous drugs	Large amount of milk, antacids and food may reduce the effects.
Calcium &Vitamin D	Diuretics	Excessive serum calcium and Vitamin D levels may develop & urinary excretion of calcium can be reduced.
Cannabis	Disulfirum	Hypomanic-like reaction is reported by concurrent use.
Carbenoxolone	Antacids	The effectiveness may be reduced by antacids.
	Antihypertensives and diuretics	Carbenoxolone may cause flide retension and BP may be raised. Hypokalaemia is reported by the concurrent use of thiazide and carbenoxolone.
	Chlorpromide, Tolbutam ide, Phenytoin, Warfarin.	Only chlorpromide is reported to cause a small reduction in serum carbenoxolone levels.
Charcoal	Other drugs	Charcoal may absorps drugs into its surface and thus reduce the availability of drugs for absorption by gut.
Chlormethiazole (clomethiazole)	Cimetidine or Ranitidine	Ranitidine appears not to interact while cimetidine is reported to cause increament of the effectiveness.
Cholestyramine	Spironolactone	Concurrent use may cause hyperchloraimic metabolic acidosis.
Cisapride	Miscellaneous drugs	Cisapride may increase the rate of absorption of diazepam and alcohol.
Clofibrate	Cholestyramine	No sigficant interaction is reported.
	Contraceptives, oral	Oral contraceptives may raise the serum cholesterol and triglyceride.
	Probenecids	Probenecids may increase the serum clofibrate levels to double.
CNS depressants	CNS depressants	Life threatening consequences may be occurred by concurrent use.
Colestipol	Clofibrate or fenofibrate	No adverse interaction is reported.
	Miscellaneous drugs	No interaction with aspirin or methyldopa. Interaction is reported in insulin-treated diabetics but is inert to those treated with phenformine and sulphonylurea.
Dimethicone	Cimetidine or doxycyclin	The bioavailability remains unaffected by dimethicone.
Dinoprostone (Prostaglandin E2)	Oxytocin	Uterine hypertonus is reported by concurrent use.
Enteral tube feeding	Antacids	Obstruction plug is reported with aluminium containing antacids.

Drugs	Interaction with	Effects
Ergot	Glyceryl trinitrate (GTN)	Ergot is reported to oppose the effects of glyceryl trinitrate.
	Macrolide antibiotics	Ergot toxicity is reported by concurrent use with erythromycin or triacetyloleandomycin. No interaction occurs with midecanycin or spiramycin.
	Tetracyclins	Ergotism is reported by concurrent use.
Ethylenedibromide	Disulfirum	Concurrent use may cause malignant tumours in man so it is advised to avoid such use.
Famotidine, Nizatidine, Roxatidine	Other drugs	No adverse effect of clinical importance is reported.
Fenfluramine	Mazindol	Cardiomyopathy is reported by concurrent use.
Folic acid	Sulphasalazine	Absorption of folic acid may be reduced by concurrent use.
Gemfibrosil	Colestipol	Gemfibrozil absorption may be reduced.
	Ispaghula (Psyllium)	No important interaction is reported.
	Rifampicin	No interaction is reported.
Glucagon	Beta-blocker	The effects of glucagon may be reduced.
Glyceryl trinitrate (GTN)	Anticholinergics	Patients having such drugs reported to have dry mouth.
Glyceryl trinitrate (GTN)	Aspirin	GTN serum levels may be enhanced resulting side-effects like hypotension and headaches.
H₂ Blockers	Antacids	The absorption of cimetidine, ranitidine and famotidine may be reduced by antacids.
	Sucralfate	The healing rate may be increased by concurrent use.
	Tobacco smoking	Healing rate is less in smokers.
Iron preparations	Antacids	The absorption of iron may be reduced by concurrent use.
Iron or Vitamin B₁₂	Chloramphenicol	Fatal bone marrow depression, reversible depression are reported.
Iron preparation	Cholestyramine	Absorption may be reduced.
	Tea	No alteration in the absorption is reported.
Liquorice	Other drugs	Pseudoaldosteronism is reported by concurrent use.
Loperamide	Cholestyramine	The effectiveness of loperanide may be reduced.
Methoxalen	Phenytoin	Phenytoin may reduce the serum methoxsalen levels.
Metyrapone	Phenytoin	The effects of metyrapone may be reduced.

Drugs	Interaction with	Effects
Oxygen (Hyperberic)	Acetazolamide, Barbiturates, Narcotics	Oxygen-induced convulsions is reported.
Paraldehyde	Disulfiram	To get rid of toxicity, concurrent use should be avoided.
Piperine	Miscellaneous drugs	Bioavailability of phenytoin and other drugs are increased.
Pirenzepine	Cimetidine	Pirenzepine increases the cimetidine-induced reduction in gastric acid secretion.
Pravestatin	Miscellaneous drugs	Bioavailability of pravestatin is reduced. No interaction with warfarin.
Retinoids	Tetracyclins, Vitamin A	Pseudotumour cerebri is reported to develop.
Roxatidine	Antacids and food	No interaction is reported.
Simvastatin	Miscellaneous drugs	No interaction is reported with beta-blockers, calcium antagonists, diuretics or NSAID's.
Sodium polystyrene sulphonate	Antacids	Metabolic alkalosis is reported.
	Sorbitol	Colonic necrosis may occur.
Somatropin (human growth hormone)	Miscellaneous hormones	Somatropin may reduce the effects of insulin and thyroid function.
Sulphinpyrazone	Flufenamic, meclofenamic or mefenamic acid	No adverse interaction is reported.
	Probenecid	Probenecid may reduce the loss in the urine.
Thyroid hormones	Anticonvulsants	Reduction in the effect of thyroxin is reported.
	Barbiturates	Reduction in the effect of thyroxin is reported.
	Cholestyramine	Concurrent use may reduce the absorption of thyroid extract, levothyroxin & triiodothyroxin.
Thyroid hormone	Levastatin	Rise in serum thyroid hormone levels is reported.
	Rifampicin (Rifampin)	The effects of thyroid hormone may be reduced.
Total parenteral nutrition	Potassium sparing diuretics	Metabolic acidosis is reported.
Trimoprostil	Antacids	No adverse interaction is reported.
Vitamin A	Aminoglycoside antibiotics	Absorption of vitamin A is reduced by meomycin.
Vitamin C (ascorbic acid)	Aspirin	The absorption of ascorbic acid is reduced by a third by concurrent use.
Vitamin D	Phenytoin	Osteomalacia is reported.
Vitamin K	Gentamycin and clindamycin	Hypothrombinaemia is reported by concurrent use.
X-ray contrast media	Calcium channel blocker	The effects may be increased by calcium channel blockers. Tachycardia is reported.
	Cholestyramine	Poor radiographic visualization is reported.
	Phenothiazine	Epileptiform reaction are reported by concurrent use.

CHAPTER IV

ADVERSE DRUG REACTIONS (ADRs)

Adverse Drug Reaction can be defined as any unintended, undesirable or unexpected effect of a prescribed medication. According to WHO definition, any noxious, unintended, undesired effect of a drug which occurs at doses used for prophylaxis, diagnosis, or therapy, excluding therapeutic failures, intentional and accidental overdose and drug abuse, and does not include adverse effects due to errors in drug administration.

History behind the Adverse Drug Reaction study : Van doeveren, professor of medicines early example of awareness of adverse drug effect when he gives the academic lecture called *remedio amorbi* in 1789 on diseases caused by treatment. **Meyler**, in his famous book on adverse drug reaction in 1951 "side effect of drugs" focused attention on Van doeveren academic lecture. Systematic attention to adverse drug reaction, including the collection of adverse drug reaction reports, was boosted by the so-called thalidomide disaster in the early 1960s. In 1971 study by **Lely**, who discovered that 19 people died from digitalis intoxication caused by a production error of the digitalis tablets, was another eye opener. Following the thalidomide disaster in early 1960s, the World health Organization set up its international drug-monitoring programme. Since 1978 the programme is being carried out by the **Uppsala monitoring centre** (UMC) in Sweden, which is responsible for the collection of data about adverse reactions from around the world. UMC is engaged in editing, updating and publishing the drug dictionary. It is maintaining and publishing the adverse reaction Terminology (WHO-ART) and carrying out special searches of the database by request. The aim is not to ban any drug as banning a drug also depends on various factors like risk-benefit ratio. UMC is attempting to ensure that the ADRs are minimized and the positive effect of the drugs are enhanced through proper usage.

Historical landmark of Advese Drug Reactions:

In:

1880	Chloroform caused Cardiac arrest.
1922	Organo-Arsenical compounds caused epidemic jaundice and fatal hepatic necrosis.
1946	Streptomycin caused deafness.
1954	Blood dyscrasias was caused by Chloramphenicol.
1961	Thalidomide caused phocomelia.
1970	Practolol caused oculomucocutaneous syndroms.
1975	Clozapine caused agranulocytosis.
1979	Triazolam caused psychosis.
1987	Ofloxacin caused psychosis.
1998	Sildenafil caused stroke, myocardial infarction, cardiac arrest and hypertension.
1993-1999	National surveillance center for ADR reported acute fulminant hepatitis was caused by Nimuselide.
2000	Cisapride caused prolonged the QT interval and caused Torsades De Pointes and ventricular tracycardia and death.
2002	Gatifloxacin induced prolongation of QTc interval leading dangerous arrhythmia, hypoglycemia.
2003	Roficoxib caused cardiac arrhythmia.

Reason for Adverse Drug Reactions:

- Over prescribtion (Polypharmacy)
- Self medicatiom
- Prior history of ADRs
- Failure to setup a therapeutic end point by the physicians
- Difference in Bioavailibility of different brands
- Patient physiological factors like age, sex, diseased colditions like hepatitis or ranal failure
- Genetic predisposition
- Drug interaction (enzyme inducting & inhibiting)

Why should we study Adverse Drug Reaction (ADR)?
We should study the ADR in order to understand the drug reaction in the following cases:

- Any drugs which are administered to patients can cause an ADR
- Peri operatively, multiple agents are administered which may lead to an adverse drug reaction.
- Fatal ADRs may cause death
- 30% of medical inpatients develop an ADR
- 3% of all hospital admissions are due to ADRs
- Risk of an allergic reaction is approximately 1-3% for most administered drugs.

Severity of Adverse drug reaction: On the basis of severity of ADR we can classify ADR under the following type:

Minor: In case of minor ADR no therapy is required, only antidote or prolongation of hospitalization is required.

Moderate: Patients with moderate ADR require changes in drug therapy, specific treatment or prolong hospital stay by at least one day.

Sever: Severe ADR is potentially life threatening which may cause permanent damage or require intensive medical treatment.

Lethal: In case of lethal drug reaction it directly or indirectly contributes to death of the patient

Classification of Adverse Effects: Adverse effects can be classified as Predictable and Unpredictable reactions.

Predictable (Type A or Augmented Reaction): This type of reaction is based on Pharmacological properties of the drug. Qualitatively normal response to the drug includes side effects, toxic effects and consequences of drug withdrawal.

Unpredictable (Type B or Bizarre Reaction): This type of effect is based on peculiarities of the patient and not on drug's known action; including allergy and idosyncrcrasy. They are less common often requiring withdrawal of the drug.

Adverse drug effects may be categorized into:

Categorization	Definition	Examples
Side effects	These are unwanted but often unavoidable Pharmacodynamic effects that occur at therapeutic dose.	Atropin used show anti secretary action
Secondary effects	These are indirect consequences of a primary action of the drug.	Suppression of bacterial flora by tetracyclines paves the way for super infections.
Intolerance	It is the appearance of characteristic toxic effects of drug in an individual at therapeutic dose.	Single dose of Triflupromazine cause muscular dystonias in some individual. Specially in childruns
Idiosyncrasy	It is the abnormal reactivity to a chemical. The drug interacts with some unique feature of individual, not found in majority of subjects and produces the uncharacteristic reaction.	Barbituratus cause excitement & mental confusions in some individuals.

Categorization	Definition	Examples
Drug allergy	It is an immunologicaliy mediated reaction producing stereotype symptoms which are unrelated to the Pharmacodynamic profile of the drug	Itching, Aplastic Anemia, Rashes, Contact Dermatitis.
Photosensitivity	It is a cutaneous reaction resulting from drug induced sensitization of the skin to UV radiation.	Local Tissue damage (Sun burn), like Erythema, Edema.
Drug dependence	It is a state in which use of drug for personal satisfaction is accorded a higher priority than other basic needs, often risks the health.	Amphetamines produce little or no physical dependences.
Withdrawal Reaction	Apart from drugs that are usually recognised as producing dependence, sudden interruption of therapy with certain other drugs also results in adverse consequence, mostly in the form of worsening of the clinical condition for which the drug was being used.	Sever hypertension, restlessness and sympathetic over activity may occur after discontinuation of Clonidine.
Teratogenicity	It refers to capacity of a drug to cause foetal abnormalities when administrated to pregnant women.	Thalidomide disaster

Definitions

Harm

Impairment of the physical, emotional, or psychological function of structure of the body and/or pain resulting there from.

Monitoring

To observe or record relevant physiological or psychological change.

Intervention

May include change in therapy or active medical/surgical treatment.

Intervention necessary to sustain life

Includes cardiovascular and respiratory support (e.g., CPR, defibrillation, intubation etc.)

NCC MERP Index for Categorizing Medication Errors

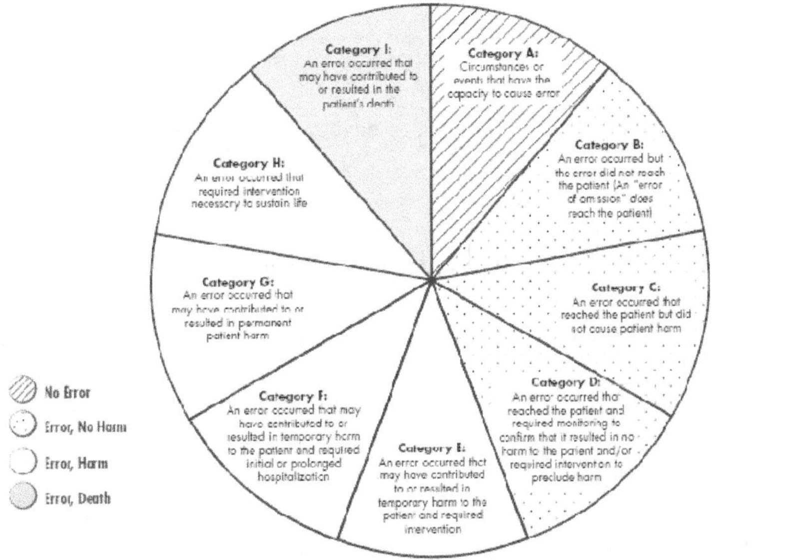

LIST OF DRUGS WITH ADR

Name of Drugs	Adverse Drug Reactions(ADR)
Acebutolol (Adrenergic)	GI upset; pruritus, urticaria, alopoecia, impotence; vertigo, fatigue;
Acetaminophen (Analgesic & antipyretic)	Nausea, upper stomach pain, itching, loss of appetite dark urine, clay-colored stools.
Acetohexamide (Anti diabetic)	Swelling, rapid weight gain, increased urination, pale or yellowed skin, dark colored urine, fever, confusion,
Acetylprocainamide (Local anaesthetic)	Headache, dizziness, fatigue; cough; somnolence, nausea; hypotension.
Acetylsaficylic acid (Analgesic)	Ringing in your ears, confusion, hallucinations, rapid breathing, seizure (convulsions); severe nausea,
Acetylcysteine (Respiratory agent)	Wheezing, tightness in chest, difficulty in breathing, Skin rash or other irritation, Clammy skin, fever,
Acrosoxacin (Quinolone antibiotic)	Nausea, vomiting, heartburn, constipation, diarrhoea, abdominal cramping, anorexia; headache, dizziness
Acetazolamide (Antiepileptic)	Paresthesias, hearing dysfunction or tinnitus, loss of appetite, taste alteration.
Actinomycin (Antiviral)	Hair loss, Nausea and vomiting, Mouth sores, Diarrhea, Skin problems (follicular acne, redness)
Acyclovir (Antiviral)	Pain, swelling, Abdominal or stomach pain, decreased frequency of urination or amount of urine.
Adrenaline (Sympathomimetis)	Abnormal or decreased touch sensation, arm, back, or jaw pain, bleeding, blistering, burning, coldness,
Ajmaline (Antiarrythmic)	Heart block; cardiac arrhythmias; eye twitching; convulsions; resp depression; hepatotoxicity; agranulocytosis
Albendazole (Anthelmintics)	Abdominal Pain, Nausea/Vomiting, Headache, Dizziness/Vertigo, Raised Intracranial Pressure,
Aldesleukin (Anticancer)	Chills, Fever, Malaise, Asthenia, Infection, Abdominal pain, Abdomen enlarged, Hypotension,
Alfentanil (Anti aesthetic)	Nausea, vomiting, heartburn, constipation, diarrhoea, abdominal cramping, anorexia; headache, dizziness
Allopurinol (Antigout)	Fever, sore throat, and headache with a severe blistering, peeling, and red skin rashnausea,
Alphaxalone (Antiaesthetic)	Depression apnoea and hypoxia, increased or decreased heart rate, and increased or decreased blood pressure.
Amlodipine (Antihypertensive)	peripheral edema , fatigue ' dizziness; palpitations; stomach pain, headache, dyspepsia,
Aminocaproic acid (Antifibrinolytic)	weakness, especially on one side of the body; sudden headache, confusion, problems with vision,
Aminopyrine (Analgesic)	Fever, asthenia, fatigue, arrhythmia, palpitation, cholestatic jaundice, hepatitis, liver enzyme abnormalities.
Aminosalicylic acid (Antimycobacterial)	Fever, skin, dermatitis, syndrome, leucopenia, agranulocytosis, hemolytic anemia,
Amitriptyline (Antidepressant)	Myocardial infarction; stroke; nonspecific ECG changes and changes in AV conduction; heart block
Amodiaquine (Antimalarial)	Dizziness or vertigo; acute renal failure, interstitial nephritis, acute tubular necrosis; electrolyte imbalances

Name of Drugs	Adverse Drug Reactions(ADR)
Amoxicillin (Antibiotic)	Headache, nausea, dizziness, vomiting, diarrhoea, black hairy tongue, maculopapular rash, urticaria, eosinophilia
Amphetamine (CNS Stimulant)	Cardiovascular Palpitations, tachycardia, elevation of blood pressure, sudden death, myocardial infarction
Amphoteracin (Antifungal)	Topical: Local irritation, pruritus and skin rash. IV infusion: Fever, chills, convulsions, malaise; nausea, vomiting
Amplicillin (Antibiotic)	GI upset, nausea, vomiting, diarrhoea; blood dyscrasias; urticaria, exfoliative dermatitis, rash; fever,
Amrinone (Inotropic agent)	GI disturbances, nausea, vomiting, thrombocytopaenia, hypotension, chest pain, hypersensitivity, myositis
Amsacrine (Antineoplastic)	Diarrhea, nausea, vomiting, stomatitis, glossitis.
Amylobarbitone (Sedative)	Hypersensitivity, dizziness, diarrhoea, nausea, vomiting, renal impairment, rash, erythema multiforme.
Anistreplase (Thrombolytic drug)	Allergic reactions; fever; nausea and vomiting; haemorrhage; hypotension; pulmonary embolism.
Antipyrine (Misc. Drug)	GI disturbances, nausea, diarrhoea, rash, bruising,
Apomorphine (Antispycotic)	Nausea and vomiting; dyskinesia; dizziness; yawning; drowsiness; transient sedation; postural hypotension
Aspirin (Analgesic & antipyretic)	GI disturbances, epigastric discomfort, prolonged bleeding time, rhinitis, urticaria; angioedema, salicylism
Astemizole (Antihistamin)	GI upset, glossitis, stomatitis, altered taste
Atenolol (AntihypertenSive)	Bronchospasm; cold extremities, fatigue, dizziness, insomnia, lethargy, confusion, headache, depression
Atracurium (Neuromuscular blocker)	Cutaneous reactions; bradycardia, transient hypotension in patients with CVS disorders; dyspnoea, bronchospasm.
Atropine (Antimuscarinic)	Dry mouth, dysphagia, constipation, flushing and dryness of skin, tachycardia, palpitations, arrhythmias, mydriasis.
Auranofin (Antiimflarnmatory)	GI disturbances (nausea, vomiting, abdominal pain, diarrhoea, pruritus, rash; dermatitis.
Aurothiomalate (Anti gout)	Skin and mucous membrane reactions; stomatitis with a metallic taste; rash with pruritus; GI disorders.
Azapropazone (Antiinflammatory)	GI disorders; hypersensitivity reactions, headache, dizziness, nervousness, depression, drowsiness,
Azathioprine (Immunosup-pressant)	Fever, chills; bone marrow depression characterised by leucopenia, thrombocytopenia or anaemia; anorexia.
Azelastin (Tropical Nasopha-ryngal Medication)	Irritation, stinging and itching of the nasal mucosa. Sneezing, nosebleeds, headache; nausea, taste disturbances.
Azlocillin (Antibiotic)	Pain at the inj site and phlebitis; electrolyte disturbances; dose-dependent coagulation defect.
Aztreonam (Antibacterial)	Phloebitis and thrombophloebitis. IM: Pain and swelling at inj site; diarrhoea, nausea, vomiting, altered taste.
Azithromycin (Antibacterial)	Mild to moderate nausea, vomiting, abdominal pain, dyspepsia, flatulence, diarrhoea, cramping; angioedema.
Bacampicillin (Antibiotic)	Hypersensitivity reactions including uticaria; fever; joint pains; rashes; angioedema.

Name of Drugs	Adverse Drug Reactions(ADR)
Bacitracin (Antibacterial)	Nausea, vomiting, hypersensitivity reactions,
Baclofen (Muscle Relaxant)	Sedation, drowsiness, ataxia, dizziness, headache, confusion, hallucinations, skin reactions, GI symptoms.
Bacmecillinam (Antibiotic)	Hypersensitivity reactions including angioedema, urticaria, rash.
Bamethan (Calcium antagonist)	Headache, dizziness, back pain, myalgia, respiratory tract disorders, asthenia/fatigue, and first dose hypotension, rash.
Barbital (Hypnotic)	Drowsiness, ataxia, paradoxical excitement.
Beclomethasone (Cortico Steroid)	Loss of skin collagen and SC atrophy; local hypopigmentation of deeply pigmented skin; dryness,
Benazepril (Anti hypertensive)	Headache, dizziness, fatigue; cough; somnolence, nausea; hypotension.
Bendrofluazide (Cardiovascular agent)	Postural hypotension; mild GI effects; impotence (reversible); electrolyte imbalance.
Benorylate (Analgesic)	Heartburn, GI disturbances, drowsiness and hypersensitivity reactions. Occasionally dizziness, tinnitus, and deafness.
Benoxaprofen (Anti inflammatory)	Dizziness or vertigo; acute renal failure, interstitial nephritis, acute tubular necrosis; electrolyte imbalances
Benperidol (Antipsychotic)	Dizziness or vertigo; acute renal failure, interstitial nephritis, acute tubular necrosis; electrolyte imbalances.
Benzafibrate (Lipid lowering agent)	GI upset; pruritus, urticaria, alopoecia, impotence; vertigo, fatigue;
Benzylpenicillin (Antibiotic)	Hypersensitivity reactions including uticaria; fever; joint pains; rashes; angioedema;
Bepridil (Calcium channel blocker)	Dizziness, nausea, dyspnea, bradycardia, oedema, palpitations, QT prolongation, CHF, nervousness, headache.
Betahistine (Antileutic)	Rash, pruritus, urticaria, dyspepsia, nausea, peptic ulcer disease, headache, dizziness, insomnia.
Betamethasone (Corticosteroid)	Sodium and fluid retention, potassium and calcium depletion. Muscle wasting, weakness, osteoporosis.
Betaxolol (Drug for Glucoma)	Topical use in eye: Mild ocular stinging and discomfort, usually transient and well-tolerated. Rarely.
Bethanidine (Antirhypertensive)	Anxiety, tachycardia, tremor, dry mouth.
Bevantolol (β_1 adrenoreceptor blocker)	Bradycardia; hypotension; heart failure, heart block; bronchospasm; fatigue; coldness of extremities; pneumonitis.
Bishydroxycoumarin (Anticoagulant)	Hair loss, Nausea and vomiting, Mouth sores, Diarrhea, Skin problems, follicular acne, redness.
Bupivacaine (Local Anesthetic)	Depression. Hypotension, bradycardia, arrhythmias and cardiac arrest.
Buprenorphme (Analgesic & antipyretic)	Sedation, nausea, dizziness, vertigo, hypotension, miosis, headache, hypoventilation, resp or CNS depression.
Bupropion (Antidepressant)	Facial oedema; nausea, dry mouth, constipation, diarrhoea, anorexia; mouth ulcer; thirst; myalgia, arthralgia.
Burimamide (Anti ulcer Drug)	Nausea, vomiting, heartburn, constipation, diarrhoea, abdominal cramping, anorexia; headache, dizziness.
Buserelin (Hormone)	GI disturbances, headache/lightheadedness, increase in menstrual bleeding, mood changes, nervousness.

Name of Drugs	Adverse Drug Reactions(ADR)
Busulphan (Antineoplastic)	GI symptoms, anorexia, wt loss, weakness, hyperpigmentation, amenorrhoea, cataracts, cough or hoarseness.
Butobarbitone (Sedative)	Drowsiness, ataxia, paradoxical excitement, confusion, headache and CNS depression; respiratory depression.
Butriptyline (Antidepressant)	Nausea, sweating, tremor, hypersensitivity reactions, behavioral, Hypersensitivity, dizziness, diarrhoea,
Cadralazine (Anti hypertensive)	Dizziness or vertigo; acute renal failure, interstitial nephritis, acute tubular necrosis;
Caffeine (CMS Stimulant)	Insomnia, restlessness, nervousness, mild delirium; nausea, vomiting, hypotension, rapid and weak pulse,
Capreomycin (Antitubercular)	Toxic nephritis, electrolyte disturbances resembling Bartter's syndrome may occur, hearing loss, tinnitus, and vertigo.
Captopril (Anti hypertensive)	Hypotension, tachycardia, chest pain, palpitations, pruritus, hyperkalaemia. Proteinuria; angioedema, skin rashes.
Carbamazepine (Anticonvulsant)	Dizziness, drowsiness, ataxia; dry mouth, abdominal pain, nausea, vomiting, anorexia; leucopenia, proteinuria.
Carbimazole (Antithyroid)	Mild leucopaenia, sore throat, mouth ulcers, fever, bruising, malaise; rarely cholestatic jaundice.
Carbenicillin (Antibacterial)	Pain at inj site and phloebitis; electrolyte disturbances; dose-dependent coagulation defect.
Carbenoxolone (Antiulcer)	Sodium and water retention, hypokalaemia. Drug Interactions, Antagonism with amiloride.
Carbocisteine (Respiratory agent)	Headache, nausea, dizziness, vomiting, diarrhoea, GI discomfort/ bleeding, black hairy tongue.
Carboplatin (Antineoplastic)	Thrombocytopenia, neutropenia, leukopenia, anaemia; nausea, vomiting, central neurotoxicity.
Carisoprodol (Muscle Relaxant)	Dizziness, drowsiness, nausea, epigastric distress, tachycardia, orthostatic hypotension, Hypersensitivity reactions
Carmustine (Antineoplastic)	GI upsets anorexia; allergic reactions, irritation; venous irritation or thrombophlebitis. Pulmonary fibrosis;
Carprofen (Antiinflammatory)	Sweating, dizziness, nausea, vomiting, dry mouth, fatigue, asthenia, somnolence, confusion, constipation, flushing
Carvedilol (Antihypertensive)	Bradycardia, AV block, angina pectoris, hypervolaemia, leucopenia, hypotension, peripheral oedema, allergy, .
Cefacetrile (Antibiotic)	Nausea, vomiting, diarrhoea, abdominal discomfort; skin rash, angioedema; elevated liver enzyme.
Cefaclor (Antibacterial)	Allergic reactions; diarrhoea, nausea, vomiting; candidiasis, eosinophilia; elevated transaminases
Cefadroxil (Antibacterial)	Nausea, vomiting, diarrhoea, abdominal discomfort; skin rash, angioedema; elevated liver enzyme values;
Cephamandole (Antibiotic)	Vomiting; diarrhoea; hypersensitivity reactions; nephrotoxicity; convulsions; CNS toxicity; pseudomembranous.
Cefapirin (Antibacterial)	Nausea;vomiting;diarrhoea; hypersensitivityreactions; nephrotoxicity; convulsions; CNS toxicity;
Cefathiamidine (Antibacterial)	Dizziness or vertigo; acute renal failure, interstitial nephritis, acute tubular necrosis; electrolyte imbalances
Cefatrizine (Antibacterial)	Nausea; vomiting; diarrhoea; hypersensitivity**reactions**; nephrotoxicity; convulsions; CNS toxicity;
Cefazaflur (Antibacterial)	Nausea, vomiting, diarrhoea, abdominal discomfort; skin rash, angioedema; elevated liver enzyme values
Cefazedone (Antibacterial)	Hypersensitivity, dizziness, diarrhoea, nausea, vomiting, renal impairment, rash, erythema multiforme.

Name of Drugs	Adverse Drug Reactions(ADR)
Cefazolin (Antibacterial)	Superinfection; nausea, vomiting, abdominal pain, anorexia, diarrhoea; rash, leukopenia, thrombocytopaenia,
Cefbuperazone (Antibacterial)	Skin rash, urticaria; eosinophilia, diarrhoea, nausea, vomiting; phloebitis; hypoprothrombinaemia; superinfection.
Cefixime (Antibacterial)	Diarrhoea, nausea, vomiting, abdominal pain; headache, dizziness, thrombocytopenia, eosinophilia.
Cefmenoxime (Antibacterial)	Nausea;vomiting; diarrhoea; hypersensitivityreactions; nephrotoxicity; convulsions;
Cefmetazole (Antibacterial)	Hypersensitivity reactions;nephrotoxicity; neutropenia; thrombocytopenia; agranulocytosis;
Cefonicid (Antibacterial)	Dizziness or vertigo; acute renal failure, interstitial nephritis, acute tubular necrosis; electrolyte imbalances
Cefoperazone (Antibacterial)	Skin rash, urticaria; eosinophilia, diarrhoea, nausea, vomiting; phloebitis; hypoprothrombinaemia; superinfection.
Ceforanide (Antibacterial)	Dizziness or vertigo; acute renal failure, interstitial nephritis, acute tubular necrosis; electrolyte imbalances
Cefotaxime (Antibacterial)	Pain at inj site; hypersensitivity **reactions**, rash, pruritus; diarrhoea, nausea, vomiting; candidiasis; eosinophilia,
Cefotetan (Antibacterial)	Stomatitis, pharyngitis, dyspnoea and neuropathy.
Cefotiam (Antibiotic)	Nausea; vomiting; diarrhoea; hypersensitivityreactions; nephrotoxicity; convulsions; CNS toxicity;
Cefoxitin (Antibacterial)	Nausea; vomiting; diarrhoea; hypersensitivityreactions;nephrotoxicity; convulsions.
Cefpimizole (Antibiotic)	Dizziness or vertigo; acute renal failure, interstitial nephritis, acute tubular necrosis; electrolyte imbalances;
Cefpiramide (Antibiotic)	Hypersensitivity reactions including uticaria; fever; joint pains; rashes; angioedema; serum sickness-like reactions.
Cefpodoxime (Antibacterial)	Anaphylactic shock; purpuric nephritis, skin rash, pruritus; diarrhoea, nausea, abdominal pain, vomiting.
Cefprozil	hypersensitivity reactions; nephrotoxicity; convulsions; CNS toxicity; hepatic dysfunction;
Cefroxadmec (Antibacterial)	Nauseavomiting; diarrhoea; hypersensitivity reactions;
Cefsulodin (Antibacterial)	Nausea; vomiting; diarrhoea; hypersensitivity reactions; nephrotoxicity; convulsions; CNS toxicity;
Cefsumide (Antibacterial)	Skin rash, urticaria; eosinophilia, diarrhoea, nausea, vomiting; phloebitis; hypoprothrombinaemia; superinfection
Ceftazidime (Antibacterial)	Hypersensitivity, dizziness, diarrhoea, nausea, vomiting, renal impairment, rash, erythema multiforme
Ceftezole	Nausea; vomiting; diarrhea; hypersensitivity ...
Ceftizoxime (Antibacterial)	Burning; rash, pruritus, fever; anorexia, nausea, vomiting, diarrhoea; rarely neutropaenia, leucopaenia, .
Ceftriaxone (Antibacterial)	Superinfection; anaphylaxis; diarrhoea; localreactions; blood dyscrasias; rash, fever, pruritus;
Cefuroxime (Antibacterial)	Cerebral irritation and convulsions; nausea, vomiting, diarrhoea, GI disturbances; erythema.
Celiprolol (Anti hypertensive)	Nausea, abdominal discomfort, diarrhoea; CHF, AV nodal block and bradycardia, palpitations; headache, fatigue,
Cephalexin (Antibiotic)	Gastrointestinal: Onset of pseudomembranous colitis may occur during or after antibacterial treatment.
Cephalexm (Antibacterial)	GI disturbances, hypersensitivity reactions, including rash, urticaria, eosinophilia, fever

Name of Drugs	Adverse Drug Reactions(ADR)
Cephaloglycm (Antibiotic)	Vomiting; diarrhoea; hypersensitivity reactions; nephrotoxicity; convulsions; CNS toxicity; pseudomembranous.
Cephaloridine (Antibacterial)	Neurotoxicity, ototoxicity, nephrotoxicity; skin rash
Cephalothin (Antibacterial)	Dizziness or vertigo; acute renal failure, interstitial nephritis, acute tubular necrosis; electrolyte imbalances
Cepnamandole (Antibacterial)	Vomiting; diarrhoea; hypersensitivity reactions; nephrotoxicity; convulsions; CNS toxicity
Cephapirm (Antibiotic)	Nausea; vomiting; diarrhoea; hypersensitivity reactions; nephrotoxicity; convulsions; CNS toxicity
Cephazolin (Antibacterial)	Superinfection; nausea, vomiting, abdominal pain, anorexia, diarrhoea; rash, leukopenia, thrombocytopaenia,
Cephradine (Antibacterial)	Dizziness or vertigo; acute renal failure, interstitial nephritis, acute tubular necrosis; electrolyte imbalances
Chloral hydrate (Hypnotic)	Gastric irritation, abdominal distention and flatulence, vertigo, ataxia, staggering gait, rashes, malaise, .
Chlorambucil (Antineoplastic)	Reversible progressive lymphocytopenia and neutropenia; GI disturbances; hepatotoxicity; skin rashes
Chloramphenicol (Antibacterial)	GI symptoms; bleeding; peripheral and optic neuritis, visual impairment, blindness; encephalopathy, confusion,
Chlorazepate (Amiolytic)	Jaundice, hepatic necrosis; extrapyramidal disorders; acute attacks of porphyria in porphyric patients, hypotension;
Chlordiazepoxide (Anxiolytic)	Physical and psychological dependence; withdrawal syndrome; impairs psychomotor performance, aggression
Chlormethiazole (Cardiovascular agent)	Nasal congestion and irritation; conjunctival irritation, headache. Rarely, paradoxical excitement, confusion
Chlormezanone (Muscle Relaxant)	Hypersensitivity, dizziness, diarrhoea, nausea, vomiting, renal impairment, rash, erythema multiforme.
Chloroquine (Antimalarial)	Retinopathy, hair loss, photosensitivity, tinnitus, myopathy (long-term therapy). Psychosis, seizures, leucopenia.
Chlorothiazide (Cardiovascular agent)	Electrolyte imbalance; hyperglycaemia; gout; dry mouth; thirst; weakness; muscle pain and cramp; seizures.
Chlorpheniramine (Antiallergic)	CNS depression, sedation, drowsiness, lassitude, dizziness. GI upsets, anorexia, or increased appetite, epigastric
Chlorpromazine (Anti psychotic)	Tardive dyskinesia (on long-term therapy). Involuntary movements of extremities may also occur. Dry mouth, constipation.
Chlorpropamide (Antidiabetic)	GI disturbances; hypoglycaemia; cholestatic jaundice; agranulocytosis, lymphocytosis, thrombocytopenia,
Chlorprothixine (Antipsychotic)	Dry mouth, constipation, urinary retention, mydriasis; agitation, insomnia, depression, convulsions,
Chlortetracycline (Antibacterial)	Hypersensitivity and photosensitivity reactions; abnormal pigmentation of the eye; myopia
Chlorthalidone (Antihypertensive)	Dyspnoea, wheeziness, bradycardia, hypotension, cold extremities, fatigue, dizziness, insomnia, lethargy,
Cias Pride (Prokinetic)	Abdominal cramps, borborygmi and loose stools (transient); rarely require discontinuation of therapy. Headache
Ciclacillin (Antibiotic)	Urticaria, candida superinfection. Potentially Fatal: Anaphylactic reaction with CV collapses esp with parenteral use.
Cilazapril (Antihypertensive)	Dizziness, headache, fatigue, GI disturbances, taste disturbances, persistent dry cough and other upper resp tract.
Cimetidine (H$_2$ antagonistic)	Diarrhoea, dizziness, tiredness, rash, headache, CNS disturbances, arthralgia, myalgia, gynaecomastia, alopecia.

Name of Drugs	Adverse Drug Reactions(ADR)
Cinnarizine (Anti vertigo)	Drowsiness, headache, GI upsets, unsteadiness, headache; rarely skin and hypersensitivity reactions, dry mouth, ..
Cinoxacin (Antibiotic)	Hypersensitivity reactions; nausea, vomiting, diarrhoea; abdominal pain; neurological effects; toxic psychoses
Ciprofloxacin (Antibacterial)	GI disturbances; headache, tremor, confusion, convulsions; rashes; joint pain; phototoxicity
Cisplatin (Antineoplastic)	Severe nausea and vomiting. Serious toxiceffects on the kidneys, bone marrows and ears. Hypomagnesaemia.
Clarithromycin (Antibacterial)	GI upset, glossitis, stomatitis, altered taste; headache, dizziness, hallucinations, insomnia, other CNS effects; rash;
Clavulanic acid (Antibacterial)	Hypersensitivity reactions, GI disturbances, pseudomembranous colitis, blood dyscrasias,
Clemastine (Antiallergic)	Drowsiness, CNS depression, dizziness, sedation; diarrhoea, nausea, vomiting; blurred vision,
Clindamycin (Antibacterial)	Diarrhoea, nausea, vomiting, abdominal pain; erythema multiforme, contact dermatitis, exfoliative and vesiculous
Clioquinol (Antibiotic)	Severe irritation or hypersensitivity.
Clobazam (Anticonvuisant)	Constipation, anorexia, nausea; dizziness, fine tremors; worsening of respiratory symptoms
Clofazimine (Antileprotics)	Anaemia, peripheral neuropathy, haemolysis and methaemoglobinaemia (dose-related).
Clofibrate (Lipid lowening agent)	Anorexia; nausea; gastric discomfort; stomatitis; headache; dizziness; vertigo; fatigue; skin reactions; alopoecia;
Clomipramine (Antidepressant)	Dryness of mouth; disturbances in micturition; drowsiness, increased sweating; sexual dysfunction; confusion.
Clomocycline (Antibiotic)	Fever, thrombophloebitis (inj). Acute anaphylactoid reactions, hyperpyrexia. Rash, erythema, pruritus, vesiculation,
Clonazepam (Anticonvuisant)	Drowsiness, fatigue, muscular hypotonia, coordination disturbances, dizziness, vertigo, anorexia
Clomdine (Antihypertensive)	Dry mouth, drowsiness, dizziness, headache, constipation, impotence, vivid dreams, urinary retention; dry, itching.
Clorazepate (Antiaxiety)	Jaundice, hepatic necrosis; extrapyramidal disorders; acute attacks of porphyria in porphyric patients,
Cloxacillin (Antibacterial)	Neutropenia, agranulocytosis; GI upsets; rash. Sore mouth or tongue. Black hairy tongue. Potentially Fatal:
Clozapine (Antipsychotic)	Drowsiness, dizziness, headache; nausea, vomiting, constipation; anxiety, confusion, fatigue, transient fever.
Cocain (Anaesthetic)	Hypertension, headache, peripheral ischaemia,
Codeine (Antiillusive)	Nausea, vomiting, constipation, dry mouth, sweating, skin rashes. Potentially Fatal: Blood dyscrasias
Colaspase (Antineoplastic)	Hypersensitivity, dizziness, diarrhoea, nausea, vomiting, renal impairment, rash, erythema multiforme,
Colchicine (Antigout)	Nausea, vomiting and abdominal pain; diarrhoea, GI haemorrhage, rashes, renal and hepatic damage.
Colistin (Antidiarrhoeals)	Superinfection; renal damage; visual disturbances; GI disturbances, dizziness, nausea, vomiting; confusion,
Cortisone (Corticosteroid)	Sodium and fluid retention. Potassium and calcium depletion. Muscle wasting, weakness, osteoporosis.
Cyclandelate (Peripheral Vasodilator)	Flushes, GI upset, nausea, tingling, tachycardia.

Name of Drugs	Adverse Drug Reactions(ADR)
Cyclizine (Antinausea/ antivertigo)	CNS depression e.g. drowsiness to deep sleep, lassitude, dizziness and incoordination.
Cyclobarbital (Barbiturates)	Dizziness or vertigo; acute renal failure, interstitial nephritis, acute tubular necrosis; electrolyte imbalances.
Cydophosphamide (Neoplastic disorders)	Congestive heart failure; leucopenia; poor wound healing; anorexia. Nausea, vomiting; alopecia.
Cyclosertne (Antitubercular)	Headache, dizziness, anxiety, confusion, irritability, paraesthesia, speech difficulties, photosensitivity, vertigo.
Cyclosporin (Immuno depressant)	Hypertension; hepatoxicity; tremor; paraesthesia, hypertrichosis, facial oedema, acne; gingival hypertrophy.
Cyproheptadine (Antiallergic)	Drowsiness, fatigue; dry mouth, GI upsets, nausea; appetite increase, wt gain.
Cyproterone (Hormone)	Inhibits spermatogenesis, reduces volume of ejaculate, causes infertility.
Cytarabine (Neoplastic disorders)	Dementia, GI disturbances, hepatic and renal dysfunction, neurotoxicity, rashes, oral and anal ulceration.
Dacarbazine (Antineoplastic)	Leucopenia, thrombocytopenia, anorexia, nausea, diarrhoea, vomiting; flu-like syndrome, myalgia,
Danazol (Gouadal Hormone)	Oedema, wt gain, sweating, acne, hirsutism, flushing, oily skin or hair, deepening of the voice, clitoral hypertrophy,
Dantrolen (Muscle Relaxant)	Fatigue, muscle weakness/pain. GI disturbances, CNS effects, tachycardia, unstable BP, dyspnoea, drowsiness
Dapsone (Antileprotic)	Anaemia, peripheral neuropathy, haemolysis and methaemoglobinaemia (dose-related), nephrotic syndrome.
Daunorubicin (Antineoplastic)	GI disturbances; stomatitis; alopoecia and dermatological reactions.
Debrisoquine (Antihypertensive)	Postural hypotension, failure of ejaculation, fluid retention, nasal decongestion, headache, .
Demeclocycline (Antibacterial)	Postural hypotension, failure of ejaculation, fluid retention, nasal decongestion, headache,
Demethylchlortetracycline (Antibiotic)	Hypersensitivity, dizziness, diarrhoea, nausea, vomiting, renal impairment, rash, erythema multiforme.
Desipramme (Antidepressant)	Psychological and physical dependence,
Desmethyldiazepam (Anxiolytic)	Fatigue, drowsiness, dizziness, prolonged reaction time, headache.
Dexamethasone (Corticosteroid)	Hypersensitivity reactions, lid itching and swelling, conjunctival erythema, increase in intraocular pressure.
Dexamphetamine (CNS stimulant)	Cardiovascular Palpitations, tachycardia.
Dextromethorphan (Steroid)	Nausea, vomiting, dry mouth, nose and throat infection.
Dextromoramide (Opioid analgesic)	Dizziness or vertigo; acute renal failure,
Dextropro-poxyphene (Analgesic & antipyretic)	Dizziness, sedation, nausea, vomiting, weakness,
Dezocine (Analgesic)	Nausea, vomiting, abdominal pain, diarrhoea; headache, dizziness, insomnia.
Diamorphine (Analgesic)	Hypersensitivity, dizziness, diarrhoea, nausea, vomiting, renal impairment, rash, erythema multiforme.
Diazepam (Anxiolytic)	Psychological and physical dependence with withdrawal syndrome, fatigue, drowsiness, sedation, ataxia, vertigo.
Diazoxide (Antihypertensive)	Hypotension; hyperglycaemia; oedema; dysgeusia; nausea; anorexia and other GI disturbances.

Name of Drugs	Adverse Drug Reactions(ADR)
Diclofenac (NSAID agent)	GI disturbances; headache, dizziness, rash; GI bleeding, peptic ulceration; abnormalities of kidney function.
Dicloxacillin (Antibacterial)	Hypersensitivity reactions including uticaria; fever; joint pains; rashes; angioedema.
Dicoumarol (Anticoagulant)	Hypoglycaemia, nausea, epigastric fullness, heartburn, Hypoglycaemic effect enhanced by dicoumarol,
Dicyclomine (Sedative)	
Didanosine (Antiviral)	Pancreatitis; peripheral neuropathy; diarrhoea, nausea, vomiting, abdominal pain; headache, fatigue, rash
Diethylpropion (Monoamine oxidase inhibitor)	Dizziness or vertigo; acute renal failure, interstitial nephritis, acute tubular necrosis; electrolyte imbalances;
Diflunisal (Analgesic)	GI disturbances or bleeding; CNS effects; hypersensitivity reactions; blood disorders.
Digitoxin (Cardiac glycoside)	Nausea, vomiting, anorexia, diarrhoea, abdominal pain, headache, facial pain, fatigue, weakness, dizziness.
Digoxin (Cardiac glycoside)	Extra beats, anorexia, nausea and vomiting.
Dihydrocodeine (Analgesic)	Nausea, vomiting, constipation, drowsiness, confusion and other CNS effects. CV effects, sweating, hypothermia.
Dihydroergotamine (Antimigrairi)	Nausea, vomiting, diarrhoea, coronary artery vasospasm, precordial pain, numbness, cramps, localised oedema.
Dilevalol (β Blocker)	Orthostatic hypotension, dizziness, fatigue, vertigo, paraesthesia, headache, nasal stuffiness, dyspnoea, diarrhea.
Diltiazem (Antihypertensive)	Headache, ankle oedema, hypotension, dizziness, fatigue, flushing, nausea, GI discomfort, gingival hyperplasia.
Diphenhydramine (Antiallergic)	CNS depression, dizziness, headache, sedation; paradoxical stimulation in children; dryness of mouth.
Diphenoxylate (Antidiarrhoeal)	GI effects; headache, drowsiness, dizziness, restlessness, euphoria, depression, numbness of the extremities.
Diphenylhydantoin (AntiConvulsion Drug)	GI effects; headache, drowsiness, dizziness, restlessness, euphoria, depression, numbness of the extremities.
Diphenylpyraline (Anti histamine)	GI disturbances or bleeding; CNS effects; hypersensitivity reactions; blood disorders; nephrotoxicity; haematuria
Dipyridamole (Antianginal)	GI disturbances, headache, dizziness, faintness, facial flushing, skin rash, liver dysfunction, angina
Disodium Cromoglycate (Anti Asthmatic Drug)	Nausea, headache, dizziness, unpleasant taste, joint pain and swelling, skin rashes, aggravation of asthma
Disopyramide (Antiarrhythmic)	Impotence, constipation, difficulty in micturition, dry mouth, blurred vision, nausea, bloating, abdominal pain, ...
Distigmine (Parasympathomimetic)	Allergic reactions, salivation, GI disturbances, resp failure.
Disulfiram (Antabuse)	Drowsiness, fatigue, lassitude, psychoticreactions, peripheral and optic neuropathies, hepatotoxicity
Dobutamine (Inotropic agent)	Increased Heart Rate, Blood Pressure, and Ventricular Ectopic Activity A 10- to 20-mm increase in systolic blood.
Domperidone (Antileutic)	Drowsiness, extrapyramidal reactions, galactorrhoea, gynaecomastia; constipation or diarrhoea, lassitude,
Dopamine (Inotropic agent)	Nausea, vomiting, tachycardia, ectopic beats, palpitation, anginal pain, hypotension, vasoconstriction, bradycardia.
Dopexamine (Vasodilator)	Dizziness or vertigo; acute renal failure, interstitial nephritis, acute tubular necrosis; electrolyte imbalances.

Name of Drugs	Adverse Drug Reactions(ADR)
Dothiepin (Anti depressant)	Cholestatic jaundice, sexual dysfunction, exacerbation of psychotic manifestation, cardiac arrhythmias, hypotension, dry mouth.
Doxapram (Respiratory Stimulant)	Dyspnoea and other respiratory problems. Muscle involvement may range from fasciculations to spasticity.
Doxazosin (Antihypertensive)	Chest pain, fatigue, headache, influenza-like symptoms, pain, hypotension, palpitation, abdominal pain, diarrhea.
Doxepin (Antidepressant)	Drowsiness, dizziness, confusion, headache, dry mouth, constipation, blurring of vision, hypotension, tachycardia.
Doxycycline (Antibiotic)	Alopecia; fever, nausea, vomiting, diarrhoea; skin rash.
Diflunisal (NSAID)	GI disturbances or bleeding; CNS effects; hypersensitivity reactions; blood disorders; nephrotoxicity; haematuria;
Doxycycline (Antibacterial)	Permanent staining of teeth; rash, superinfection; nausea, GI upsets, glossitis; dysphagia; photosensitivity.
Droperidol (Antidopaminergic)	Dry mouth, constipation, micturition difficulty, blurred vision, mydriasis, delirium, agitation, catatonic-like states.
Dihydrogesterone (Gonadal Hormone)	Dizziness, nausea, headache, fatigue, emotional lability, irritability; abdominal pain and distention;
Edrophonium (Anticholinestarase inhibitor)	Muscle weakness, paralysis, muscle atrophy
Entosuximide (Anti epileptic)	Blood toxicities and disorders; headache, fatigue, lethargy, drowsiness, dizziness, ataxia, hiccup and mild euphoria
Emetine (Anti amoebic Drug)	Drowsiness, extrapyramidal reactions, galactorrhoea, gynaecomastia; constipation or diarrhoea, lassitude, decreased libido, skin rash
Enalapril (Antihypertensive)	Initial hypotension may be severe and prolonged. Dizziness, headache, fatigue, persistent dry cough
Encainide (Antiarrythmic)	Asthenia, fever, nausea, diarrhea, dry mouth
Enoxacin (Antibiotic)	GI disturbances; CNS effects; hypersensitivity-type reactions; reversible arthralgia; hepatic effects
Enxaparin (Anti coagulant)	hrombocytopenia, mild bleeding, inj site irritation, pain and ecchymoses, hypersensitivity and erythema
Enoximone	Fatigue, palpitations, tachycardia, nausea, diarrhea
Epanolol (β-adrenoreceptor antagonist)	Diarrhoea, dizziness, pruritus, skin rashes, GI tract infections, chest pain, headache, nausea, pain, anxiety
Ephedrine (Respiratory agent)	Anxiety, tachycardia, tremor, dry mouth, hypertension, cardiac arrhythmias, impaired circulation to the extremities
Epirubicin (Antineoplastic)	Myelosuppression; cardiotoxicity, alopoecia; mucositis; hyperpyrexia; lethargy; amenorrhoea; nausea and vomiting
Ergometrine (Obstetrics Drug)	Nausea, vomiting, abdominal pain, headache, dizziness, rashes, hypertension, bradycardia, arrhythmia
Ergonovine (Uterine Stimulant)	Diarrhoea, vomiting, headache, asthenia
Ergotamine (Antimigrain)	Muscle cramps, stiffness, tiredness. Numbness and tingling of extremities. Nausea, vomiting, diarrhoea
Erythromycin (Antibiotic)	Rash, urticaria; nausea, vomiting, GI discomfort; ototoxicity; central neurotoxicity; agranulocytosis,
Eserine (AntiCholinesterase inhibitor)	Dry mouth, dysphagia, constipation, flushing and dryness of skin, tachycardia, palpitations, arrhythmias, mydriasis

Name of Drugs	Adverse Drug Reactions(ADR)
Esmolol (Antiarrhythmic)	Hypotension, bradycardia, heart failure, local irritation, diaphoresis, peripheral ischaemia, dizziness, somnolence.
Estramustine (Antineoplastic)	Gynaecomastia, fluid retention and CV effects, GI disturbances, hepatic dysfunction, loss of libido, hypersensitivity.
Ethacrynic acid (Cardiovascular agent)	Fluid and electrolyte imbalance, nausea, diarrhoea, blurred vision, headache, dizziness, hypotension.
Ethambutol (Antitubercuiar drug)	Retrobulbar neuritis with a reduction in visual acuity, constriction of visual field, central or peripheral scotoma.
Ethanol (Alcohol)	Loss of judgement, emotional lability, visual impairment, slurred speech, ataxia.
Ethinyloestradiol (Gonadal Hormone)	Menstrual irregularities; headache, dizziness.
Ethosuximide (Anticonvulsant)	Blood toxicities and disorders; headache, fatigue, lethargy, drowsiness, dizziness, ataxia, hiccup and mild euphoria.
Etidocaine (Antiaesthetic)	Dizziness, paraesthesia, drowsiness, confusion.
Etintidine (Antispasmodic)	Nausea, vomiting, dry mouth, constipation, allergic reactions.
Ethyl biscoumacetate (Anticoagulant)	Headache, asthenia, tremor, palpitations, nausea, diarrhea.
Etodolac (NSAID)	GI disturbances; CNS effects; hypersensitivityreactions. Rash, pruritus; neuromuscular and skeletal weaknesses.
Etomidate (Anaesthetic)	Excitatory phenomena eg, involuntary myoclonic muscle movements, convulsions; hypersensitivity reactions, pain.
Etoposide (Antineoplastic agent)	Nausea, vomiting, anorexia, diarrhoea, stomatitis; reversible alopoecia; rarely, disturbances of liver dysfunctio
Famciclovir (Antiviral)	Dizziness, headache, diarrhoea, constipation, nausea, vomiting, hallucinations, confusion, pruritus
Famotidine (H$_2$ antagonist)	Headache, dizziness, constipation, diarrhoea, nausea, rash, GI discomfort, fatigue, gynaecomastia, impotenc
Felbamate (Antiseizure agent)	Somnolence, headache, fever, dizziness, insomnia, fatigue, nervousness, anorexia, nausea, vomiting, constipation
Felodipine (Anti hypertensive)	Flushing, headache, peripheral oedema, tachycardia, palpitation, dizziness, fatigue. Ankle swelling
Fenbufen (Antiinflammatory)	GI disorder; skin rashes; CNS disorders; erythema multiforme; photosensitivity; haematuria; renal failure
Fenfluramine (Monoamine)	Urticaria, GI upsets, palpitations, tachycardia
Fenoprofen (Antiinflammatory)	GI disorders, cholestatic jaundice, occult blood in stools; headache; itching; fluid retention; dizziness, somnolence
Fenoterol (Respiratory agent)	Fine tremor of skeletal muscle, palpitations, tachycardia, nervous tension, headaches, peripheral vasodilatation
Fentanyl (Neuromuscular blocker)	Nausea, vomiting; bradycardia, oedema, CNS depression, confusion, dizziness,drowsiness, headache, sedation
Finasteride (Anti prostate)	Testicular pain. Hypersensitivity reactions e.g. swelling of lips and face, urticaria, rashes
Flecamide (Aptiarrythemic)	Dizziness, visual disturbances, lightheadedness and other CNS **effects**, nausea, vomiting, headache, tremor
Floxuridine (Antineoplastic)	Rash; alopoecia; GI disorders, taste disturbances

Drugs	Ionization constant (pKa)	Partition Coefficient (log p)	Oral Absorption (%)	Bio Availability (%)	Tmax	Volume Distribution (l/kg)	Protein Binding (%)	Half Life (hours)	Clearance (ml/min)	Urinary Excretion (%)
Metoprolol (Antihypertensive)	9.7	-0.1	>95	50	1-2	6	12	2-5	1000	<5
Metronidazole (Antibacterial/ antifungal)	2.5	0								
Mexiletine (Antiarrythmatic)	9	2,6	>90	90	5-8		70	7-25	500	10-20
Mezlocillin (Antibiotic)			Poor			0.25	35	1	200	60-70
Mianserin (Antidepressant)	7.1	4.3	Good	30	2	6-45	90-95	6-39	320	5
Miconazole (Antibacterial/ antifungal)	6.7	6D				20	92-99	24	760-	<1
Midazolam (Anxiolytic)	6.2	3.7	iv			1.3-2.2	>94	2-5	700-1700	<1
Midodrine (Antihypertensive)		-0.4								
Milrinone (Inotropic Agent)				380		0.32	70	0.8	6.1	85
Mifepristone (Anti progesterone)		4.9								
Minocycline (Antibacterials)	2.8	-1.4				1.5	70	15	120	<10
Minoxidil (Hair growth)		1.4				3	<5	3-4	600	<20
Misonidazole (Radiosensitizer)		-0.4								
Misopristol (Prostaglandin E1 (PGE1) analog)		2.9								
Mitomycin (Antineoplastic)	10.9	-0.4	iv							10
Mitotane (Antineoplastic)		5.6	<50							<10
Mitoxantrone (Antineoplastic)		Iv						43		Low
Moclobemide (Monoamine oxidase inhibitor)		2A		60						

Name of Drugs	Adverse Drug Reactions(ADR)
Glibenclamide (Oral Antidiabetic)	Hypoglycaemia; cholestatic jaundice; agranulocytosis; aplastic anaemia; haemolytic anaemia. Blood dyscrasias.
Glibornuride (Antidiabetic)	GI disturbances; metallic taste; skin rashes, pruritus, and photosensitivity; facial flushing; hypoglycaemia.
Gliclazide (Oral Antidiabetic)	GI disturbances, skin reaction, leucopenia, thrombocytopenia, agranulocytosis, haemolytic anaemia, cholestati.
Glipizide (Oral Antidiabetic)	GI upsets, diarrhoea, nausea; allergic skinreactions, leucopenia, thrombocytopenia, agranulocytosis.
Gliquidone (Antidiabetic)	GI disturbances; metallic taste; skin rashes, pruritus, photosensitivity; facial flushing; hypoglycaemia
Glutethimide (Hypnotic)	Orthostatic hypotension, dizziness, fatigue, vertigo, paraesthesia, headache
Glyburide (Antidiabetic)	Blood dyscrasias (reversible), liver dysfunction, hypoglycaemia, GI symptoms, allergic skin reactions
Glycerin (Antianginal/ coronary vasodilator)	Facial flushing, dizziness, tachycardia, throbbing headache and tolerance. Large doses can cause vomiting, Headache, nausea, diarrhoea, thirst, mental confusion.
Glycopyrronium (Antisparmodic)	Xerostomia; loss of taste, nausea, vomiting, constipation, reduced sweating; urinary hesitancy and retention.
Glymidine (Antidiabetic)	Fluid and electrolyte disorders e.g. acidosis, electrolyte loss, marked diuresis, urinary retention, and oedema.
Goserelin (Hormone)	Vaginal bleeding and dryness, arthralgia, paraesthesias, increase in menstrual bleeding, hot flushes,
Gold sodium (Thiomalate)	Skin and mucous membrane reactions; stomatitis with a metallic taste; rash with pruritus.
Granisetron (Antiemetic)	Headache; sensation of flushing; constipation; hypersensitivity reactions; chest pain; dizziness.
Griseofulvin (Antifungal)	Oral thrush; GI distress, taste perversion; dizziness, confusion, headache, depression, insomnia, fatigue.
Guanabenz (Antihypertensive)	Weight Gain, Dizziness, orthostatic hypotension, palpitation, headache, weakness, fatigue, hyperkalaemia, chest pain
Guanadrel (Antihypertensive)	Cardiac abnormalities, hypertension;
Guanethidine (Antihypertensive)	Severe postural and exertional hypotension, diarrhoea, dizziness, syncope, muscle weakness, lassitude, angina.
Guanfecine (Antihypertensive)	Drowsiness, dry mouth, dizziness, headache, constipation, depression, anxiety, fatigue, nausea, anorexia.
Guanoxan (Antihypertensive)	Dizziness or vertigo; acute renal failure, interstitial nephritis, acute tubular necrosis; electrolyte imbalances.
Haloperidol (Antipsychotic)	Tardive dyskinesia; extrapyramidal reactions. Anxiety, drowsiness, depression, anorexia, transient tachycardia.
Heparin (Anticoagulant, Antithrombosis)	Slight fever, headache, chills, nausea, vomiting, constipation, epistaxis, bruising, slight haematuria, skin necrosis
Heroin (Opioid Analgesic)	Nausea, vomiting, dry mouth, constipation, allergic reactions.
Hexobarbital (Sedative)	GI disturbances, visual impairment and irritation; increase serum concentrations of digoxin, cyclosporin, terfenadine.
Homatropine (Anticholinergic Drug)	Blurred vision; photophobia; increased intraocular pressure.
Hydralazine (Antihypertensive)	Tachycardia; palpitations; angina pectoris; haemolytic anaemia; paralytic ileus; severe headache; GI disturbances.

Name of Drugs	Adverse Drug Reactions(ADR)
Hexobarbital (Sedative)	GI disturbances, visual impairment and irritation; increase serum concentrations of digoxin, cyclosporin, terfenadine.
Hydralazine (Antihypertensive)	Tachycardia; palpitations; angina pectoris; haemolytic anaemia; paralytic ileus; severe headache; GI disturbances.
Hydrochlorothiazide (Diuretic)	Volume depletion and electrolyte imbalance, dry mouth, thirst, lethargy, drowsiness, muscle pain
Hexobarbital (Sedative)	GI disturbances, visual impairment and irritation; increased serum concentrations of digoxin, cyclosporin, terfenadine.
Hydralazine (Antihypertensive)	Tachycardia; palpitations; angina pectoris; haemolytic anaemia; paralytic ileus; severe headache; GI disturbances.
Hydrochlorothiazide (Diuretic)	Volume depletion and electrolyte imbalance, dry mouth, thirst, lethargy, drowsiness, muscle pain and cramps.
Hydralazine (Antihypertensive)	Tachycardia; palpitations; angina pectoris; haemolytic anaemia; paralytic ileus; severe headache; GI disturbances.
Hydrochlorothiazide (Diuretic)	Nebivolol Headache, fatigue, parasthesias, dizziness, dry mouth, thirst, lethargy, drowsiness, muscle pain and cramps.
Hydrocortisone (Corticosteroid)	Sodium and fluid retention. Potassium and calcium depletion. Muscle wasting, weakness, osteoporosis.
Hydroxizime (Anxiolytic, Sedatives)	CNS depression, paradoxical CNS stimulation, dry mouth, thickened respiratory secretions, constipation.
Hydroxychloroquine (Antiprotozoal)	Retinopathy, hair loss, photosensitivity, tinnitus, Psychosis, seizures.
Hydroxyprogesterone (Gonadal Hormone)	GI disturbances, increased appetite, wt gain or loss, oedema, acne, allergic skin rashes, urticaria,
Hydroxyurea (Antineoplastic)	GI disturbances, renal impairment, pulmonary oedema, dermatological reactions, headache, and dizziness.
Hydroxizine (Anxiolytic)	CNS depression, paradoxical CNS stimulation, dry mouth, thickened respiratory secretions, constipation.
Hyoscine (Antinausea)	Flushing, postural hypotension, tachycardia, fibrillation. Rarely psychotic reactions. Dizziness.
Ibuprofen (NSAID agent)	Dyspepsia, vomitting, abdominal pain, heart burn, nausea, diarrhoea, epigastric pain, edema, fluid retention.
Idoxuridine (Antinausea)	Irritation; inflammation of the eye or eyelids; pain; photophobia; pruritus; conjunctivitis; oedema.
Ifosfamide (Antineoplastic)	Confusion, alopoecia, nausea, vomiting, phloebitis, somnolence, depression, hallucinations.
Imipenem (Antibiotic)	Skin rashes, urticaria, eosinophilia, fever, nausea, vomiting, diarrhoea, tooth or tongue discoloration .
Imipramine (Antidepressant)	Sinus tachycardia, AV/bundle-branch block, postural hypotension, dry mouth, wt loss/gain, constipation.
Indapamide (Antihypertensive)	Headache, dizziness, weakness, drowsiness, fatigue, agitation, nervousness, anorexia, nausea, vomiting, pain.
Indomethacin (NSAID agent)	Dyspepsia, nausea, abdominal pain, and diarrhea. Constipation, anorexia, flatulence, gastroenteritis,
Indoramin (Antihypertensive Drug)	Rash, pruritus, urticaria, dyspepsia, nausea, peptic ulcer disease, headache, dizziness, insomnia.
Interferon (Antiviral)	Depressive illness, suicidal behaviour, irritability, insomnia, anxiety. Flu-like symptoms. Headache,

Name of Drugs	Adverse Drug Reactions(ADR)
Interferon (Antiviral)	Flu-like symptoms; alopecia; hypersensitivity reactions; nausea; anorexia; myelosuppression;
Indoramin (Antiadrenegic)	Loss of judgement, emotional lability, visual impairment.
Insulin (Pancreatic Hormone)	Hypoglycaemia, insulin resistance, lipoatrophy, oedema; pruritus; rash.
Ipratropium (Antiasthamatic)	Dry mouth, urinary retention, buccal ulceration, paralytic ileus, headache, nausea, constipation.
Iprindole (AntiDepressant)	Hypersensitivity, dizziness, diarrhoea, nausea, vomiting, renal impairment, rash, erythema multiforme.
Iproniazid (Monoamine oxidase inhibitor)	Skin rash, urticaria; eosinophilia, diarrhoea, nausea, vomiting; phloebitis; hypoprothrombinaemia; superinfection.
Isocarboxazid (Monoamine oxidase inhibitor)	Vertigo; acute renal failure, interstitial nephritis, acute tubular necrosis; electrolyte imbalances, dizziness, diarrhoea, nausea, vomiting, renal impairment, rash.
Isoniazid (Antituberculars)	Peripheral neuritis, optic neuritis; psychotic reactions, convulsions, nausea, vomiting, fatigue, epigastric distress.
Isoprenaline (Antiasthamatic)	Nervousness, restlessness, insomnia, anxiety, tension, blurring of vision, fear, excitement.
Isosorbide dinitrate (Antianginal)	Hypotension, tachycardia, flushing, headache, dizziness, palpitation, syncope, confusion. Nausea, vomiting.
Isosorbide mononitrate (Antianginal)	Hypotension, tachycardia, flushing, headache, dizziness, palpitation, syncope, confusion. Nausea,
Isoxsuprine (Peripheral Vasodilator)	Hypotension, dizziness, palpitation, nausea, vomiting, abdominal distress, severe rash, flushing, tachycardia.
Isotretinoin (Anti acne agent)	Dryness of mucous membranes, dryness of skin with scaling, fragility, erythema, cheilitis, pruritus,
Isradipine (Calcium antagonist)	Dizziness; flushing; headache; hypotension; peripheral oedema; tachycardia; palpitations; GI disturbances.
Itraconazole (Antifungal)	Dyspepsia, abdominal pain, nausea, vomiting, diarrhoea; menstrual disorders; constipation, rash, pruritus.
Kanamycin (Antibacterial)	Pain, inflammation, bruising, haematoma at inj site; GI disturbances; malabsorption of fat, , loose feces
Ketamine (Anaesthetics)	severe confusion, hallucinations, unusual thoughts, extreme fear, Less serious side effects may include,
Ketanserin (Antihypertensive)	Sedation, fatigue, lightheadedness, dizziness, headache, dry mouth, GI disturbances, oedema
Ketazolam (Anticonvulsant)	Diarrhoea, depression, sedation, hyperacusis, rebound insomnia, tension, photophobia, severe anxiety,
Ketoconazole (Antifungal)	GI disturbances e.g. nausea and vomiting; rash, dermatitis, burning sensation, pruritus; headache, dizziness, allergic reactions.
Ketoprofen (NSAIDs)	HTN; GI symptoms e.g. dyspepsia, discomfort, nausea, diarrhoea; pain and tissue damage at inj site (IM).
Ketorolac (Analgesic & antipyretic)	Swelling of face, fingers, lower legs, ankles, feet, weight gain, Bruising, high blood pressure, skin rash or itching.
Labetalol (Antihypertensive)	Orthostatic hypotension, dizziness, fatigue, vertigo, paraesthesia, headache, nasal stuffiness, dyspnoea, diarrhea.
Lanatoside C (Cardiovascular agent)	Nausea, vomiting, anorexia, diarrhoea, abdominal pain, headache, facial pain, fatigue, weakness, dizziness.
Latamoxef (Antibiotic)	Hypoprothrombinaemia, serious bleeding episodes, fever, pain at inj site, diarrhoea, cutaneous eruption.

Name of Drugs	Adverse Drug Reactions(ADR)
Leucovorin (Antineoplastics)	Allergic sensitization, including anaphylactoid reactions, urticaria, GI toxicity, seizures, syncope, hypersensitivity.
Levallorphan (Opoid Antidote)	Respiratory depression, apnea, rigidity, and bradycardia, respiratory arrest, circulatory depression,
Levamisole (Anthelmintic)	Nausea, vomiting, diarrhoea, abdominal pain, dizziness and headache, fever, influenza-like syndrome, arthralgia.
Levobunolol (Antiglucoma)	Ocular stinging, burning, blepharoconjunctivitis, decreased heart rate, decreased BP, iridocyclitis, headache.
Levodopa (Antirigidity/antitremor)	Abnormal thinking, agitation, anxiety, clenching or grinding of teeth, clumsiness or unsteadiness,
Levorphanol (Analgesic)	Nausea, vomiting, constipation, dizziness, headache, fatigue, dry mouth, sweating, and itching, allergic reaction.
Levonorgestre (Progestin agent)	Menstrual irregularities; headache, dizziness; breast discomfort; gynaecomastia; depression.
Lidoflazine (Antianginal)	
Lignocain (Anaesthetics)	Flushing, redness of the skin, small red or purple spots on the skin, swelling at the site of application.
Lincornycm (Antibacterial)	Hypotension (IV); vertigo; dermatitis, erythema multiforme, rash, urticaria; colitis, diarrhoea, glossitis, nausea
Liothyroine (Thiroid agent)	Arm, back or jaw pain, changes in appetite, chest pain, chest tightness, cold clammy skin, confusion, diarrhea,
Lisinopril1 (Antihypertensive)	KIdney disease, liver disease, heart disease or congestive heart failure, diabetes, Marfan syndrome,
Lisuride (Misc. Drug)	Confusion, drowsiness, delirium, memory disturbance, visual hallucination
Lithium (Antidepressant)	Heart disease, kidney disease, underactive thyroid, hyponatremia.
Lodoqumol (STD agent)	
Lofepramine (Anti depressant)	Hypotension, cardiac arrhythmias, convulsion, coma, urinary retension, palpitations, metabolic acidosis,
Lomefloxacin (Antibacterial)	Nausea, abdominal pain or discomfort, diarrhoea; headache, dizziness, insomnia; rash, pruritus, photosensitivity.
Loperamide (Antidiarrhoeal)	Bloating, constipation, loss of appetite, stomach pain, nausea and vomiting, skin rash.
Loracarbef (Antibiotic)	Diarrhoea, nausea, vomiting, abdominal pain; headache; skin rashes; abnormalities in haematological parameters.
Loratidine (Antiallergic)	Diarrhea, epistaxis, pharyngitis, flu-like symptoms, fatigue, stomatitis, tooth disorder, Headache, somnolence, fatigue, dry mouth.
Lorazepam (Sedative)	Drowsiness, relaxed, calm, sleepiness, abdominal pain, aggressive, angry, agitation, anxiety, attack, assault, or force, black, tarry stools.
Lorcainide (Antiarrythmic)	
Lormustine (Antineoplastic)	Ulmonary infiltrates pulmonary fibrosis, nausea, vomiting, hepatotoxicity, nephrotoxicity, stomatitis, alopecia.
Lornoxicam (Antiinflammatory)	Abdominal pain, diarrhoea, dizziness, dyspepsia, nausea, vomiting; headache, haematologic disorders.
Lovastatin (Lipid lowering agent)	Bladder pain, cloudy urine, chest tightness, cough, painful urination, difficulty with moving, fever, headache, joint pain.
Lymecycline (Antiinflammatory)	GI disturbances, hypersensitivity & photosensitivity

Name of Drugs	Adverse Drug Reactions(ADR)
Lysergide (Recreational Drug)	
Maprotiline (Antidepressants)	Vomiting, epigastric distress, diarrhea, bitter taste, tingling, motor hyperactivity, akathisia, seizures, restlessness, nightmares, hypomania.
Mazindol (Monoarnine oxidase inhibitor)	Nervousness, agitation, dizziness, drowsiness, depression, psychosis, vertigo, insomnia, dryness of mouth.
Mebendazole (Anthelmintics)	Nausea, vomiting, diarrhea, and abdominal pain, Rash, pruritus, urticaria.
Mecamyramine (Anti Hypertention)	Nausea, vomiting, anorexia, glossitis, and dryness of mouth, dizziness, postural hypotension, convulsions, choreiform movements, tremor.
Mecillinam (Antibiotic)	Hypersensitivity reactions including angioedema, urticaria, rash, serum sickness-like reactions, haemolytic anemia.
Meclizine (Antihistamine, H1 antagonist)	Drowsiness, dry mouth, blurred vision.
Medazepam (Anxiolytic)	Fatigue, drowsiness, dizziness, prolonged reaction time, headache, coordination disorders, confusion.
Medifoxamine (Antidepressant)	Hypertension, hypotension, hyperprolactinaemia leading to galactorrhea, constipation, depression, headache.
Medigoxin (Cardiac glycoxide)	Extra beats, anorexia, nausea and vomiting. Diarrhoea in elderly, confusion, dizziness, drowsiness, restlessness
Medroxy-progesterone (Gonadai Hormone)	Depression, fluid retention, fatigue, insomnia, dizziness, headache, nausea, breast tenderness, wt gain/loss.
Mefenamic acid (Analgesic, antipyretic)	Abdominal pain, dyspepsia, constipation, diarrhoea, nausea, GI ulcers, oedema, bronchospasm, headache.
Mefloquin (Antimalanal)	Dizziness, myalgia, nausea, fever, headache, vomiting, chills, diarrhea, skin rash, abdominal pain, fatigue
Mefruside (Diuretic)	Electrolyte imbalance, hyperglycaemi,; gout, dry mouth, thirst, weakness, muscle pain and cramp, seizures.
Mepacrine (Anti Protozoal Drug)	Dizziness, headache; nausea, vomiting, reversible yellow discolouration of the skin, conjunctiva.
Meperidine (Narcotic analgesic)	Weakness, headache, disorientation, respiratory depression, delirium, seizures, tremors, dizziness,
Melphalan (Antineoplastic)	Diarrhoea, stomatitis, vomiting; haemolytic anaemia, vasculitis, pulmonary fibrosis, hepatic disorders.
Mepacrine (Antimalarial)	Dizziness, headache; nausea, vomiting; reversible yellow discolouration of the skin, conjunctiva, psychosis, CNS stimulation, convulsions.
Mepenzolate (Antispasmodic)	Dizziness, drowsiness, headache, weakness, nausea, vomiting, constipation, bloatedness, weakness, loss of taste.
Mepivacaine (Anaesthetic)	Hives, itching, skin redness, nausea, sweating, feeling hot, fast heartbeats, sneezing, difficult breathing,
Meprobamate (Hypnotic)	Drowsiness, blurred vision, diarrhea, dizziness, false sense of well-being, headache, nausea, vomiting, unusual tiredness, weakness.
Meptazinol (Analgesic)	Nausea, vomiting, constipation, diarrhoea, stomach pains, indigestion, dizziness, vertigo, drowsiness,
Mercaptopurine (Antineoplastic)	Nausea, vomiting, anorexia, diarrhea, skin rashes, alopecia, and hyperpigmentation.
Mesalazine (Antiinflammatory)	Abdominal pain, eructation, nausea, diarrhea, dyspepsia, ulcerative colitis, vomiting, constipation,
Metaraminol (Cardiovascular agent)	Apprehension, anxiety, restlessness, tremor, weakness, faintness, dizziness, headache, precordial pain.

Name of Drugs	Adverse Drug Reactions(ADR)
Metformin (Oral antidiabeticl)	Vomiting, abdominal pain, nausea, dyspnea, hypothermia, hypotension, and bradycardia, flatulence, abdominal pain.
Methadone (Respiratory agent)	Confusion, disorientation, dysphoria, euphoria, seizures, sleepiness or insomnia, and dizziness, confusion.
Methaqualone (Hypnotic)	Dizziness, nausea, vomiting, diarrhea, abdominal cramps, fatigue, itching, rashes, sweating, dry mouth, headache, insomnia, tremors.
Methicillin (Antibiotic)	Neutropenia, leukopenia, thrombocytopenia, rash, eosinophilia, pruritus, fever, chills, and myalgias, pain at injection site.
Methimazole (Anti thyroid drug)	Stomach upset, nausea, vomiting, mild rash, headache, drowsiness, dizziness, nausea, vomiting, or stomach upset, itching, minor skin rash.
Methocarbamol (Muscle Relaxant)	Diarrhea, difficulty swallowing, dizziness, fast heartbeat, feeling of warmth, fever, headache, itching, joint or muscle pain.
Methohexitone (Anaesthetic)	Gangrene, Thrombosis, Bronchospasm, Cardiovascular collapse, Local pain.
Methotrexate (Antineoplastic)	Nausea, vomiting, diarrhea, pharyngitis, stomatitis, anorexia, hematemesis, melena, gastrointestinal ulceration and bleeding, enteritis.
Methoxamine (Anti Hypotensive Drug)	Excessive BP elevations particularly with high dosage, ventricular ectopic beats, reflex bradycardia nausea.
Methotrimeprazine (Antipsychotic)	Drowsiness, dry mouth or constipation, dry mouth, skin rash.
Methylamphetamine (CNS Stimulation)	Dry mouth, unpleasant taste, diarrhea, constipation, anorexia, weight loss, restlessness, dizziness, insomnia, euphoria, dyskinesia, dysphoria, tremor, and headache.
Methyldopa (Antihypertensive)	Slow heart rate, yellowed skin, fever, confusion or weakness, nausea, upper stomach pain, itching,
Methylphenobarbitone (Barbiturates)	Dizziness, clumsiness, sleepiness, staggering walk, drowsiness, vomiting, tiredness, nausea,
Methylprednisolone (Corticosteroid)	Hypokalemia, ulceration, insomnia to nervousness, restlessness, mania, catatonia, depression, delusions, hallucinations, violent behavior.
Methyltestosterone (Hormone)	Oedema, headache, anxiety, depression; acne, male-pattern baldness, seborrhoea; hypercalcaemia.
Methyprylone (Sedative)	Skin rash, fever, depression, ulcer or sores in mouth, respiration depression, double vision etc.
Methysergide (Analgesic)	Malaise, fatigue, weight loss, backache, low grade fever, urinary obstruction, dyspnea, tightness, pain in the chest, insomnia, drowsiness.
Metoclopramide (Prokinetic)	Extrapyramidal symptoms, restlessness, drowsiness, anxiety, diarrhoea, hypotension, hypertension, headache.
Metocurine (Muscle relaxant)	Release histamine, has cardiovascular side effects.
Metolazone (Diuretic)	Chest pain, palpitation, necrotising angiitis, orthostatic hypotension, syncope, venous thrombosis, vertigo.
Metoprolol (Antihypertensive)	Asthma, COPD, sleep apnea, liver disease, congestive heart failure, problems with circulation, thyroid disorder, pheochromocytoma.
Metronidazole (Antibacterial/ antifungal)	Convulsive seizures, encephalopathy, aseptic meningitis, Headache, dizziness, omiting, abdominal discomfort.
Mexiletine (Antiarrythmatic)	Dysphagia, salivary changes, altered taste, changes in oral mucosa, hiccups, peptic ulcer disease, tremor, dizziness, and difficulties with coordination.
Mezlocillin (Antibiotic)	Diarrhoea, nausea, vomiting, pseudomembranous enterocolitis, hypersensitivity *reactions*
Mianserin (Antidepressant)	Drowsiness, liver dysfunction and jaundice, gynaecomastia; convulsions, hypomania, hypotension, hypertension.
Miconazole (Antibacterial/ antifungal)	Oral discomfort, oral pain, dry mouth, glossodynia, loss of taste, altered taste, tongue ulceration, mouth ulceration, tooth disorder

Name of Drugs	Adverse Drug Reactions(ADR)
Midazolam (Anxiolytic)	Nausea, vomiting, and hiccups, alterations in blood pressure, arrhythmias, ventricular irritability.
Midodrine (Antihypertensive)	Cardiac awareness, pounding in the ears, headache, and blurred vision, dizziness, skin hyperesthesia, insomnia.
Milrinone (Inotropic agent)	Ventricular arrhythmias, sustained and nonsustained ventricular tachycardia, ventricular & arterial fibrillation, headaches, tremor, dizziness.
Mifepristone (Anti pregesterone)	Uterine cramping, uterine hemorrhage, vaginitis, leukorrhea, pelvic pain, abdominal pain, nausea, vomiting, diarrhea, dyspepsia.
Minocycline (Antibacterials)	Liver disease, kidney disease, asthma, sulfite allergy.
Minoxidil (For hair growth)	Sinus tachycardia, provocation of angina, edema, weight gain, nausea and vomiting, contact dermatitis, desquamative, bullous rashes.
Misonidazole (For radiation therapy)	Neurotoxicity, hypertension
Misopristol (PGE$_1$ agonsit)	Diarrhoea, abdominal pain, dyspepsia, constipation, flatulence, nausea, vomiting, abnormal vaginal bleeding.
Mitomycin (Antineoplastic)	Hemolytic-uremic syndrome, microangiopathic hemolytic anemia, nephropathy, marrow depression.
Mitotane (Antineoplastic)	Anorexia, nausea, vomiting, diarrhea, hypersialorrhea, dizziness, vertigo, weakness, muscle tremors, headache.
Mitoxantrone (Antineoplastic)	Arrhythmia, oedema, ECG changes, pain, fatigue, fever, headache; alopecia, nail bed changes, amenorrhoea.
Moclobemide (Monoamine oxidase inhibitor)	Tachycardia, hypotension, dizziness, headache, drowsiness, sleep disturbances, agitation, nervousness, sedation.
Molindone (Antipsychotic)	Orthostatic hypotension, tachycardia, arrhythmia; extrapyramidal *reactions*, mental depression.
Monosialoganglioside (Transferase enzyme)	
Moricizine (Antiarrythemic)	Atrial and ventricular arrhythmias, heart failure, hypotension, syncope, vomiting or diarrhea, abdominal discomfort, anxiety, fatigue.
Morphine (Analgesic)	Convulsions, nausea, vomiting, dry mouth, constipation, urinary retention, headache, vertigo, palpitations
Moxalactam (Antibiotic)	Vomiting, headache, dizziness, oral vaginal candidiasis, pseudomembranous colitis,
Mustine (Antineoplastic)	Nausea and vomiting are dose-limiting. Anorexia and diarrhea have also been reported. Hypersensitivity side effects, cardiac irregularities.
Nabilone (Antinausea)	Nasal congestion and irritation; conjunctival irritation
Nabumetone (NSAID)	Drowsiness, insomnia; reduced sexual ability; bradycardia, palpitation, oedema, CHF, reduced peripheral.
Nadolol (β_1-adrenoreceptor antagonist)	Hypersensitivity reactions, local reactions, renal, hepatic, or nervous system effects with high dosage.
Nafcillin (Antibiotic)	Nausea and epigastric pain, rash, hepatitis or hepatic failure, hearing loss.
Naftidrofuryl (Cerebral vasodialator)	Chest pain, difficult breathing, difficulty swallowing, fainting, fast, pounding, irregular heartbeat,
Nalbuphine (Analgesic)	Sedation, dizziness, vertigo, miosis, headache; nausea, vomiting, dry mouth; itching, burning, urticaria.
Nalidixic acid (Antibacterial)	Nausea, vomiting, diarrhoea, abdominal pain; photosensitivity reactions, allergic rash, urticaria, pruritus; visual disturbances.
Nalorphine (Opioid Antagonist)	Drowsiness, respiratory depression, miosis, dysphoria, lethargy.
Naloxone (Opioid Antagonist)	Stomach cramps, body aches, convulsions, diarrhea, difficult breathing, excessive crying, fast, pounding, irregular heartbeat, fever.

Name of Drugs	Adverse Drug Reactions(ADR)
Naltrexone (Opioid Antagonist)	Abdominal pain, nausea, vomiting; anxiety, insomnia, lethargy, headache, musculoskeletal pain; anorexi.
Naproxen (NSAID)	Belching, bruising, difficult breathing, headache, itching skin, large, flat, blue, purplish patches in the skin, shortness of breath, skin eruptions, stomach pain.
Natamycin (Antiinfective)	Allergic reaction, change in vision, chest pain, corneal opacity, dyspnea, eye discomfort, eye edema, eye hyperemia, eye irritation, eye pain, foreign body sensation, paresthesia, and tearing.
Nefopam (Analgesic, antipyretic)	Nausea, vomiting, sweating, drowsiness, insomnia, urinary retention, dizziness, hypotension, tremor, paraesthesia
Neomycin (Antibacterial)	Any loss of hearing, clumsiness, diarrhea, difficulty in breathing, dizziness, drowsiness, decreased frequency urine, increased amount of gas, increased thirst.
Neostigmine (Neuromuscular agent)	Twitches of the muscle visible under the skin, blurred vision, changes speech, chest pain, confusion, cough, difficult breathing, and difficulty in moving.
Netilmicin (Antibacterial)	Headache, malaise, visual disturbances, disorientation, tachycardia, hypotension, palpitations, thrombocytosis,
Nicardipine (Calcium antagonist)	Dizziness, flushing, headache, hypotension, peripheral oedema, tachycardia, palpitations, nausea, dyspepsia, dry mouth.
Nicitinic acid (Anticoagulant)	Darkening of urine, light gray-colored stools, loss of appetite, severe stomach pain, yellow eyes or skin.
Nicotine (Para sympathomimetic)	Headache, cold and flu-like symptoms; insomnia; nausea; myalgia and dizziness; palpitations; dyspepsia, hiccups
Nicoumalone (Anticoagulant)	
Nifedipine (Antihypertensive)	Bloating or swelling of the face, arms, hands, lower legs, cough, difficult breathing, dizziness,
Nilvadipine (Calcium antagonist)	Headache, peripheral oedema, dizziness, fatigue, Jaundice, Confusion, Dyspepsia, Anxiety, Chest pain.
Nimodipine (Cardiovascular agent)	Cirrhosis or other liver disease, heart disease, high or low blood pressure.
Nisoldipine (Calcium channel blocker)	Dizziness, headache, peripheral oedema, palpitations, pharyngitis, vasodilatation, sinusitis, chest pain, nausea
Nitrazepam (Hypnotic)	Hypotension, palpitation; agitation, aggressiveness, amnesia, ataxia, confusion, delusions, disorientation
Nitrendipine (Antihypertensive)	Hypotension, flushing, oedema, dizziness, palpitation, fatigue, headache, nausea, bloating, diarrhoea
Nitrofurantoin (Antibacterial)	Changes in facial skin color, chest pain, chills, cough, fever, hives, hoarseness, itching.
Nitroglycerine (Vasodilator)	Bloating or swelling of the face, arms, hands, lower legs, or feet, difficult breathing, feeling faint, dizzy, lightheadedness, feeling of warmth or heat, headache.
Nizatidine (Antiulcer)	Headache, dizziness.
Noradrenaline (Sympathom imetic)	Hypertension, headache, peripheral ischaemia, bradycardia, arrhythmias, anxiety, skin necrosis.
Northiondrone (Hormone)	Menstrual abnormalities, amenorrhea, frequent, irregular, prolonged, or infrequent bleeding, nausea, weight changes, breast changes, headache.
Norethisterone (Gonadal Hormone)	Mental depression, cholestatic jaundice, porphyria, epilepsy, migraine, headache, breast discomfort, dizziness
Norfloxacin (Antibacterial)	Nausea, vomiting, heartburn, constipation, diarrhoea, abdominal cramping, anorexia; headache, dizziness
Nortriptyline (Antidepressant)	Abdominal pain, agitation, anxiety, black, tarry stools, bleeding gums, blood in the urine or stools, blurred vision.

Name of Drugs	Adverse Drug Reactions(ADR)
Noscapine (Antitussive, Expectorant)	Loss of coordination, hallucinations , loss of sexual drive, swelling of prostate, loss of appetite, dilated pupils, increased heart rate, chest pains.
Novobiocin (Antibiotic)	Nausea, diarrhoea, vomiting, irritation or soreness of the mouth or rectal area; dyspnoea, eosinophilia
Nystatin (Antifungal)	Diarrhoea, GI distress, nausea and vomiting. vaginal pessaries/cream: May damage latex contraceptives
Octretide (Growth Hormone inhibitor)	Gallbladder abnormalities, diarrhea, loose stools, nausea and abdominal discomfort, sinus bradycardia,
Oestradiol (Hormone)	Allergic reaction, difficulty breathing, swelling face, lips, tongue, or throat, vaginal bleeding, chest pain,
Ofloxacin (Antibacterial)	Nausea, vomiting, abdominal pain, diarrhea, headache dizziness, insomnia, hallucination, leucopenis, eosinophilla.
Omeprazole (Proton Pump inhibitor)	Diarrhea, nausea, fatigue, constipation, vomiting, flatulence, acid regurgitation, taste prevention, arthralgia, myalgia, urticaria, dizziness.
Ondansetron (Antiemetic, antinauseant)	Headache, fatigue, constipation, drowsiness, fever, dizziness, anxiety, cold sensation, pruritus, rash, diarrhea.
Orciprenaline (Antiasthamatic)	Tachycardia, nervousness, increased serum glucose, increased potassium levels, tremor, palpitation, headache.
Ornidazole (Antibacterial)	Somnolence, headache nausea, vomiting, dizziness, tramor, rigidity, poor co coordination, tiredness, vertigo, skin reactions.,
Orphenadrine (Antirigidity, antitremor)	chest pain, chills, cough, fever, hallucinations, headache, shortness of breath, troubled breathing, tightness in chest, skin rash, hives, itching, redness, sores, ulcers mouth.
Ouabain (Cardiac glycoside)	Nausea and vomiting pulse irregularities.
Oxacillin (Antibiotic)	Nausea ,vomiting, diarrhea, gastrointestinal irritation, neutropenia, leukopenia, thrombocytopenia, bone marrow depression, hypersensitivity reactions
Oxamniquine (Anthelmintic)	Allergic reaction, seizures, headache, dizziness, drowsiness, abdominal pain, decreased appetite, vomiting.
Oxaprozin (NSAID)	Skin rash, Bloating, bloody or black, burning upper abdominal pain, cloudy urine, constipation, itching skin, loss of appetite, nausea or vomiting, pale skin
Oxazepam (Anxiolytic, sedative)	Cyncope, oedema, drowsiness, ataxia, dizziness, vertigo, memory impairment, headache, lethargy, amnesia, rash, euphoria.
Oxprenolol (β-adrenoreceptor antagonist)	Pulmonary oedema, postural hypotension, Prolonged PR interval, sinus arrest, palpitation, chest pain, hot flashes, syncove, vertigo.
Oxybutynin (Anticholinerigic)	Dry mouth, constipation, nausea, abdominal pain, blurred vision, headache, dizziness, drowsiness, diarrhea, insomnia.
Oxypentifylline (Antiulcer)	Nausea, vomiting, dizziness, headache, flushing; angina, palpitations; occasional cardiac arrhythmias; hepatitis
Oxyphenbutazone (NSAID)	Weakness, Headache, Drowsiness, Irritability, Diarrhea, Heart burn, Brushing, Weight loss, Loss of appetite.
Oxytetracycline (Antibacterial)	Anorexia, nausea, vomiting, diarrhea, glssistis, dysphagia, photosensitivity, oesphageal irration & ulceration, nephrotoxicity.
Paclitaxel (Antineoplastic)	Neutropenia, leucopenia, thrombocytopenia, anemia, bleeding, hypersensitivity reactions, bradycardia, abnormal ECG, nausea vomiting.
Pafenolol (Antihypertensive)	Orthostatic hypotension, dizziness, fatigue, vertigo, paraesthesia, headache, nasal stuffiness, dyspnoea, diarrhea.
Pamidronate (Nutritional supplement)	Anorexia, dyspepsia, nausea, abdominal pain, vomiting, metastates, fatigue, arthralgia, myelgia,
Pancuronium (Neuromuscular blocker)	Tachycardia, induce miosis, excessive salivation, rashes, itchiness, wheezing, BP increased, cardiac output increased,

Name of Drugs	Adverse Drug Reactions(ADR)
Papaverine (Anti Spasmodic)	Allergic reaction, low fever, nausea, stomach pain, loss of appetite, dark urine, clay-colored stools, jaundice, warmth, redness, or tingly feeling in your face, swelling, pain.
Paracetamol (Analgesic, antipyretic)	Nausea, allergic reaction, skin rashes, acute renal tubular necrosis, blood dyscrasias, lever damage.
Paraldehyde (Antiepileptic)	Coughing, skin rash, redness, swelling, pain at injection site, yellow eyes or skin, cloudy urine, confusion, decreased urination, muscle tremors, restlessness, irritability.
Pargyline (MAO inhibitor)	Vertigo, Muscle twitching, Blurred vision, Dizziness, Headache, Vomiting, Fever, Insomnia, and Sweating.
Paroxetine (Anti depressant)	Insomnia, headache, dizziness, decreased libido, nausea, xerostomia, constipation, diarrhea, weakness, tramor.
PAS (Antituberculosis)	
Pefloxacin (Antibacterial)	Nausea, vomiting gastric pain, dizziness, insomnia, allergic skin reaction, thrombocytopenia, leukopenis, photosensation.
Pelrinone (PDE inhibitor)	headache, tremors, easy bruising or bleeding, chest pain, bronchospasm, low potassium, eadache; tremors
Pemoline (Monoamine oxidase inhibitor)	insomnia, nervousness, headache, drowsiness, weight loss, nausea, vomiting, abdominal pain,
Penbutolol (β-adrenoreceptor antagonist)	headache, fatigue, dizziness, nausea, uneven heartbeats;
Penicillamine (Antigout)	Nausea, anorexia, vomiting, oral ulceration, stomatitis, fever and skin reaction, loss of test, thrombocytopenia, neutropenis.
Pentaerythritoltn (Antianginal)	Cardiovascular: Flushing, postural hypotension, headache, lightheadedness, dizziness, neuromuscular & skeletal weakness, Drug rash, exfoliative dermatitis.
Pentamidine (Antimicrobial)	Headache, disorientation, hallucinations, dizziness, confusion, fatigue, neuralgia, chest pain, ECG abnormalities, syncope, vasodilation, vasculitis, phlebitis, hypertension, palpitations, arrhythmias, severe hypotension, pharyngitis
Pentazocine (Analgesic, antipyretic)	Physical dependence, sedation, dizziness, euphoria, alteration of mood, resp depression, visual hallucination, disorientation, confusion.
Pentobarbitone (Sedative)	Residual sedation, drowsiness, lethargy, vertigo, nausea, vomiting, headache, Behavioral problems, impaired memory, tics, dyskinesias, nystagmus.
Pentoxifylline (Peripheral vasodilator)	Nausea, vomiting, dizziness, headache, flushing, angina, palpitation, jaundice, blood dyscrasias reported, agitation, sleep disturbances.
Pergolide (Misc. agent)	Anxiety, bloody or cloudy urine, confusion, difficult or painful urination, frequent urge to urinate, hallucinations uncontrolled movements of the body,
Pencyazine (Antipsychotic)	Drowsiness, dizziness, dry mouth, nausea, vomiting, constipation, diarrhea, uncontrolled muscle movements, patches on skin, weight gain, decreased libido.
Permdopril (Anti hypertensive)	Hypertension, cough, headache, asthenia and dizziness, back pain
Perphenazine (Antipsychotic)	Hanges in BP, orthostatic hypotension, changes in heart rate, dizziness; extrapyramidal symptoms, dizziness.
Pethidine (Analgesic)	Hypotension; fatigue, drowsiness, dizziness, nervousness, headache,
Phenathicillin (Antibiotic)	Nausea, vomiting, dizziness, headache, flushing; angina, palpitations; occasional cardiac arrhythmias; hepatitis
Phenelzine (MAO inhibitor)	Dizziness, dry mouth, headache, lethargy, sedation, insomnia, anorexia, weight gain, nausea, vomiting, diarrhea, tramor, hyperthermia, sweting.
Phenformin (Oral antidiabetic)	Metallic taste, wt loss, skin *reactions*, acute pancreatitis, Lactic acidosis, CV adverse effects

Name of Drugs	Adverse Drug Reactions(ADR)
Phenindamine (Respiratory agent)	Drowsiness, dizziness, headache, loss of appetite, stomach upset, visual disturbances, irritability, dry mouth.
Phenindione (Anticoagulant)	Haemorrhage. Skin rash, pyrexia, diarrhoea, vomiting, and sore throat. Rarely, skin necrosis.
Pheniramine (Antiallergics)	Oral sedation, hypersensitivity reaction, lassitude, dizziness, tinnitus, inability to concentrate, incoordination, irritability, insomnia, trammors.
Phenobarbitone (Anticonvulsant)	Brabycardia, hypotension, drowsiness, lethargy, CNS excitation or depression, impaired judgment, hangover effect.
Phenoxy-Mepenicillin (Antibiotic)	Nasal congestion, slight GI irritation, miosis, postural hypotension with dizziness, fatigue.
Phentermine (Monoamine oxidase inhibitor)	Reduced-calorie diet, behavior change, lose weight, overweight, heart disease, diabetes, high blood pressure.
Phenylbutazone (Antiinflammatory)	Tachycardia, hypotension, myocarditis, atrial fibrillation, atrial flutter, angina, CHF, myocardial depression.
Phenylethyl-malonamide	Drowsiness, ataxia; nausea, vomiting, hepatic.
Phenylephrine (Mydriatic / cycloplegic)	Anxiety, reflex bradycardia, tachycardia, arrhythmias, headache, cold extrimetis, hypertension, nausea, vomiting, fever, weakness, sweting.
Phenylpro-panolamine (Anticonvulsant)	Hypertension, epilepticseizures, hallucinations, dizziness, headache, nausea, palpitation.
Phenytoin (Antiepileptic)	Hypersensitivity, lack of appetite, headache, dizziness, tremor, insomnia, GI disturbances, acne, hirsutism.
Pholcodine (Respiratory agent)	Dizziness, occasional drowsiness, nausea, vomiting, constipation, rash, sputum retention, excitation, confusion,
Physostigmine (AChE inhibitor)	heart failure, high or low blood pressure, ever had a heart attack, asthma, a stomach ulcer or stomach spasms, Epilepsy, hyperthyroidism, parkinson's disease.
Pimozide (Antipsychotic)	Extra pyramidal reaction, insomnia, drowsiness, dizziness, ECG changes, dry mouth, constipation, urinary difficulty.
Pinacidil (Antihypertensive)	Tachycardia, palpitation, edema, dizziness, headache, nausea, palpitation, tachycardia, rashes, increased intracranial pressure.
Pindolol (β-adrenoreceptor antagonist)	Bradycardia, hypotension, peripheral oedema, heart failure, bronco spasm, fatigue, dizziness, insomnia, dizzarre dreams.
Pipecuronium (Neuromuscular Blocker)	Transient hypotension, bradycardia,
Piperacillin (Antibiotic)	GI disturbances, hypersensitivity reactions, eosinophillia, hyponatraemia, hypokalaemia, inj site related reaction like painerythema & induration.
Piperazine (Anthelmintic)	Nausea, vomiting, colic, abdominal pain, diarrhea, urticaria, skin rashes, headache, bronchospasm, dizziness, mystagmus.
Pipothiazine (Antipsychotic)	Dyskinesia, leucopenia, agranulocytosis, hypothermia, leucocytosis, cardiovascular symptoms, extrapyramidal effects, haemolytic anemia.
Pipothiazine (Antipsychotic)	Parkinsonian symptoms, dystonia, akathisia, tardive dyskinesia. Interference with temp regulation.
Piracetam (Cognitive enhancer)	Hyperkinesia, nervousness, depression, diarrhoea, rashes. CNS stimulation, sleep disturbances, dizziness.
Pirbuterol (Cerebral activator)	Headache, dizziness, lightheadedness, insomnia, tremor or nervousness, sweating, nausea, vomiting, or diarrhea, or dry mouth, allergic reaction.
Pirenzepine (Antimuscarinic)	Dry mouth, blurred vision, drowsiness, dizziness, nausea, heartburn, diarrhea, constipation, bitter taste, decreased sexual ability or desire, bad breath

Name of Drugs	Adverse Drug Reactions(ADR)
Piretanide (Diuretic)	Thrombocytopenia, ototoxicity, hypotension, dehydration, leucopenia, hyponatremia, urinary retention, gout, cardiac arrhythmia, renal failure, hypotension.
Piroxicam (NSAID)	GI disturbances, peptic ulcer, GI bleeding, headache, dizziness, blurred vision, tinnitus, skin rashes &pruritus.
Pirprofen (Antiinflammatory)	GI disturbances, peptic ulcer, headache, dizziness, blurred vision, tinnitus, skin rashes and pruritus.
Pivampicillin (Antibiotic)	Hypersensitivity *reactions* including urticaria; fever; joint pains; rashes; angioedema; serum sickness-like *reactions*
Pivmecillinam (Antibiotic)	Hypersensitivity *reactions* including uticaria; fever; joint pains; rashes; angioedema; serum sickness-like *reactions,* gastrointestinal disturbances.
Pizotifen (Analgesic)	Sedation, dry mouth, drowsiness, increased appetite and weight gain. CNS depression; headache, psychomotor impairment, antimuscarinic *effects*; GI disturbances.
Polymixin B (Antibacterial)	Dizziness, paraesthesia, muscle weakens, atexia, confusion, drowsiness, psuchoses, convulsion, coma, neuromuscular block.
Polythiazide (Diuretic)	Abdominal or stomach pain, black, tarry stools, bleeding, gums, bloating, blood in urine or stools,
Practolol (β-adrenoreceptor antagonist)	Bronchoconstriction, cardiac failure, cold extremities, fatigue and depression, hypoglycaemia, oculomucocutaneous syndrome.
Pravastain (Hypolipidemic agent)	GI symptoms, headache, insomnia, chest pain, rash, fatigue, dizziness, myalgia, hypersensitivity, anaphylaxis, angioedema.
Prazepam (Hypnotic)	Drowsiness, sedation, muscle weakness and ataxia; less frequently vertigo, headache, confusion, depression.
Praziquantel (Anthelmintic)	Headache, drowsiness, dizziness, malasia, abdominal discomfort, nausea vomiting, diarrhea, rashes, urticaria.
Prazosin (Antihypertensive)	Postural hypotension, syncope, palpitation, lack of energy, nausea, oedema, chest pain, dyspnoea, constipation, vomiting.
Prednisolone (Cortico steroid)	Cushing's syndrome, & growth, retardation in childn; osteoporosis, fractures, peptic ulceration; glaucoma cataracts, hyperglycemia, pancreatitis.
Prednisone (Corticosteroid)	Insomnia, nervousness, increased appetite, indigestion, dizziness, headache, hirsutism
Prenalterol (Cerebral vasodialator)	
Prenyleamine (Calcium channel blocker)	Liver damage, parkinson's disease
Primaquine (Antimalarial)	Nausea, vomiting, epigastria distress, abdominal cramps, leucopenia, leucocytosis, agranulocytosis, haemolytic anemia, thrombocytopaenia.
Primidone (Anticonvulsant)	Drowsiness, ataxia, nausea, vomiting, visual disturbances, rashes, nystagmus, vertigo, hypersensitivity.
Prilocaine (Local Anesthetic)	Methemoglobinaemia; cyanosis, restlessness, excitement, nervousness, paraesthesias, dizziness, tinnitus, blurred vision.
Probenecid (Antigout drug)	Mild nausea, vomiting, stomach pain, loss of appetite, headache, dizziness, hair loss, warmth or tingly feeling.
Procaine (Local Anesthetic)	GI upsets; diarrhoea; flatulence; abdominal pain; nausea; vomiting. Hypersensitivity *reactions*
Procarbazine (Antincoplastic)	Severe hypotension, ventricular fibrillation and asystole with rapid IV admin. *Drug*-induced SLE syndrome.
Prochlorperazine (Antiemetic, antinauseants)	Allergic reaction, chest pain or slow or irregular heartbeats, dizziness, drowsiness, anxiety, nausea or vomiting, seizures.

Name of Drugs	Adverse Drug Reactions(ADR)
Procyclidine (Antirigidity, antitremor)	GI disturbances, anorexia, nausea and vomiting; bone marrow depression; leukopenia and thrombocytopaenia
Progabide (Antiepileptic)	Cholestatic jaundice, cardiac arrhythmia, orthostatic hypotension, leucopaneia, thrombocytopaenis, dry mouth, blurring of vision, glaucoma.
Progesterone (Gonadal Hormone)	Excitability, dizziness, hallucination, dry mouth, blurred vision, constipation, urinary retention, agitation, confusion.
Proguanil (Antimalarial)	Dizziness, headaches, dependence; drowsiness, sedation, ataxia.
Promazine (Antipsychotic)	GI disturbance, appetite, fluid retension, oedema, acne, skin rash, urticaria, depression, headache, fever, fatigue.
Promethazine (Anti emetic, antin-auseants)	Nausea, vomiting, abdominal pain, headache, diarrhea, weakness, loss of appetite, and dizziness, ever, mouth sores.
Propafenone (Antiarrythmatic)	Drowsiness, dystonia, akathisia, dyskinesia, Fever, altered consciousness, autonomic dysfunction, insomnia, nausea, vomiting, constipation
Propantheline (Prokinetics)	CNS depressions, paradoxical excitation in childn, dryness of mouth, blurring of ision, retension of urine, constipation, trachucardia.
Propofol (Anaesthetics)	Dizziness, visual disturbances, vertigo dry mouth, headache, GI disturbances, alternation in test, allergic skin, rashes.
Propranolol (β blocker)	Dry mouth, thrust, difficulty in swallowing, skin dryness, flashing, reduced sweating, heat stroke, constipation, nausea.
Propylthiouracil (Thyroid agent)	Involuntary muscle movements, nausea, vomiting, headache, fever, pain, burning or stinging at inj site, apnoea.
Protriptyline (Antidepressant)	Transient hypertension, hypertension, dizziness, flashing, fatigue, drowsiness, weakness, seizures, nausea, vomiting.
Pyrantel (Anthelmintic)	Black, tarry stools, chest pain, chills, cough, fever, painful or difficult urination, shortness of breath, sore throat, sores, ulcers, or white spots on the lips or in the mouth.
Pyrazinamide (Antituberculers)	Myocardial infarction, stroke, heart block, arrhythmias, particularly orthostatic hypotension, hypertension,
Pyridostigmine (AcheE inhibitor)	Anorexia, nausea, vomiting, abdominal cramps, drowsiness, insomnia, diarrhea, headache, dizziness, rash.
Pyrimethamine (Antiprotozoal)	Fever, irritation or soreness of tongue, skin rash, black, tarry stools, bleeding or crusting sores on lips, blood in urine or stools, chest pain, chills.
Quazepam (Hypnotic)	Drowsiness, dizziness, anxiety, dry mouth, hyperventilation, increased muscle spasm, irregular heartbeats, irritability, nervousness, nightmares, restlessness.
Quinacrine (Anthelmintic)	Abdominal pain, stomach cramps, diarrhea, fever, headache, loss of appetite, pelvic pain, vaginal itching, nausea and vomiting.
Quinalbarbitone (Barbiturate)	Somnolence, Impaired motor functions, Impaired coordination, Impaired balance, Dizziness, Anxiety, Confusion, Agitation, irritability, or excitability, Headache
Quindine (Antiarrythmic)	Diarrhea, loss of appetite, muscle weakness, nausea or vomiting, abdominal pain and/or yellow eyes, confusion,
Quinine (Antimalarial)	Muscle weakness, nausea vomiting, diarrhea, cinchonism symptoms including impaired hearing, headache, blurred vision, dizziness, vomiting.
Quinapril (Antihypertensive)	cough, dizziness, fatigue, nausea, vomiting, hypotension, allergic reaction, feeling light-headed, fainting, fever, chills, body aches, flu symptoms;
Ramipril (Antihypertensive)	Nausea, vomiting, diarrhea, dizziness, fatigue, headache, abdominal pain, cough,
Ranitidine (H2 receptor antagonist)	Headache, dizziness, hepatitis, thrombocytopenic.
Reproterol (Respiratory agent)	Fine tremor of skeletal muscle, palpitations, muscle cramps, tachycardia, nervous tension, headache,
Reserpine (Antihypertensive)	Nasal congestion, headache, CNS disorders, Gi disturdance, Brest engorgement, galactorrhoea, gynaecomastia, decreased libido.
Ribavirin (Antiviral)	Increased serum bilirubin and uric acid, haemolytic anemia, reticulocytosis, anorexia, dyspepsia, nausea, vomiting, irritability.

Name of Drugs	Adverse Drug Reactions(ADR)
Rifabutin (Antibiotic)	Diarrhea, fever, heartburn, indigestion, loss of appetite, nausea, skin itching and rash.
Rifampicin (Antftuberculers)	GI disturbances, pseudomembranous colitis, abnormalities of liver function, liver disorders, influenza like symptoms, skin reactions.
Rimantadine (Anti viral)	Nausea, vomiting, abdominal pain, diarrhoea, dyspepsia, xerostomia, taste alteration, anorexia, headache
Rimiterol (Respiratory agent)	Fine tremor of skeletal muscle, palpitations, muscle cramps, tachycardia, nervous tension, headache,
Risperidone (Antipsychotic)	Agitation, anxiety, dizziness, headache, somnolence, orthostatic hypotension, constipation, dyepepsia, nausea, vomiting.
Roxatidine (Antihyperacidic agent)	Occasional headache, GI disturbances, gynaecomastia, alopecia, blood dyscrasias, pancreatitis, sleep disturbances, restlessness, dizziness.
Roxithromycin (Antibacterial)	Nausea, vomiting, abdominal pain, diarrhea, weakness, malaise, anorexia, constipation, dyspepsia, hepatitis, rashes.
Salbutamol (Antiasthamic)	Fine skeletal muscle tremor esp hands, tachycardia, palpitations, muscle cramps, headache,
Salicylate (Analgesic)	GI disorders, fatigue, hypersensitivity *reactions*, skin eruptions, haemolytic anaemia, weakness, dyspnoea.
Salsalate (Antiinflammatory)	GI symptoms, hypersensitivity *reactions*, skin eruptions, angioedema, weakness, rhinitis and dyspnoea.
Salicylazo-sulfapyridine (Anti inflammatory Drug)	
Scopolamine (Antimuscarnic)	Dry mouth, dyshidrosis, tachycardia, bradycardia, urinary retention, hallucinations, and agitation.
Secbutobarbitone (Barbiturate)	Facial flushing, palpitations, chest pain
Secobarbital (Hypnotic)	Unwanted sleepiness, trouble waking up, dizziness, excitation, headache, tiredness, loss of appetite, nausea, or vomiting.
Selegiline (Antirigidity& antitremor)	Hallucination, dizziness, confusion, anxiety, dreams, palpitations, syncope, irritability, restlessness, nausea, vomiting, dry mouth.
Semustine (Antincoplastic)	Bone marrow suppression, stomach ache, hemorrhagic cystitis, diarrhea, darkening of the skin, alopecia, changes in color and texture of the hair, and lethargy.
Sertraline (Antidepressant)	Nausea, vomiting, anorexia, dyspepsia, constipation, diarhoea, dry mouth, vomiting, ejaculation failure, increased sweating.
Simvastatin (Lipid lowering agent)	Headache, nausea, flatulence, heartburn, abdominal pain, diarrhea, dysgeusia, hypensensitivity.
Succinylsulfathiazole (Anti Microbial)	Allergic reactions, vomiting, diarrhea.
Sodium cromoglycate (Antiasthmatic)	Nausea, headache, dizziness, unpleasant test, joint pain and swelling, skin rashes, aggravation of asthma, pulmonary inflitates.
Sotalol (Antihypertensive)	Fatigue, vertigo, dyspnea, bradycardia, headaches, occasionally edema, nausea, diarrhea, hypotension.
Spectinomycin (Antibacterial)	Dizziness; nausea; urticaria; chills; fever; headache, insomnia, mild to moderate pain after inj.
Spironolactone (Antidiuretic)	Numbness or tingly feeling, muscle pain or weakness, slow, fast, or uneven heart rate, feeling drowsy, restless, shallow breathing, tremors, confusion.
Streptokinase (Anticoagulant)	Fever, chills, back pain, abdominal pain, nausea, vomiting, arthythmia, brushing, rash, pruritus, allergic reaction.
Streptomycin (Antibacterial)	Glddiness, vertigo, tinnitus, atexia, hypersensitivity reaction, ototoxicity & nephrodoxicity, anaphylactic shock, aplastic anemia & agranulocytosis.
Streptozocin (Antineoplastic)	Swelling of feet or lower legs, unusual decrease in urination, Nausea and vomiting, anxiety, nervousness, chills, cold sweats, pale skin.

Name of Drugs	Adverse Drug Reactions(ADR)
Sufentanil (Anaesthetic)	GI disturbances. Difficulty with micturition, ureteric or biliary spasm; dry mouth; sweating; headache, facial flushing.
Sulfadiazine (Anti Microbial)	Nausea, vomiting, anorexia, diarrhea, hypersensitivity, skin reacn, lumber pain, haematoria, olguria, anuria, cryslatization in urine.
Sulfadimethoxine (Anti Microbial)	Anemia, lethargic, vomiting, loss of appetite, joint pain, kidneydamage.
Sulfafurazole (Anti Microbial)	Nausea, vomiting, anorexia, diarrhoea, hypersensitivity *reactions*, SLE, serum sickness-like syndrome.
Sulfamethiazole (Anti Microbial)	Nausea, vomiting, anorexia, diarrhoea, hypersensitivity reactions, blood disorders, serum sickness-like syndrom
Sulfamethox-ypyridazine (Anti MIcrobial)	Dizziness or vertigo; acute renal failure, interstitial nephritis, acute tubular necrosis; electrolyte imbalances.
Sulfamethoxazole (Anti Microbial)	Loss of appetite, nausea, vomiting, bleeding, aplastic anemia, jaundice, hepatic necrosis, mouth sores, joint aches, severe skin rashes, itching,
Sulfametopyrazine (Antibacterial)	Nausea, vomiting, anorexia, diarrhoea
Sulfasalazine (Anti Microbial)	Headache, anorexia, nausea, vomiting, diarrhea, abdominal discomfort, photosensitivity, crystalluria, slaining of contact lens, alopecia,
Sulfathiazole (Anti Microbial)	Localized irritation, allergy, Stevens-Johnson syndrome
Sulfaurea (Antibacterial)	Irritation, stinging, burning of the skin, allergic reactions, bloody diarrhea, fever, joint pain, red, swollen
Sulfinopyrazone (Antigout)	Nausea, vomitting, diarrhoea, skin rashes, renal impairment or failure, salt and water retention, blood dyscrasia
Sulfisoxazole (Antimicrobial)	Anxiety, blurred vision, changes in menstrual periods, chills, cold sweats, coma, confusion, cool, pale skin,
Sulindac (Antiinflammatory)	Acid or sour stomach, belching, constipation, headache, heartburn, nausea or vomiting, skin rash, stomach pain.
Sulipride (Antipsychotic)	Postural hypotension, hyperprolactinaemia, weight gain, sedation, insomnia, extrapyramidal symptoms.
Sulphadiamidine (Antibacterial)	Nausea, vomiting, anorexia, diarrhoea, hypersensitivity reactions, SLE, serum sickness-like syndrome
Sulphadiazine (antibacterial)	Rash, fainting, blood in the urine, difficult or painful urination, yellowing of the skin or eyes, ringing in the ears, difficulty breathing, sore throat, chills, skin rash.
Sulphadoxine (Antiprotozole)	Fever, increased sensitivity of skin to sunlight, irritation or soreness of tongue, skin rash, Black, tarry stools, chest pain.
Sulphaguanidine (Antibacterial)	GI effects, hypersensitivity reactions, nephrotoxic reactions, CV effects, hypoglycaemia, hypothyroidism, neurological reactions
Sulphamethoxazole (Antibacterial)	Loss of appetite, nausea, vomiting. Patient's allergic, bleeding, aplastic anemia, jaundice, hepatic necrosis, mouth sores, joint aches, severe skin rashes, itching.
Sulphasazine (antigout)	Aching of joints, fever, and headache, increased sensitivity of the skin to sunlight, skin rash, itching, vomiting, back, leg, or stomach pains.
Sulphinpyrazone (Antigout)	Nausea, vomitting, diarrhoea, skin rashes, renal impairment or failure, salt and water retention, blood dyscrasia
Sultinpyrazole (Anti MIcrobial)	
Sumatriptan (Antimigrain)	Transient hypertension, hypotension, dizziness, flashing, fatigue, drowsiness, weakness, seizures, nausea, vomiting, parasethesia.
Sutamicillin (Antibiotic)	
Tacrine (AchE inhibitor)	Dizziness, headache, nausea, vomiting, diarrhoea, myalgia, ataxia.

Name of Drugs	Adverse Drug Reactions(ADR)
Tacrolimus (AChE inhibitor)	Tremor, headache, paraesthesias, nausea, vomiting, diarrhea, hypertension, blood dyscrasias, leucocytosis, inpaired ranal function.
Talampicillin (Antibiotic)	Diarrhea, allergic reactions, severe stomach pain, unusual bruising or bleeding, jaundice.
Tamoxifen (Antineoplastic)	Hot flashes, oedema, fluid retension, dry skin, veg bleedind, veg discharge, pruritus valve, GI upsets, nausea, vomiting.
Temazepam (Anxiolytic)	CNS depression, somnolence, dizziness, fatigue,ataxia, lethargy, impairment of memory and learning, reduced alertness,
Teniposide (Anticancer)	Reversible alopoecia, nausea, vomiting, diarrhoea, mucositis, rash, fever, neurotoxicity, hepatic or renal problem.
Tenoxicam (NSAIDs)	GI upsates including epigastric pain & gastritis, nausea, vomiting, hypersensitivity reacn, headache, dizziness, sleep disturbances.
Terazocin (Antihypertensive)	Orthoseaeic hypotension, syncope, dizziness, fatigue, somnolence, peripheral oedema, headache, nasal congestion.
Terbutaline (Bronchodilator)	Fine skeletal muscle tremor esp hands, flashes, dizziness, anxiety, swelling, nausea, vomiting, lethargy, tinnitus, trachycardia.
Terconazole (Antiprotozoal)	Asthenia, fever, chills, nausea, vomiting, myalgia, arthralgia, malaise, hypersensitivity, anaphylaxis, face edema, dizziness, bronchospasm, skin rash.
Terfenadine (Antiallergic)	Drowsiness or dizziness, headache, nervousness, nausea, diarrhea, abdominal discomfort, dry mouth, dry skin or itchiness.
Testosterone (Gonadal Hormone)	Fluid & electrolyte reacn, increased vascularity of skin, hypercalcemia, impaired glucose toleracce, increased bone growth.
Tetrabenazine (Antirigidity & Antitremor)	Body aches, pain, chills, cough, difficulty in breathing, difficulty with swallowing, discouragement, drowsiness, ear congestion, fear or nervousness, fever, irritability
Tetracycline (Anti Biotic)	Oesophageal ulceration, nausea, vomiting, oral candidiasis, diarrhea, epigasteic burning, sore throat, black hairy tongue, pancreatitis.
Tetrayhdrocannabinol (Hallucinogen)	Photosensitivity reaction, dry mouth, hepatitis, thrombocytopenia, generalized edema, depression, pruritus,
Thalidomide (Immunomodulator)	Severe and irreversible peripheral neuropathy, constipation dizziness, orthostatic hypotension, drowsiness.
Theobromine (Bronchodilator)	Nausea, vomiting, dizziness, headache, flushing
Theophylline (Bronchodilator)	Nausea, vomiting, abdominal pain, headache, diarrhea, insomnia, dizziness, anxiety, restlessness, tremor.
Thiabendazole (Anthelmintic)	Confusion, diarrhea, hallucinations, irritability, loss of appetite, nausea, vomiting, numbness or tingling in the hands or feet.
Thiamphenicol (Antibiotic)	Hypersensitivity, GI disturbances, stomatitis, glossitis, encephalopathy, mental depression and headache
Thioguanine (Antineoplastic)	Black, tarry stools, blood in urine or stools, cough or hoarseness, fever, chills, lower back or side pain, painful or difficult urination, pinpoint red spots on skin.
Thiopental (Sedative)	Coughing, hiccupping, sneezing, muscle twitching, laryngospasm, bronchospasm, tissue necrosis, burning pain.
Thioridazine (Antipsychotic)	Drowsiness, dry mouth, blurred vision, dizziness, sedation, antimuscarinic affects, postural hypotension, akathisia,
Thiotepa (Antineoplastic)	GI disturbances; fatigue, weakness, headache and dizziness; hypersensitivity *reactions*; blurred vision
Thymoxamine (Calcium antagonist)	Hypersensitivity, dizziness, diarrhoea, nausea, vomiting, renal impairment, rash, erythema multiforme
Thyroxine (Thyroidal Hormone)	Chest pain or discomfort, decreased urine output, difficult or labored breathing, difficulty with swallowing, dilated neck veins, extreme fatigue, fainting, and fever.

Name of Drugs	Adverse Drug Reactions(ADR)
Tiapamil (Calcium antagonist)	CNS disturbances, dizziness; visual disturbances (blurred or yellowish vision); arrhythmia
Tiaprofenic acid (Antiinflammatory)	Drowsiness, dizziness, headache, stomach upset, nausea, diarrhea, trouble sleeping, irritability,constipation, dry mouth.
Ticarcillin (Antibiotic)	Hypersensitivity *reactions*, GI disturbances, pseudomembranous colitis, blood dyscrasias,
Ticlopidine (Anticoagulant)	Diarrhea, nausea, dyspepsia, bleeding pupura, skin rash, increase in serum cholesterol concentration, hepatitis.
Timolol (Antiglucoma)	Fatigue, headache, coldness of extremist, paraesthesia, GI synptoms, Dyspnoea, Skin rash, alopecia, dry mouth, bradicardia.
Tinidazole (Antibacterial)	Metallic test, nausea, headache, vomiting, dark urine, flushing, anorexia, diarrhea, tiredness, transient leucopenis.
Tobramycin (Antibacterial)	Nausea, vomiting, dizziness, acute renal failure, intestinal nephritis, acute tubular necrosis, electrolyte inbalances, purpura.
Tocainide (Antiarrythmic)	Dizziness, lightheadedness, loss of appetite, nausea, blurred vision, confusion, headache, nervousness.
Tolazoline (Vasodilator)	Piloerection, headache, flushing, nausea, vomiting, diarrhoea, epigastric pain, tachycardia, cardiac arrhythmias.
Tolazamide (Antidiabetic)	Abdominal, stomach pain, chills, clay colored stools, dark urine, diarrhea, difficulty swallowing, dizziness,
Tolbutamide (Hypoglycemic Drug)	Hypoglycemia, nausea, vomiting, epigastric fullness, heartburn, headache, allergic skin reactions, jaundice.
Tolfenamic acid (Anti inflammatory)	Dysuria especially in males; diarrhoea, nausea, epigastric pain, vomiting, dyspepsia, erythema, headache.
Tolmetin (Anti inflammatory)	Nausea, dyspepsia, diarrhoea, flatuence, vomiting, headache, GI bleed, hypersensitivity *reactions*, asthenia.
Tolrestat (Antidiabetic)	
Torasemide (Antihypertensive)	Electrolyte disturbances, hypokalemia, dehydration, dry mouth, headache, dizziness, hypotension, weakness, drowsiness, and confessional states.
Tranexamic acid (Anti Fibirolic)	Diarrhea, nausea, vomiting, disturbance in coloue vision, giddiness, hypertension.
Tranylcypromine (Antidepressant)	Absence of or decrease in body movement, actions that are out of control, agitation, anxiety, black, tarry stools, bleeding gums, blood in the urine or stools, chest pain.
Trazodone (Antidepressant)	Drowsiness, dizziness, restlessness, confutional state, nausea, vomiting, wt loss, weakness, dry mouth, constipation, diarrhea.
Triamcinolone (Corticosteroid)	
Triamterene (Cardiovascular agent)	Photosensitivity reactions, increase in uric acid concentrations, megaloblastic anemia, thrombocytopenia, hyperkalaemia.
Triancinolone (Corticosteroid)	HPA exis suppression, intracranial hypertension, cushings syndrome, growth reduction in children, osterprosis, feactures.
Triazolam (Anxiolytic)	Somnolence, dizziness, feeling of lightness, coordination problems, tachycardia, tiredness, confusional states, memory impairment, cramps, depression.
Trichloroethanol (Sedative)	Gastric irritation, abdominal distention and flatulence
Trifluoperazine (Anti Psychotic)	Heart disease high blood pressure, angina, severe asthma, emphysema, glaucoma, seizures, pheochromocytoma, Parkinson's disease, hypocalcemia.
Trimeprazine (Respiratory agent)	Hypoglycemia, Depression, Hypotension, Tachycardia, Respiratory failure, Hypoventilation, .
Trimethoprim (Anti Bacterial)	Abdominal, stomach pain, black, tarry stools, blistering, peeling, or loosening of the skin, changes in skin color, chest pain, chills, cough or hoarseness, dizziness.

Name of Drugs	Adverse Drug Reactions (ADRs)
Trimipramine (Antidepressant)	Dry mouth, accommodation disturbances, tachycardia, constipation, hesitancy of micturation, drowsiness, sweating.
Tripolidine (Respiratory agent)	CNS depression, headache, psychomotor impairment, dry mouth, thickened resp tract secrations, blurred vision, urinary difficulty or retension.
Tubocurarine (Neuro muscular blocking agent)	Anaphylactoid reactions, apnea, cardiovascular collapse, ganglionic blockage, postoperative respiratory failure, urticaria, erythema.
Urapidil (Antihypertensive)	Dizziness, nausea, headache, fatigue, orthostatic hypotension, palpitations.
Valproate (Antiepileptic)	Asthenia, nausea, diarrhea, abdominal pain, thrombocytopenia, weight gain, peripheral edema, tremor, insomnia.
Vancomycin (Antibacterial)	Otoloxicity, nephrotoxicity, eosinophilla, urticaria, thrombopholoebitis, tryeresensivity reacns, stevens Johnson syndrome.
Vecuronium (Neuromuscular blocker)	Muscle weakness, paralysis, muscle atrophy, hypersensitivity reactions, ulticiria & aerythema, anaphylaxis, resp failure.
Venlafaxine (Antidepressant)	Nausea, vomiting, anorexia, dry mouth constipation, orthostatic hypotension, tramor, sweating, rash, anxiety, dizziness, fatigue.
Verapamil (Antihypertensive)	Bradicardia, CHF, MI, AV block, worsening heart failure, transient asystole, hypotension, pulmonary edema, nausea, fatigue.
Vidarabine (Antiviral)	Rritation; pain; superficial punctate keratitis; photophobia; lachrymation; blockage of lachrymal duct, allergic reactions.
Vigabartrin (Antiepileptic)	headache, somnolence, fatigue, dizziness, convulsion, nasopharyngitis, weight increased, upper respiratory tract infection, visual field defect, depression,tremor, nystagmus.
Viloxazine (Antidepressant)	Headache, nausea, vomiting, drowsiness, tremor, ataxia, antimuscarinic *side effects* (e.g. dry mouth, constipation)
Vinblastin (Anti Cancer)	Alopecia, constipation, malaise, stomatitis, dose-limiting bone marrow suppression
Vincristine (Anti Cancer)	Hyperuricaemia, bronchospasm, azopernia, amenorrhoea, alopecia, leucopenia, urinary dysfunction, abdominal cramps, vomiting, diarrhea, severe constipation.
Vindesine (Antiepileptic)	Alopoecia. Granulocytopaenia (dose-limiting); thrombocytopenia, neurotoxicity. Malaise, dizziness, weakness
Warfarin (Anticoagulant)	Hypersensitivity, rash, alopecia, diarrhea, drop in haematocrit, skin necrosis, jaundice, nausea, vomiting, hepatic dysfunction, pancreatitis.
Xamoterol (Cardiac stimulant)	Hypotension, bronchospasm, dizziness, headache, palpitation, rashes, muscle cramps.
Xipamide (Antidiuretic)	GI disturbances, hypokalaemia, hyperuricaemia, nocturia, dizziness, impaired glucose metabolism.
Zalcitabin (Reverse transcriptase inhibitor)	Peripheral neuropathy (numbness, sharp shooting pain), oral and esophageal ulceration; hypersensitivity reacn
Zidovudine (Antiviral)	Nausea, vomiting, severe headache, myalgia,insomnia, vomiting, anorexia, diarrhea, asthenia, dizziness, test prevension, convulsions.
Zimeldine	
Zolpidem (Anxiolytic)	Amnesia, drowsiness, dizziness, diarthoea, nausea, vomiting, abnormal thinking and behavior, back pain, ataxia, confusion.
Zopiclone (Hypnotic)	Metallic or bitter affertaste, imitibility, confusion, depressed mood, aggressiveness, incoordination, anterograde anemia, drowsiness.
Zuclopenthixol (Antipsychotic)	Drowsiness, blurred vision, tachycardia, nausea, dizziness, headache, excitement, postural hypotension

ADR of Commonly used some Herbs

Name of Herbs	Toxic effect or system affected	Adverse drug reaction	Intended use
Ephedra (Ephedrine)	Cardiovascular	Hypertension, cardiac arrhythmia, restlessness, anxiety, tremors, MI, cerebrovascular events, renal stones, seizures.	Herbal weight loss.
Liquorice (Liquorice root)	Pseudoaldosteronism (sodium and water retention)	Water retention	Treatment of peptic ulcer, flavouring agent, hypertension, heart failure.
Comfrey	Hepatotoxic	Liver damage, lung damage, and cancer	Repairing of bones and muscles, Prevention of kidney stones.
Chan Su	Cardiovascular	Cardiac arrest, atrial fibrillation	Tonic for heart
Borage Oil	Hepatocarcinogenic	Nausea, headaches and gastrointestinal upset	Source of essential fatty acid, rheumatoid arthritis, hypertension.
Calamus	Carcinogenic	Ulcers, gas, upset of stomach	Psychoactive
Chaparral	Hepatotoxic, nephrotoxic, carcinogenic	Stomach pain, nausea, diarrheal, weight loss, fever	General cleansing tonic, arthritis remedy, weight loss product
Gingko Biloba	Blood vessels	Spontaneous bleeding	Alzheimer's disease, dementia
Sweet clover	Skin	Photosensitivity	Leg pain, heaviness, night cramps
Paprika	Blood vessels	Headache	Preparation of spice
Senna Leaf	Immunity	Hives	Purgative
Kava	Immunity	Hives	Anxiety, insomnia, epilepsy
Chast tree fruit	GIT	Diarrhoea	Premenstrual syndrome, Premenstrual dysphoric disorder
St John Wort	GIT	GIT disturbance, allergic reaction, fatigue, dizziness, confusion, dry mouth.	Mild to moderate depression, anxiety and insomnia

REFERENCES FOR FURTHER READING

1. Br Med J 1983, **286**, 1043.
2. Ann Interm Med 1973, **78**, 541.
3. Drugs 1983, **25**, 290.
4. Antimicrob Ag Chemother 1980, **18**, 738.
5. Br J Anaesth 1986, **58**, 512.
6. Lancet 1984, **1**, 1318.
7. Clin Pharmacokinet 1983, **8**, 187.
8. New Engl J Med 1985, **312**, 897.
9. Drugs 1981, **22**, 363.
10. Clin Neuropharmac 1990, **13**, 559.
11. Curr Ther Res 1970, **12**, 551.
12. Med Lett 1987, **29**, 59.
13. Br Med J 1987, **294**, 1504.
14. Anesthesia 985, **40**, 121.
15. Hosp Formulary 1991, **26**, Suppl A, 2.
16. Clin Pharmac Ther 1977, **22**, 316.
17. Ann Interm Med 1981, **94**, 454.
18. Drug Ther Bull 1976, **14**, 55.
19. Drugs of the Future 1990, **15**, 282.
20. Ann Interm Med 1981, **95**, 328.
21. Med Lett 1981, **23**, 109.
22. Drugs 1985, **29**, 236.
23. Med Lett 1981, **23**, 71.
24. Ann Pharmacother 1990, **23**, 757.
25. Clin Pharmacokinet 1984, **9**, 261.
26. Clin Pharmacokinet 1988, **15**, 1.
27. Lancet 1985, **2**, 805.
28. Drugs 1981, **22**, 337.
29. Med Lett 1986, **28**, 41.
30. Clin Pharmac Ther 1983, **34**, 79.
31. New Engl J Med 1986, **314**, 349.
32. Pharmacotherapy 1985, **5**, 78.
33. Br J Clin Pharmac 1974, **1**, 41.
34. Br J Clin Pharmac 1984, **18**, 559.
35. Br Med J 1988, **296**, 307.
36. Arzneim Forsch 1983, **33**, 381.
37. Drugs 1990, **40**, 75.
38. Anaesthesiol 1984, **61**, 328.
39. Br J Hosp Med, 1985, **33**, 138.
40. Med J Aust 1984, **140**, 73.
41. Eur J Clin Pharmac 1981, **20**, 147.
42. Diabetic 1985, **34**, 1306.
43. Drugs 1989, **38**, 778.
44. Ann Interm Med 1982, **97**, 755.
45. Antimicrob Ag Chemother 1984, **26**, 493.
46. Pharmacotherapy 1982, **2**, 313.
47. Eur J Clin Pharmac 1991, **40**, 363.
48. Lymphology 1979, **12**, 85.
49. Arzneim Forsch 1968, **18**, 1212.
50. Drug Ther Bull 1986, **24**, 1.
51. Br J Clin Pract 1987, **41**, 967.
52. Br Med J 1984, **288**, 1344.
53. Rheumatol Rehab 1978, **17**, 254.
54. Drug Ther Bull 1974, **12**, 12.
55. Eur J Clin Pharmac 1981, **21**, 209.
56. Drugs 1986, **31**, 266.
57. Postgrad Med J 1976, **52**, 501.
58. Clin Pharmac Ther 1986, **39**, 313.
59. Eur J Clin Pharmac 1990, **40**, 75.
60. J Clin Pharmac 1978, **18**, 249.
61. Drugs 1988, **5**, 1.
62. Curr Med Res Opin 1987, **10**, 390.
63. Eur J Clin Pharmac 1984, **27**, 619.
64. Br J Clin Pharmac 1987, **23**, 623P.
65. Cancer 1977, **40**, 2772.
66. Eur J Clin Pharmac 1990, **39**, 569.
67. New Engl J Med 1979, **300**, 473.
68. J Pharm Sci 1973, **62**, 1776.
69. Clin Tr J 1983, **20**, 115.
70. Ann Interm Med 1984, **100**, 78.
71. New Engl J Med 1975, **293**, 486.
72. Br J Clin Pharmac 1983, **16**, 285S.
73. Drugs 1984, **28**, 485.
74. Int J Clin Pharmac Biopharm 1978, **16**, 54.
75. Drugs 1984, **28**, 426.
76. Clin Pharmacokinet 1980, **5**, 340.
77. Br Med J 1982, **284**, 1830.
78. Lancet 1985, **2**, 1236.
79. Am J Kid Dis 1983, **3**, 155.
80. Br Med J 1983, **286**, 1980.
81. Br Clin Pharmac 1977, **4**, 91.
82. Arzneim Forsch 1985, **35**, 623.
83. Clin Pharmac Ther 1993, **33**, 355.
84. Tubercle 1972, **53**, 47.
85. Br Med J 1985, **290**, 180.
86. Clin Pharmacokinet 1986, **11**, 177.
87. Handbook of Clin. Pharm. Data 1992, **ed.1**, P-131.
88. Eur J Resp Dis 1986, **69**, 160.
89. Gastroenterology 1978, **74**, 7.

90.	Lancet 1990, **335**, 1107.
91.	Cancer Treat Rev 1985, **12**, Suppl A, 73.
92.	Martindale **29**[th] **edn.**, 1231.
93.	New Engl J Med 1980, **303**, 1323.
94.	Clin Pharma Ther 1981, **29**, 257.
95.	Clin Pharmac Ther 1984, **35**, 301.
96.	Curr Med Res Opin 1981, **7**, 168.
97.	Drugs 1986, **32**, 1.
98.	Chematherapy (Basle) 1976, **22**, 274.
99.	Chin Med J 1979, **92**, 26.
100.	Drugs 1980, **20**, 137.
101.	Drugs of Today 1976, **12**, 171.
102.	Arzneim Forsch 1979, **29**, 361.
103.	Chemotherapy (Tokyo) 1982, **30**, 212.
104.	Jpn J Antibiot 1987, **40**, 1537.
105.	Drugs 1987, **34**, 188.
106.	Antimicrob Ag Chemother 1990, **34**, 1944.
107.	Drugs 1986, **32**, 222.
108.	Drugs 1981, **22**, 423.
109.	Drugs 1987, **34**, 41157.
110.	Handbook of Clin. Pharm. Data 1992, **ed.1**, 131.
111.	J Antimicrob Chemother 198, **11**, Suppl A1.
112.	Drugs 1979, **17**, 1.
113.	J Antimicrob Chemother 1990, **26**, Suppl, 41.
114.	Int J Clin Pharmac Ther Tokyo 1990, **28**, 435.
115.	Clin Pharmacokinet 1984, **3**, 373.
116.	J Antibiot 1976, **29**, 444.
117.	Med Lett 1985, **27**, 85.
118.	J Antimicrob Chemother 1982, **10**, Suppl C1.
119.	Med Lett 1984, **26**, 15.
120.	J Card Pharmac 1986, **Suppl 4**, S75.
121.	Eur J Clin Pharmac 1979, **16**, 4.
122.	Postgrad Med J 1983, **Suppl 5**, 1.
123.	Br J Opthalm 1973, **57**, 421.
124.	Med Lett 1986, **28**, 33.
125.	Ann Interm Med 1985, **103**, 70.
126.	Drugs 1986, **31**, 449.
127.	Clin Pharmacokinet 1987, **12**, 136.
128.	Clin Pharmac Ther 1977, **21**, 355.
129.	New Engl J Med 1987, **316**, 52.
130.	Antimicrob Ag Chemother 1975, **7**, 153.
131.	Eur J Clin Pharmac 1979, **15**, 171.
132.	Eur J Clin Pharmac 1978, **13**, 267.
133.	Eur J Clin Pharmac 1980, **17**, 275.
134.	Eur J Drug Met Pharmacokinet 1991, **16**, 43.
135.	Br J Clin Pharmac 1983, **15**, 471.
136.	Br Med J 1983, **286**, 1535.
137.	New Engl J Med 1983, **308**, 1275.
138.	Am J Kid Dis 1983, **3**, 155.
139.	Drugs 1981, **22**, 211.
140.	Pian 1978, **5**, 367.
141.	Br J Derm 1976, **95**, 317.
142.	Pharmacotherapeutica 1983, **3**, 475.
143.	Am J Kid Dis 1983, **3**, 155.
144.	Drugs 1991, **41**, 799.
145.	Gastroenterology 1985, **89**, 522.
146.	Drug Ther Bull 1981, **19**, 27.
147.	Clin Pharmac Ther 1976, **19**, 119.
148.	Chemotherapy 1990, **36**, 385.
149.	Ann Interm Med 1984, **100**, 704.
150.	Ther Drug Monit 1984, **6**, 424.
151.	J Int Med Res 1983, **11**, 92.
152.	Drug Intell Clin Pharm 1970, **4**, 332.
153.	Analyt Prof Drug Subs 1989, **18**, 57.
154.	Br J Clin Pharmac 1987, **23**, 137.
155.	Ann Int Med 1982, **97**, 788.
156.	J Am Med Ass 1985, **254**, 2097.
157.	Drugs 1990, **39**, 136.
158.	J Am Med Ass 1980, **243**, 2513.
159.	J Clin Psychiat 1986, **47**, 238.
160.	Br J Clin Pharmac 1983, **15**, Suppl 4, 4555.
161.	Br Med J 1987, **294**, 42.
162.	New Engl J Med 1991, **324**, 746.
163.	Drug Met Diposit 1975, **3**, 1.
164.	J Pharm Pharmac 1986, **38**, 264.
165.	New Engl J Med 1986, **314**, 1001.
166.	J Antimicrob Chemother 1986, **18**, 293.
167.	J Org Chem 1986, **51**, 4323.
168.	New Engl J Med 1968, **279**, 596.
169.	J Pharm Sci 1975, **64**, 1576.
170.	J Clin Oncol 1988, **6**, 1377.
171.	Antimicrob Ag Chemother 1987, **31**, 969.
172.	Med J Aust 1986, **145**, 146.
173.	Lancet 1984, **2**, 517.
174.	Arzneim Forsch 1973, **23**, 1550.
175.	Br Clin Pharmac 1979, **8**, 219.
176.	Gut 1982, **23**, A447.
177.	Scot Med J 1979, **24**, 147.
178.	Lepr rev 1983, **54**, 139.
179.	Sem Oncol 1984, **Suppl 3**, 2.
180.	Br Med J 1977, **1**, 422.
181.	Br J Clin Pharmac 1983, **16**, 245.
182.	J Clin Psychiat 1984, **45**, 3.
183.	Br J Clin Pharmac 1981, **12**, 434.
184.	Eur J Clin Pharmac 1984, **27**, 123.
185.	Lancet 1984, **1**, 1449.
186.	Drug Ther Bull 1983, **21**, 17.
187.	Clin Anaesth 1983, **1**, 159.
188.	New Engl J Med 1984, **310**, 1213.
189.	New Engl J Med 1983, **309**, 354.

190. Clin Pharmacokinet 1977, **2**, 198.
191. Drugs 1988, **35**, 244.
192. Drug Intell Clin Pharm 1984, **18**, 530.
193. Br Med J 1985, **291**, 1014.
194. Curr Med Res Opin 1979, **6**, Suppl 1, 107.
195. Drugs 1980, **19**, 84.
196. New Engl J Med 1973, **289**, 1063.
197. Clin Pharmacokinet 1985, **10**, 1.
198. Int J Pharmac Ther Toxicol 1981, **19**, 372.
199. Br Med J 1983, **286**, 675.
200. Ann Interm Med 1980, **92**, 387.
201. J Clin Pharmac 1988, **28**, 644.
202. Eur J Clin Pharmac 1983, **24**, 635.
203. Br J Clin Pharmac 1981, **11**, 305.
204. New Engl J Med 1987, **316**, 1247.
205. Arzneim Forsch 1957, **7**, 15.
206. Clin Pharmac Ther 1984, **36**, 520.
207. Ann Interm Med 1983, **99**, 490.
208. Drugs 1982, **2**, 360.
209. Br J Anaesth 1986, **58**, 151.
210. Arzneim Forsch 1968, **18**, 479.
211. J Clin Psychiat 1980, **41**, 64.
212. Br J Clin Pharmac 1975, **2**, 180 P.
213. Am J Cardiol 1987, **59**, IG.
214. J Clin Psychopharmac 1985, **5**, 102.
215. Eur J Clin Pharmac 1985, **28**, 205.
216. Br J Clin Pharmac 1983, **16**, 245.
217. Martindale 1989, **29th edn.**, 735.
218. Lancet 1977, **2**, 982.
219. Br J Anaesth 1986, **58**, 825.
220. Drugs 1986, **31**, 198.
221. Am J Cardiol 1986, **58**, 74C.
222. J Antimicrab Chemother 1984, **14**, Suppl C, 1.
223. Drugs 1989, **38**, Suppl 2, 18.
224. Clin Pharm 1985, **4**, 393.
225. Cancer Treat Rep 1984, **68**, 679.
226. Drugs 1983, **26**, 364.
227. Br Med J 1977, **2**, 36.
228. Drugs 1987, **33**, 392.
229. Practitioner 1984, **228**, 725.
230. Am J Kid Dis 1983, **3**, 155.
231. Eur J Clin Pharmac 1973, **6**, 133.
232. Clin Pharmacokinet 1980, **5**, 1.
233. Neurol Clin 1986, **4**, 601.
234. Eur J Clin Pharmac 1978, **13**, 365.
235. Eur J Clin Pharmac 1988, **34**, 101.
236. Lancet 1983, 24.
237. Clin Pharmacokinet 1987, **12**, 223.
238. Drugs 1986, **32**, 197.
239. Drugs of Today 1989, **25**, 589.
240. Drugs 1981, **21**, 1.
241. Curr Med Res Opin 1979, **6**, Suppl 1, 15.
242. Clin Pharmac Ther 1980, **27**, 286.
243. Analyt Prof Drug Subs 1978, **7**, 319.
244. Eur J Clin Pharmac 1987, **32**, 529.
245. Clin Pharmac Ther 1990, **48**, 262.
246. Lancet 1986, **2**, 440.
247. Eur J Clin Pharmac 1987, **32**, 403.
248. Eur J Clin Microb 1988, **7**, 364.
249. Drugs 1983, **25**, 41.
250. Arzneim Forsch 1971, **21**, 1133.
251. Curr Ther Res 1969, **11**, 533.
252. J Clin Pharmac 1985, **25**, 400.
253. Fundam Clin Pharmac 1990, **4**, 643.
254. Eur J Clin Pharmac 1983, **24**, 261.
255. Psychopharmacologie 1976, **27**, 1.
256. Lancet 1978, **1**, 1217.
257. Clin Pharmac Ther 1977, **21**, 355.
258. Drugs 1979, **18**, 417.
259. Br Med J 1977, **2**, 1541.
260. Drugs & Aging 1991, **1**, 104.
261. Lancet 1985, **2**, 648.
262. Clin Pharmacokinet 1979, **4**, 170.
263. Drugs 1985, **29**, 57.
264. Am J Kid Dis 1983, **3**, 155.
265. Am J Cardiol 1984, **4**, 908.
266. New Engl J Med 1986, **314**, 801.
267. New Engl J Med 1987, **317**, 1237.
268. Antimicrob Ag Chemother 1981, **20**, 515.
269. Mayo Clin Proc 1985, **60**, 439.
270. Drugs 1984, **27**, 301.
271. Clin Pharmacokinet 1984, **3**, 473.
272. Martindale 1989, **29th edn.**, 390.
273. New Engl J Med 1975, **292**, 250.
274. Pharmacotherapy 1985, **5**, 43.
275. Drugs 1983, **34**, 391.
276. Br Med J Pharmac 1983, **16**, 523.
277. Martindale 1989, **29th edn.**, 391.
278. Lancet 1983, **2**, 415.
279. Pharmatherapeutica 1983, **3**, 441.
280. Drugs 1983, **26**, 212.
281. Clin Pharmac Ther 1973, **14**, 204.
282. Clin Nephrol 1973, **1**, 14.
283. Am J Cardiol 1986, **57**, IE.
284. J Clin Psychiat 1983, **44**, 440.
285. Clin Pharmac Ther 1980, **28**, 804.
286. Lancet 1984, **1**, 496.
287. J Pediat 1984, **105**, 799.
288. J Clin Pharmac 1978, **18**, 190.
289. Curr Res Ther 1984, **35**, 715.

290. Antibiot Chemother 1962, **12**, 583.
291. New Engl J Med 1977, **296**, 67.
292. New Engl J Med 1985, **313**, 1571.
293. Clin Pharmac Ther 1969, **10**, 395.
294. J Int Med Res 1986, **14**, 53.
295. Prescr J 1981, **21**, 159.
296. Lancet 1985, **2**, 496.
297. Clin Pharmacokinet 1990, **18**, 346.
298. Drugs 1984, **28**, 189.
299. Eur J Clin Pharmac 1990, **38**, 343.
300. Br J Clin Pharmac 1976, **3**, 489.
301. J Am Med Ass 1983, **128**, 24.
302. J Am Med Ass 1986, **255**, 20905.
303. Therapie 1984, **39**, 509.
304. Med Lett 1986, **28**, 51.
305. Tubercle 1984, **65**, 211.
306. Prescribers J 1983, **23**, 32.
307. Drugs 1982, **23**, 165.
308. Drugs Ther Bull 1984, **22**, 7.
309. Drug Ther Bull 1980, **18**, 34.
310. Clin Pharmac Ther 1990, **48**, 590.
311. Antimicrob Ag Chemother 1980, **18**, 158.
312. Ann Intern Med 1983, **98**, 171.
313. Drugs 1987, **34**, 98.
314. Clin Pharmac Ther 1986, **40**, 56.
315. Drug Ther Bull 1980, **18**, 94.
316. Br J Clin Pharmac 1985, **19**, 211.
317. Med Lett 1986, **28**, 61.
318. Clin Pharmac Ther 1986, **39**, 89.
319. Br J Clin Pharmac 1982, **13**, Suppl 1.
320. Pharm J 1982, **1**, 15.
321. Eur J Drug Met Pharmacokinet 1982, **7**, 247.
322. Am J Opthalm 1985, **99**, 18.
323. New Engl J Med 1984, **310**, 1357.
324. Res Com Chem Path Pharmac 1983, **41**, 3.
325. Drug Ther Bull 1983, **21**, 27.
326. Br Med J 1983, **286**, 1332.
327. Develop Pharmac Ther 1990, **14**, 148.
328. Handbook of Clin. Pharm. Data 1992, **ed.1**, 131.
329. Med Lett 1988, **30**, 41.
330. Eur Neutrol 1983, **22**, 240.
331. Clin Pharmacokinet 1980, **5**, 385.
332. Br Clin J Pract 1986, **40**, 59.
333. Antimicrob Ag Chemother 1988, **32**, 617.
334. J Am Med Ass 1986, **255**, 757.
335. Drugs 1989, **37**, 42.
336. Br J Clin Pharmac 1982, **14**, 141P.
337. Drugs 1984, **27**, 29.
338. J Am Med Ass 1973, **225**, 32.
339. Drug Exp Clin Res 1990, **16**, 57.
340. Clin Pharmac Ther 1973, **14**, 852.
341. Med Lett 1981, **23**, 58.
342. Acta Neurol Scand 1979, **60**, 250.
343. Br J Clin Pharmac 1982, **13**, 829.
344. Pharmacotherapy 1985, **5**, 1.
345. Arch Neurol 1972, **27**, 129.
346. Br J Anaesth 1975, **47**, 464.
347. Hum Psychopharmac 1988, **3**, 195.
348. Clin Pharmac Ther 1977, **22**, 280.
349. Contraception 1977, **16**, 605.
350. Curr Med Res Opin 1979, **5**, 754.
351. Eur J Clin Pharmac 1987, **32**, 173.
352. Arzneim Forsch 1967, **17**, 653.
353. Ann Interm Med 1984, **101**, 14.
354. Med Lett 1988, **291**, 23.
355. Toxicol Appl Pharmac 1971, **18**, 185.
356. Br J Anasthes 1985, **57**, 1006.
357. Drugs 1979, **17**, 198.
358. Postgrad Med J 1985, **61**, Suppl 2.
359. New Engl J Med 1987, **317**, 447.
360. Clin Pharmac Ther 1986, **40**, 287.
361. Drug Ther Bull 1986, **24**, 38.
362. Can Med Ass J 1968, **99**, 868.
363. Can Med Ass J 1983, **128**, 24.
364. Br Med J 1982, **282**, 630.
365. Br J Clin Pharmac 1982, **14**, 333.
366. Antimicrob Ag Chemother 1978, **14**, 566.
367. Clin Med 1966, **73**, 41.
368. Anesthesiol 1985, **62**, 567.
369. Drugs 1990, **39**, 489.
370. Postgrad Med J 1984, **60**, 881.
371. J Pharmac Exp Ther 1976, **198**, 264.
372. Martindale 1989, **29th edn.**, 404.
373. New Engl J Med 1990, **322**, 1459.
374. J Clin Pharmac 1973, **13**, 142.
375. J Pharm Sci 1985, **74**, 1001.
376. Br J Hosp Med 1984, **31**, 142.
377. Clin Pharmacokinet 1983, **8**, 523.
378. J Clin Pharmac 1985, **25**, 369.
379. Pharm res 1990, **7**, 953.
380. Pharmacotherapeutica 1986, **4**, 525.
381. Drugs 1990, **40**, 374.
382. Antimicrob Ag Chemother 1984, **25**, 556.
383. Br J Clin Pharmac 1983, **15**, 263 S.
384. Drugs 1982, **24**, 85.
385. Anasthesia 1986, **41**, 482.
386. Arzneim Forsch 1976, **2**, 2145.
387. Can Med Ass J 1968, **99**, 849.
388. Lancet 1977, **2**, 515.
389. Human Toxicol 1985, **4**, 425.

390. J Am Med Ass 1981, **245**, 1123.
391. New Engl J Med 1984, **310**, 649.
392. Ann Interm Med 1986, **105**, 67.
393. Int Clin Psychopharmac 1987, **2**, 165.
394. J Clin Pharmac 1981, **21**, 351.
395. Stroke 1989, **20**, 1143.
396. Am J Cardiol 1990, **65**, 26D.
397. Ther Drug Monit 1991, **13**, 1.
398. Arch Dis Childhood 1986, **61**, 727.
399. Drugs 198, **30**, 127.
400. Drug Ther Bull 1988, **26**, 41.
401. Br J Clin Pharmac 1985, **19**, 37.
402. Drug Ther Bull 1988, **26**, 25.
403. Drugs 1983, **26**, 191.
404. New Engl J Med 1991, **324**, 384.
405. Drugs 1990, **40**, 91.
406. Pharmatherapeutica 1983, **3**, 441.
407. Drugs 1980, **19**, 249.
408. J Antimicrob Chemother 1987, **31**, 605.
409. Anaesthesiology 1979, **51**, 222.
410. Drug Ther Bull 1982, **20**, 11.
411. J Am Coll Cardiol 1984, **4**, 908.
412. Drugs 1984, **27**, 148.
413. Br J Clin Pharmac 1983, **16**, 491.
414. New Engl J Med 1982, **307**, 1618.
415. Cardiov Drug Rev 1988, **6**, 97.
416. Drugs 1989 , **37**, 669.
417. J Am Call Cardiol 1985, **6**, 47.
418. Clin Pharmac Ther 1985, **38**, 697.
419. Eur J Clin Pharmac 1985, **28**, 473.
420. Antimicrob Ag Chemother 1977, **12**, 655.
421. Clin Pharmac Ther 1990, **47**, 724.
422. J Am Med Ass 1986, **255**, 2905.
423. Clin Pharmacokinet 1991, **20**, 15.
424. Drugs 1985, **30**, 482.
425. Antimicrob Ag Chemother 1980, **18**, 158.
426. Lancet 1987, **2**, 856.
427. Am J Med 1989, **87**, Suppl 5A, 24.
428. New Engl J Med 1991, **324**, 915.
429. Cancer Treat Rev 1987, **14**, 333.
430. J Forens Sci 1974, **19**, 193.
431. Lancet 1985, **1**, 1386.
432. Toxicol Appl Pharmac 1971, **20**, 44.
433. Trans Roy Soc Trop Med Hyg 187, **81**, 55.
434. Drugs 1978, **16**, 358.
435. Eur J Clin Pharmac 1975, **8**, 3.
436. New Engl J Med 1985, **313**, 800.
437. Drugs 1987, **34**, 50.
438. Drug Ther Bull 1984, **22**, 88.
439. Mayo Clin Proc 1987, **62**, 906.
440. J Nucl Med 1985, **26**, 1135.
441. Br Med J 1987, **295**, 595.
442. Drugs 1983, **25**, 290.
443. Am J Obs Gyn 1962, **84**, 1778.
444. Neuropsychobiology 1985, **13**, 31.
445. Arch Intern Med 1984, **144**, 1888.
446. Eurt J Clin Microb 1987, **6**, 521.
447. J Med Chem 1988, **31**, 814.
448. Curr Ther Res 1980, **27**, 429.
449. Br J Clin Pharmac 1977, **4**, 135.
450. Arthris Rheum 1982, **25**, 111.
451. Clin Pharmac Ther 1980, **28**, 436.
452. Drug Alc Depend 1985, **14**, 313.
453. Digestion 1973, **8**, 448.
454. Angiology 1986, **37**, 555.
455. Arzneim Forsch 1986, **154**, 431.
456. Arzneim Forsch 1967, **17**, 159.
457. Clin Pharmac Ther 1990, **47**, 397.
458. Drugs of Today 1978, **14**, 120.
459. Br J Clin Pharmac 1982, **14**, 385.
460. Med J Aust 1987, **146**, 634.
461. Int J Clin Pharmac Ther Tox 1985, **23**, 59.
462. J Paediatr 1975, **86**, 459.
463. J Clin Pharm Ther 1988, **13**, 5.
464. Am J Kid Dis 1983, **3**, 155.
465. Lancet 1982, **2**, 140.
466. Pharmacotherapeutica 1983, **3**, 300.
467. Clin Pharmacokinet 1978, **3**, 369.
468. Circulation 1977, **56**, 385.
469. Drugs 1984, **27**, 328.
470. Drug Ther Bull 1984, **22**, 70.
471. Br J Clin Pharmac 1979, **7**, 533.
472. New Engl J Med 1983, **34**, 440.
473. J Antimicrob Chemother 1982, **9**, 489.
474. Pharm J 1988, **240**, 367.
475. Br med J 1984, **289**, 734.
476. Br Med J 1985, **290**, 1173.
477. Drugs 1985, **29**, 489.
478. Eur J Clin Pharmac 1985, **28**, 305.
479. Drugs 1986, **32**, 509.
480. Drug Ther Bul 1981, **19**, 78.
481. Antimicrob Ag Chemother 1978, **13**, 90.
482. Drugs 1972, **3**, 159.
483. J Antimicrob Chemother 1987, **20**, Suppl 8, 157.
484. Clin Pharmac Ther 1977, **21**, 105.
485. Br Med J 1973, **2**, 177.
486. J Clin Pharmac 1984, **24**, 446.
487. J Antimicrob Chemother 1985, **15**, 1.
488. Clin Pharmac Ther 1980, **27**, 779.
489. J Endocrinol 1959, **18**, 278.

490. J Cardiov Pharmac 1987, **10**, 38.
491. Br Med J 1985, **291**, 23.
492. Am J Kid Dis 1983, **3**, 155.
493. Lancet 1976, **2**, 376.
494. Lancet 1981, **1**, 450.
495. Clin Phrmac Ther 1984, **35**, 285.
496. Lancet 1979, **2**, 1249.
497. Martindale 1989, **29th edn.,** 763.
498. Eur J Clin Pharmac 1985, **28**, 73.
499. Acta Neurol Scand 1984, **69**, 200.
500. Br Med J 1980, **80**, 825.
501. Med J Aust 1975, **2**, 342.
502. Br J Hosp Med 1984, **31**, 354.
503. Clin Pharmacokinet 1991, **21**, 1.
504. Prescribers J 1984, **24**, 106.
505. Postgrad Med J 1985, **61**, Suppl 3, 105.
506. Clin Pharmac Ther 1983, **34**, 440.
507. Handbook of Clin. Pharm. Data 1992, **ed.1**, 131.
508. New Engl J Med 1982, **307**, 1037.
509. Med Lett 1986, **28**, 9.
510. Tubercle 1984, **65**, 1.
511. Clin Pharmac Ther 1980, **28**, 78.
512. Trans Roy Soc Trop Med Hyg 1975, **69**, 139.
513. Pharmacotherapy 1990, **10**, 1.
514. Ann Inter Med 1980, **93**, 286.
515. Am Heart J 1978, **96**, 829.
516. Br Med J 1986, **293**, 11.
517. Eur J Clin Pharmac 1986, **31**, 9.
518. Curr Ther Res 1986, **40**, 74.
519. New Engl J Med 1990, **323**, 1672.
520. Clin Tr J 1973, **10**, 3.
521. Clin Pharmac Ther 1973, **14**, 325.
522. Antimicrob Ag Chemother 1985, **28**, 467.
523. Br Med J 1984, **288**, 1595.
524. Drugs 1988, **35**, Suppl 3, 48.
525. Br Med J 1984, **289**, 1032.
526. Lancet 1986, **1**, 242.
527. Br J Derm 1986, **115**, Suppl 31, 63.
528. Clin Pharmac Ther 1986, **39**, 420.
529. Martindale 1989, **29th edn.,** 766.
530. Br J Psychiat 1983, **142**, 508.
531. Ann Interm Med 1980, **93**, 286.
532. Gut 1981, **22**, 55.
533. Br J Clin Pharmac 1990, **29**, 277.
534. Eur J Clin Pharmac 1984, **27**, 345.
535. Am Heart J 1978, **96**, 389.
536. Br Med J 1970, **1**, 614.
537. Gut 1983, **24**, A596.
538. Circulation 1984, **70**, 1118A.
539. Br J Anaesthes 1987, **59**, 1147.
540. Martindale 1989, **29th edn.,** 310.
541. Eur J Rheumatol Inflamm 1978 , **1**, 3.
542. Drug Ther Bull 1984, **22**, 31.
543. Lancet 1972, **2**, 210.
544. Martindale 1989, **29th edn.,** 305.
545. Chemotherapy 1969, **14**, 195.
546. Clin Pharmacokinet 1980, **5**, 405.
547. Eur J Obs Gyn Biol 1977, **7**, 383.
548. Clin Pharmac Ther 1985, **37**, 36.
549. Ann Interm Med 1984, **3**, 377.
550. J Antimicrob Chemotherb 1982, **10**, 49.
551. Lancet 1988, **1**, 1309.
552. Age of Aging 1989, **18**, 223.
553. Br J Vener Dis 1982, **58**, 180.
554. Pharmac Ther 1984, **25**, 127.
555. Eur J Clin Pharmac 1990, **38**, 153.
556. Drugs 1987, **34**, 289.
557. Prescribers J 1986, **32**, 159.
558. Drug Ther Bull 1985, **23**, 7.
559. J Clin Psychiat 1978, **39**, 81.
560. Ann Interm Med 1981, **95**, 328.
561. Br Med J 1987, **294**, 141.
562. Br J Clin Pharmac 1983, **15**, 604P.
563. Br J Opthal 1980, **64**, 30.
564. Scand J Haemat 1984, **33**, 453.
565. Eur J Clin Pharmac 1985, **28**, 543.
566. Curr Ther res 1977, **21**, 720.
567. Can Med Ass J 1980, **244**, 2065.
568. Curr Med Res Opin 1982, **8**, 158.
569. Handbook of Clin. Pharm. Data 1992, **ed.1**, 131.
570. Clin Ther 1983, **5**, 595.
571. Drugs 1988, **35**, Suppl 1.
572. J Antimicrob Chemother 1987, **19**, 363.
573. Drugs 1986, **31**, 517.
574. Br Med J 1982, **285**, 84.
575. Drugs 1982, **24**, 85.
576. Eur J Clin Pharmac 1983, **24**, 643-705.
577. New Engl J Med 1986, **315**, 41.
578. Am J Kid Dis 1983, **3**, 155.
579. Rheumatol Rehabil 1978, **17**, 150.
580. Drugs 1991, **41**, Suppl 3, 14.
581. Drugs 1985, **29**, 236.
582. Arch Dis Psychiat 1985, **42**, 962.
583. Drugs 1981, **21**, 401.
584. Eur J Clin Pharmac 1983, **24**, 453.
585. Eur J Clin Pharmac 1985, **29**, 85.
586. Drugs 1981, **22**, 81.
587. Ann Interm Med 1980, **93**, 284.
588. Curr Ther Res 1980, **28**, 650.
589. Br Med J 1982, **284**, 1508.

590. Drugs 1989, **38**, Suppl 1, 17.
591. Antimicrob Ag Chemother 1979, **15**, 651.
592. Br J Anaesthes 1980, **52**, 893.
593. Drugs 1990, **40**, Suppl 4, 21.
594. Lancet 1986, 511.
595. Acta Odontol Scand 1985, **43**, 47.
596. Anaes Analg 1985, **64**, 212.
597. Ann Interm Med 1980, **93**, 875.
598. Clin Pharmac Ther 1980, **27**, 690.
599. Neurology 1987, **37**, 184.
600. Curr Med res Opin 1977, **5**, 217.
601. New Engl J Med 1978, **298**, 1101.
602. New Engl J Med 1980, **303**, 585.
603. Drug Intell Clin Pharm 1980, **14**, 28.
604. New Engl J Med 1991, **324**, 1865.
605. Clin Pharmac Ther 1990, **48**, 628.
606. New Engl Med 1987, **316**, 557.
607. Int J Psycopharmac 1990, **5**, 147.
608. Mol Pharmac 1974, **10**, 759.
609. Drugs 1985, **29**, 531.
610. Clin Pharmacokinet 1982, **7**, 93.
611. Clin Pharmacokinet 1981, **6**, 21 5.
612. Clin Pharmacokinet Ther 1989, **46**, 182.
613. Eur J Clin Pharmacol 1983, **25**, 253.
614. Clin Pharmacokinet 1991, **20**, 123.
615. Invest Urol 1979, **17**, 149.
616. Br J Clin Pharmac 1985, **19**, 363.
617. Clin Pharmac Ther 1975, **17**, 701.
618. J Antimicrob Chemother 1983, **12**, Suppl 8, 29.
619. Pharm Sci 1977, **66**, 447.
620. J Pharm Pharmac 1984, **36**, 202.
621. Eur J Clin Pharmac 1986, **30**, 705.
622. Clin Pharmac Ther 1978, **23**, 414.
623. Cancer Res., 1990, **50**, 2017.
624. Clin Pharmac 1987, **6**, 275.
625. Clin Pharmacokinet 1986, **11**, 343.
626. Postgred Med J 1972, **48**, Suppl 2, 1.
627. Clin Therap 1991, **13**, 100.
628. Clin Pharmac Ther 1977, **22**, 545.
629. Clin Pharmac 1977, **17**, 704.
630. Pharm Acta Helv 1973, **48**, 181.
631. Antimicrob Ag Chemother 1985, **27**, 774.
632. Antimicrob Ag Chemother 1984, **25**, 458.
633. Clin Pharmac Ther 1969, **10**, 401.
634. Aust J Pharma 1981, **62**, 403.
635. Clin Pharmacokinet 1985, **10**, 353.
636. Clin Pharmacokinet 1984, **9**, 136.
637. Clin Pharmacokinet 1985, **10**, 257.
638. Br J Clin Pharmac 1986, **22**, 21.
639. Br J Clin Pharmac 1097, **23**, 127.
640. Drugs 1979, **18**, 169.
641. Clin Pharmacokinet 1983, **8**, 17.
642. Clin Pharmacokinet 1976, **1**, 297.
643. Clin Pharmacokinet 1987, **13**, 91.
644. Drug Met Disposit 1977, **5**, 579.
645. Clin Pharmacokinet 1977, **2**, 93.
646. Br J Clin Pharmacol 1991, **31**, 143.
647. Clin Pharmac Ther 1979, **26**, 275.
648. Clin Pharmacokinet 1980, **5**, 424.
649. Drugs 1984, **28**, 38.
650. Drugs 1983, **25**, Suppl 2.
651. Anaes Analg 1986, **65**, 743.
652. Eur J Clin Pharmac 1984, **26**, 613.
653. Clin Pharmacokinet 1986, **11**, 133.
654. Eur J Clin Pharmac 1987, **32**, 303.
655. Int J Derm 1981, **20**, 461.
656. Arzneim Forsch 1981, **31**, 1184.
657. J Antimicrob Chemother 1983, **1**, B101.
658. Antimicrob Ag Chemother 1983, **21**, 681.
659. Clin Pharmacokinet 1993, **25**, 370.
660. Clin Pharmacokinet 1994, **26**, 99.
661. J Antimicrob Chemother 1981, **8**, Suppl C, 41.
662. Ann Int Med 1967, **67**, 151.
663. Analyt Prof Drug Subs 1985, **14**, 527.
664. Eur J Clin Pharmac 1982, **23**, 249.
665. Arzneim Forsch 1981, **31**, 843.
666. Med J Aust 1987, **146**, 37.
667. Drugs. 1991, **42**, 511.
668. Clin Pharmac Ther 1977, **23**, 385.
669. Br Med J 1973, **3**, 347.
670. Scand J Rheumatol 1976, Suppl **13**, 9.
671. J Pharm Sci 1979, **68**, 850.
672. Martindale 1989, **29**[th] **edn.**, 714.
673. Eur J Clin Pharmac 1980, **17**, 305.
674. Clin Pharmacokinet 1976, **1**, 297.
675. Qun J Cardiol 1985, **55**, 8c.
676. Drugs 1983, **25**, 77.
677. Eur J Clin Pharmac 1983, **25**, 643.
678. Eur J Clin Pharmac 1986, **31**, 231.
679. Clin Pharmac Ther 1975, **17**, 363.
680. Drugs 1988, **35**, 1.
681. Arzneim Forsch 1983, **33**, 745.
682. Arzneim Forsch 1985, **35**, 149.
683. J Chromatogr 1987, **403**, 263.
684. Cancer Chemother Pharmac 1978, **1**, 177.
685. Drugs 1991, **41**, 130.
686. Clin Pharmacokinet 1985, **10**, 248.
687. Pharmacokinet Biopharm 1976, **4**, 1.
688. Biopharm Drug Disposit 1982, **3**, 337.
689. Eur J Clin Pharmac 1979, **15**, 275.

690. Br J Clin Pharmac 1982, **14**, 49.
691. Br J Clin Pharmac 1983, **16**, Suppl 2, 200S.
692. J Chromatogr 1978, **157**, 65.
693. Eur J Clin Pharmac 1985, **28**, 317.
694. Clin Pharmacokinet 1987, **12**, 440.
695. Clin Pharmacokinet 1987, **13**, 191.
696. Clin Pharmacokinet 1983, **8**, 332.
697. Eur J Clin Pharmacol, 1981, **21**, 127.
698. Br J Med 1987, **295**, 96.
699. Clin Pharmac Ther 1983, **34**, 86.
700. Eur J Clin Pharmac 1976, **10**, 263.
701. Arzneim Forsch 1974, **24**, 93.
702. Eur J Drug Met Pharmacokinet 1985, **10**, 147.
703. Eur J Clin Pharmac 1989, **37**, 525.
704. Tubercle 1972, **53**, 47.
705. Clin Pharmacokinet 198, **10**, 377.
706. Clin Pharmacokinet 1978, **3**, 128.
707. Handbook of Clin Pharm Data 1992, **ed. 1**, P131.
708. Antimicrob Ag Chemother 1980, **17**, 608.
709. Drugs 1976, **11**, 245.
710. Eur J Clin Pharmac 1991, **40**, 387.
711. Cancer Res 1984, **44**, 1693.
712. Martindale 1989, **29ᵗʰ edn.**, 1231.
713. Clin Pharmacokinet 1983, **8**, 202.
714. J Pharm Sci 1980, **69**, 1245.
715. Eur J Clin Pharmac 1983, **25**, 95.
716. Clin Pharmacokinet 1994, **26**, 335.
717. J Pharm Sci 1975, **64**, 1899.
718. Analyt Prof Drug Subs 1980, **9**, 107.
719. Drugs 1986, **32**, Suppl 3, 1.
720. J Pharmacokinet Biopharm 1978, **6**, 153.
721. J Pharm Sci 1975, **64**, 1899.
722. Antimicrob Ag Chemother 1972, **1**, 54.
723. Antimicrob Ag Chemother 1976, **9**, 800.
724. J Clin Pharmac 1977, **17**, 128.
725. Arzneim Forsch 1979, **29**, 361.
726. Antimicrob agents Chemother 1981, **19**, 613.
727. Chemotherapy (Tokyo) 1982, **30**, 212.
728. Clin Pharmac Ther 1985, **38**, 590.
729. Antimicrob Ag Chemother 1982, **21**, 141.
730. Antimicrob Ag Chemother 1985, **28**, 544.
731. Drugs 1986, **3**, 222.
732. Antimicrob Ag Chemother 1981, **19**, 298.
733. Antimicrob Ag Chemother 1982, **21**, 323.
734. Pharmacokinet Biopharm 1985, **13**, 121.
735. Drugs 1985, **30**, 382.
736. Antimicrob Ag Chemother 1982, **22**, 958.
737. Analyt Prof Drug Subs 1982, **11**, 195.
738. Antimicrob Ag Chemother 1980, **26**, 802.
739. Antimicrob Ag Chemother 1984, **25**, 221.
740. J Antimicrob Chemother 1990 , **26**, Suppl E, 21.
741. Drugs 1993, **45**, 295.
742. Pharmacokinet Biopharm 1982, **10**, 15.
743. Antimicrob Ag Chemother 1984, **25**, 579.
744. J Antibiot 1976, **29**, 444.
745. Antimicrob Ag Chemother 1990, **34**, 2307.
746. Antimicrob Ag Chemother 1976, **10**, 1.
747. Drugs 1985, **29**, 281.
748. Drugs 1984, **27**, 469.
749. J Antimicrob Chemother 1979,5, 183.
750. Drugs 1987, **34**, 438.
751. Postgrad Med J 1983, **59**, Suppl 5, 16.
752. J Pharm Sci 1975, **64**, 1899.
753. J Infect Dis 1978, **137**, Suppl May, S80.
754. Chemotherapy 1977, **23**, 389.
755. Clin Pharmac Ther 1980, **27**, 550.
756. Clin Pharmac Ther 1975, **18**, 215.
757. Clin Pharmac Ther 1973, **14**, 147.
758. Eur J Clin Pharmac 1984, **27**, 111.
759. J Clin Pharmac 1972, **12**, 74.
760. Eur J Clin Pharmac 1985, **28**, 229.
761. Clin Pharmacokinet 1978, **3**, 381.
762. Human Toxicol 1983, **2**, 361.
763. Arzneim Forsch 1986, **36**, 1116.
764. Br J Clin Pharmac 1987, **23**, 467.
765. Pharm J 1981, **2**, 265.
766. Analyt Prof Drug Subs 1973, **7**, 43.
767. Clin Pharmacokinet 1983, **3**, 14.
768. Eur J Clin Pharmac 1980, **18**, 165.
769. J Aanalyt Toxicol 1983, **7**, 29.
770. Br J Clin Pract 1968, **22**, 37.
771. Eur J Clin Pharmac 1980, **17**, 203.
772. Drug Dev Res 1986, **8**, 225.
773. Antimicrob Ag Chemother 1981, **19**, 1086.
774. Am J Med 1989, **87**, (Suppl 6) Br Med J, 45.
775. Clin Pharmacokinet 1991, **20**, 218.
776. Drugs 1983, **26**, 44.
777. Antimicrob Ag Chemother 1979, **31**, 956.
778. Clin Pharmacokinet 1983, **8**, 202.
779. Clin Pharmacokinet 1993, **25**, 189.
780. Antimicrob Ag Chemother 1982, **21**, 681.
781. Arzneim Forsch 1978, **28**, 1017.
782. Medicamenta 1973, **61**, 177.
783. J Pharm Sci 1973, **62**, 1929.
784. Drugs 1980, **20**, 161.
785. Drug Met Disposit 1981, **9**, 521.
786. Clin Pharmacokinet 1978, **3**, 425.
787. Clin Pharmacokinet 1991, **20**, 93.
788. New Engl J Med 1985, **312**, 1121.

789.	Drugs 1976, **12**, 321.
790.	Eur J Clin Pharmac 1983, **24**, 21.
791.	Eur J Clin Pharmacol 1979, **15**, 175.
792.	J Paedraitr 1984, **105**, 829.
793.	Eur J Clin Pharmac 1988, **34**, 445.
794.	Analyt Prof Drug Subs 1986, **15**, 151.
795.	Arzneim Forsch 1978, **28**, 308.
796.	J Pharma Pharmac 1983, **35**, 762.
797.	Eur J Drug Met Pharmacokinet 1989, **14**, 317.
798.	J Clin Pharmac 1982, **22**, 321.
799.	Med J Aust 1987, **146**, 37.
800.	Arzneim Forsch 1962, **12**, 853.
801.	Analyt Prof Drug Subs 1977, **6**, 83.
802.	Eur J Clin Pharmac 1976, **9**, 440.
803.	Clin Pharmacokinet 1991, **20**, 194.
804.	Arzneim Forsch 1975, **222**, 1769.
805.	J Clin Pharmac 1983, **26**, 358.
806.	Analyt Prof Drug Subs 1980, **9**, 155.
807.	Arzneim Forsch 1976, **26**, 914.
808.	Clin Pharmac Ther 1971, **12**, 944.
809.	Eur J Cancer 1972, **8**, 85.
810.	Int Med Res 1977, **5**, Suppl 3, 18.
811.	J Am Med Ass 1975, **231**, 862.
812.	Clin Pharmacokinet 1986, **11**, 299.
813.	Eur J Clin Pharmac 1985, **29**, 127.
814.	Drugs 1985, **29**, 342.
815.	Ther Drug Monit 1982, **4**, 115.
816.	Am J Psychiat 1985, **142**, 155.
817.	J Clin Pharmacol 1988, **28**, 853.
818.	Eur J Clin Pharmac 1983, **24**, 103.
819.	Clin Pharmac Ther 1978, **23**, 585.
820.	J Pharm Sci 1977, **66**, 1047.
821.	Drugs 1983, **26**, 70.
822.	J Clin Pharmac 1979, **19**, 205.
823.	Drug Met Rev 1975, **4**, 39.
824.	Clin Pharmacokinet 1978, **3**, 72.
825.	Clin Pharmacokinet 1977, **2**, 198.
826.	Drugs 1980, **20**, 24.
827.	Antimicrob Ag Chemother 1976, **10**, 441.
828.	Br J Med 1985, **291**, 1014.
829.	Clin Pharmacokinet 1993, **24**, 101.
830.	Drug met Rev 1975, **4**, 267.
831.	Drugs 1980, **19**, 84.
832.	Clin Pharmacokinet 1985, **10**, 514.
833.	Clin Pharmacokinet 1980, **5**, 137.
834.	Br J Med 1985, **290**, 1287.
835.	Clin Pharmac Ther 1981, **30**, 673.
836.	Clin Pharmac Ther 1989, **46**, 648.
837.	Eur J Drug Met Pharmacokinet 1991, **16**, 75.
838.	Clin Pharmac Ther 1974, **16**, 1066.
839.	Clin Pharmac Ther 1972, **13**, 407.
840.	Br J Clin Pharmac 1979, **7**, 81.
841.	Drug Intell Clin Pharma 1984, **18**, 869.
842.	Clin Pharmacokinet 1986, **1**, 214.
843.	Martindale 1990, **29ᵗʰ edn.**, 1329.
844.	J Pharm Pharmac 1990, **42**, 806.
845.	Clin Pharmac Ther 1978, **24**, 537.
846.	Eur J Drug Met Pharmacokinet 1981, **6**, 61.
847.	Am J Hosp Pharm 1979, **36**, 881.
848.	Br J Clin Pharmac 1986, **21**, 393.
849.	Clin Pharmacokinet 1983, **8**, 179.
850.	Br J Clin Pharmac 1976, **3**, 123.
851.	Br J Clin Pharmac 1982, **13**, 699.
852.	Clin Pharmacokinet 1985, **10**, 365.
853.	Clin Pharmacokinet 1988, **15**, 15.
854.	Eur J Drug Met Pharmacokinet 1983, **8**, 43.
855.	Clin Pharmacokinet 1977, **2**, 344.
856.	Martindale 1989, **29ᵗʰ edn.**, 1397.
857.	Clin Pharmac Ther 1976, **19**, 813.
858.	Martindale 1989 , **29ᵗʰ edn.**, 403.
859.	Clin Pharmacokinet 1985, **10**, 377.
860.	Drugs 1987, **34**, 519.
861.	J Antimicrob Chemother 1986, **18**, Suppl D7.
862.	Thromb Heamost 1994, **71**, 305.
863.	Clin Pharmacokinet 1987, **13**, 91.
864.	Drugs 1989, **38**, Suppl 2, 10.
865.	Drugs 1978, **15**, 3.
866.	Cancer Treat Rep 1982, **66**, 1819.
867.	Clin Pharmacokinet 1985, **10**, 334.
868.	J Antimicrob Chemother 1987, **20**, 467.
869.	J Clin Pharmac 1986, **26**, 44.
870.	Med Lett 1982, **24**, 74.
871.	Drugs 1985, **29**, 57.
872.	Clin Pharmac Ther 1977, **22**, 615.
873.	Gen Pharmac 1990, **21**, 267.
874.	Br J Clin Pharmac 1092, **13**, 325.
875.	Clin Pharmacol. 1982, **3**, 174.
876.	Br J Anaes 1975, **47**, 213.
877.	Clin Pharmacokinet 1991, **20**, 218.
878.	Drugs Ther Bull 1987, **25**, 11.
879.	Clin Pharmacokinet 1987, **12**, 79.
880.	Human Toxixol 1986, **5**, 136.
881.	Antimicrob Chem Chemother 1993, **4**, Suppl 1, 47.
882.	Drugs 1989, **38**, 560.
883.	Clin Pharmacokinet 1993, **24**, 441.
884.	Drugs 1987, **34**, Suppl 3.
885.	Drugs 1981, **21**, 1.
886.	Drugs 1975, **10**, 241.
887.	Drugs 1977, **13**, 241.

888. J Pharm Sci 1979, **68**, 1456.
889. Br J Anaes 1986, **58**, 950.
890. Pharmacotherapy 1993, **13**, 309.
891. Eur J Clin Pharmac 1991, **40**, 155.
892. Martindale 1989, **29th edn.**, 628.
893. Eur J Clin Pharmac 1985, **27**, 713.
894. Antimicrob Ag Chemother 1985, **28**, 648.
895. Clin Pharmacokinet 1983, **8**, 17.
896. Analyt Prof Drug Subs 1974, **3**, 281.
897. Analyt Prof Drug Subs 1982, **11**, 313.
898. Br J Clin Pharmac 1986, **22**, 421.
899. Clin Pharmacokinet 1986, **11**, 18.
900. Clin Pharmacokinet 1983, **8**, 202.
901. Clin Pharmacokinet 1994, **26**, 201.
902. Eur J Clin Pharmac 1980, **18**, 355.
903. Eur J Clin Pharmac 1983, **25**, 709.
904. Clin Pharmacokinet 1976, **1**, 426.
905. Drugs 1979, **18**, 417.
906. Arzneim Forsch 1970, **20**, 1689.
907. Martindale 1989, **29th edn.**, 1400.
908. Antimicrob Ag Chemother 1989, **33**, 742.
909. Clin Pharmac Ther 1983, **34**, 644.
910. Drugs 1992, **43**, 123.
911. Clin Pharmacokinet 1979, **4**, 279.
912. Clin Pharmac Ther 1971, **12**, 793.
913. Clin Pharmacokinet 1993, **24**, 441.
914. Z Kardiol 1989, **78**, Suppl 15, 20.
915. Drugs 1990, **39**, 597.
916. Drugs 1988, **36**, 314.
917. Clin Pharmacokinet 1979, **4**, 170.
918. Clin Pharmacokinet 1984, **9**, 473.
919. Arzneim Forsch 1972, **22**, 2153.
920. Drugs 1984, **27**, 301.
921. Drugs 1979, **18**, 329.
922. Arzneim Forsch 1975, **2**, 1455.
923. Clin Pharmac Ther 1971, **12**, 849.
924. Drugs of Today 1989, **25**, 689.
925. Clin Pharmacokinet 1983, **8**, 410.
926. J Pharm Pharmac 1974, **26**, 352.
927. Arzneim Forsch 1964, **14**, 394.
928. Biopharm Drug Dispos 1984, **5**, 101.
929. Drugs 1991, **41**, 254.
930. Eur J Clin Pharmacol 1994, **46**, 159.
931. Analyt Prof Drug Subs 1979, **8**, 219.
932. Clin Pharmac Ther 1980, **27**, 44.
933. Drugs 1985, **30**, 22.
934. Eur J Clin Pharmac 1979, **15**, 121.
935. Clin Pharmac Ther 1979, **25**, 283.
936. Xenobiotica 1990, **20**, 1357.
937. Int Pharmacopsychotherap 1982, **17**, 238.

938. Clin Pharmacokinet 1980, **5**, 204.
939. Clin Pharmacol Ther 1988, **43**, 436.
940. Clin Pharmacokinet 1982, **7**, 185.
941. Clin Pharmacokinet 1979, **4**, 63.
942. Analyt Prof Drug Subs 1983, **12**, 277.
943. J Pharm Sci 1979, **68**, 1456.
944. Eur J Clin Pharmac 1985, **28**, 357.
945. Martindale 1989, **29th edn.**, 1401.
946. Drugs 1984, **28**, 324.
947. Postgrad Med J 1975, **51**, Suppl 7, 76.
948. J Pharm Sci 1984, **73**, 561.
949. Biopharm Drug Disposit 1990, **11**, 507.
950. Cancer Res 1989, **49**, 2415.
951. Clin Pharmac Ther 1976, **19**, 365.
952. Drugs 1992, **44**, 408.
953. Curr Ther Res 1984, **36**, 228.
954. Clin Pharmacokinet 1987, **13**, 254.
955. Clin Pharmacokinet 1981, **6**, 245.
956. Clin Pharmacokinet 1990, **19**, 390.
957. Pharm Res 1993, **10**, 567.
958. Xenobiotica 1990, **20**, 1357.
959. Clin Pharmacokinet 1985, **10**, 303.
960. Br J Pharmac 1972, **46**, 958.
961. J Am Pharm Ass Sci Ed 1953, **42**, 457.
962. Analyt Prof Drug Subs 1973, **2**, 295.
963. Clin Pharmacokinet 1979, **4**, 401.
964. J Pharma Pharmac 1974, **26**, 265.
965. Clin Pharmac Ther 1985, **38**, 140.
966. Clin Pharmacokinet 1988, **15**, 32.
967. J Paediatr 1981, **98**, 146.
968. Clin Pharmacokinet 1992, **23**, 42.
969. Eur J Clin Pharmac 1987, **32**, 361.
970. Hand Book of Clin Pharm Data **1st ed.** 1992, P-131.
971. Clin Pharmacokinet 1979, **4**, 170.
972. Clin Pharmacokinet 1987, **12**, 79.
973. Drugs 1990, **40**, 903.
974. Clin Pharmacokinet 1983, **8**, 233.
975. Clin Pharmacokinet 1983, **8**, 17.
976. Clin Pharmacokinet 1987, **12**, 214.
977. Drugs Exp Clin Res 1985, **11**, 479.
978. Clin Pharmacokinet 1984, **9**, 157.
979. Clin Pharmac Ther 1977, **21**, 647.
980. Drugs 1983, **26**, 279.
981. Clin Pharm 1988, **7**, 52.
982. Biopharm Drug Disposit 1986, **7**, 71.
983. Drugs 1987, **34**, 648.
984. Eur J Clin Pharmac 1980, **17**, 215.
985. Res Comm Chem Path Pharmac 1983, **41**, 3.
986. Clin Pharmacokinet 1995, **28**, 203.

987. Br Med J 1981, **282**, 400.
988. Clin Pharmacokinet 1987, **13**, 91.
989. Clin Pharmac Ther 1981, **29**, 808.
990. Pharm Data 1992, **ed.1**, 131.
991. Eur J Clin Pharmac 1987, **32**, 11.
992. Eur J Clin Pharmac 1991, **40**, 399.
993. Ther Drug Monit 1980, **2**, 73.
994. J Pharm Sci 1966, **55**, 730.
995. Drug Ther Bull 1983, **21**, 99.
996. Biopharm Drug Disposit 1990, **11**, 543.
997. J Clin Pharmac 1979, **19**, 211.
998. Drugs, 1993, **45**, 716.
999. J Clin Pharmac 1987, **27**, 530.
1000. Clin Pharmacokinet 1981, **6**, 89.
1001. Clin Pharmac Ther 1979, **26**, 187.
1002. Clin Pharmacokinet 1983, **8**, 202.
1003. Postgrad Med J 1990, **66**, Suppl 4, S28.
1004. Clin Pharm 1988, **7**, 21.
1005. Clin Pharmac Ther 1978, **24**, 233.
1006. Drugs 1977, **13**, 321.
1007. J Clin Pharmac 1972, **12**, 453.
1008. Clin Pharmac Ther 1981, **30**, 551.
1009. Antimicrob Ag Chemother 1983, **23**, 827.
1010. Martindale 1989, **29th edn.**, 456.
1011. Br J Clin Med 1977, **4**, 51.
1012. Eur J Clin Pharmac 1990, **39**, 169.
1013. Eur J Clin Pharmac 1977, **12**, 387.
1014. Chemotheraoia 1986, **5**, 159.
1015. Curr Ther Res 1968, **10**, 592.
1016. Clin Pharmacokinet 1985, **10**, 187.
1017. Eur J Clin Pharmac 1980, **17**, 59.
1018. Clin Pharmacokinet 1982, **7**, 421.
1019. Clin Pharmac Ther 1979, **26**, 737.
1020. Toxicol Appl Pharmac 1978, **44**, 225.
1021. J Pharm Sci 1972, **61**, 1663.
1022. Br J Anaes 1979, **51**, 481.
1023. Chemotherapie 1964, **9**, 20.
1024. Drugs 1985, **30**, 285.
1025. Clin Pharmacokinet 1986, **11**, 87.
1026. New Engl J Med 1983, **308**, 1005.
1027. Clin Pharmacokinet 1985, **10**, 285.
1028. Clin Pharmacokinet 1986, **5**, 572.
1029. Br J Clin Pharmac 1981, **12**, 235.
1030. Clin Pharmacokinet 1986, **11**, 87.
1031. J Pharmacokinet Biopharm 1978, **6**, 111.
1032. Rev Infect Dis 1985, **7**, 287.
1033. Handbook of Clin Pharm Data 1992, **ed.1**, 131.
1034. Martindale 1990, **29th edn.**, 1235.
1035. Clin Pharmacokinet 1987, **1**, 1.
1036. Clin Pharmacokinet 1984, **9**, 335.
1037. Clin Pharmac Ther 1976, **19**, 435.
1038. Clin Pharmacokinet 1982, **7**, 221.
1039. Merck Index 1989, **11th edn.**, 919.
1040. J Pharm Sci 1985, **74**, 375.
1041. J Pharm Sci 1972, **61**, 1746.
1042. Arch Int Pharmavcodyne Ther 1956, **106**, 388.
1043. Headache 1976, **16**, 96.
1044. Drugs 1983, **25**, 451.
1045. Anaesthesiology 1986, **64**, 72.
1046. Clin Pharmac Ther 1974, **16**, 322.
1047. Br J Clin Pharmac 1981, **11**, 287.
1048. Clin Pharmacokinet 1983, **8**, 43.
1049. Br J Clin Pharmac 1978, **6**, 103.
1050. J Antimicrob Chemother 1975, **1**, 39.
1051. Drugs 1978, **16**, 273.
1052. Clin Pharmacokinet 1983, **8**, 17.
1053. Anaesthesiol 1984, **61**, 27.
1054. Arch Int Pharmacodyn Ther 1979, **238**, 96.
1055. Drugs 1988, **36**, 158.
1056. Drugs 1988, **35**, 187.
1057. J Antimicrob Chemother 1977, **3**, 247.
1058. Drugs 1978, **22**, 257.
1059. Human Toxicol 1984, **3**, 29.
1060. Dig Dis Sci 1985, **30**, Suppl 126S.
1061. Clin Pharmac Ther 1983, **34**, 259.
1062. Martindale 1989, **29th edn.**, 643.
1063. Cancer Treat Rev 1983, **10**, (Suppl), Br Med J, 23.
1064. Eur J Clin Pharmar 1985, **28**, 89.
1065. Clin Ther 1985, **7**, 169.
1066. Clin Pharmac Ther 1991, **50**, 141.
1067. Drugs 1990, **40**, 138.
1068. Clin Pharmacokinet 1986, **11**, 505.
1069. Clin Pharm 1984, **3**, 351.
1070. Br J Derm 1982, **107**, Suppl 22, 25.
1071. Clin Pharmac Ther 1977, **22**, 85.
1072. Drugs 1988, **35**, 504.
1073. J Clin Pharmac 1979, **19**, 712.
1074. Gastroenterology, 1977, **73**, 1388.
1075. Eur Toxicol 1969, **11**, 40.
1076. Drugs 2983, **26**, 191.
1077. J Clin Pharmac 1982, **22**, 490.
1078. Qun. Emerg. Med., 1983, **12**, 438.
1079. Drugs 1988, **35**, 192.
1080. Drugs 1990, **40**, 91.
1081. Analyt Prof Drug Subs 1981, **10**, 513.
1082. Drugs 1980, **19**, 249.
1083. Clin Pharmac Ther 1983, **34**, 644.
1084. Anesthesiology 1983, **59**, 220.
1085. Eur J Clin Pharmac 1983, **24**, 643.

1086.   Postgrad Med J 1984, **60**, Suppl 4.
1087.   Clin Pharmacokinet 1978, **3**, 425.
1088.   Clin Pharm Ther 1993, **53**, 316.
1089.   Br Clin Pharmac 1981, **12**, 621.
1090.   Drugs 1985, **30**, 182.
1091.   J Clin Pharmac 1987, **27**, 293.
1092.   Pharmac Res 1987, **4**, Suppl 2.
1093.   Clin Pharm Bull 1985, **33**, 3456.
1094.   Drugs 1987, **34**, 578.
1095.   Br J Clin Pharmac 1977, **4**, 709.
1096.   Drugs 1987, **33**, 134.
1097.   J Antimicrob Chemother 1986, **17**, 333.
1098.   Clin Pharmacokinet 1988, **15**, 32.
1099.   Drug Met Disposit 1986, **14**, 175.
1100.   Clin Pharmac Ther 1979, **26**, 669.
1101.   Pharmacology of Conceptive steroids, 1994, **136**.
1102.   Br J Clin Pharmac 1978, **24**, 448.
1103.   J Antimicrob Chemother 1984, **13**, Suppl B59.
1104.   Br J Clin Pharmac 1985, **19**, 832.
1105.   Arzneim Forsch 1979, **29**, 967.
1106.   Analyt Prof Drug Subs 1977, **6**, 341.
1107.   Clin Pharmacokinet 1993, **25**, 375.
1108.   Med Lett 1986, **28**, 119.
1109.   Drugs 1987, **34**, Suppl 1, 21.
1110.   Eur J Clin Pharmac 1990, **39**, 195.
1111.   Eur J Clin Pharmac 1987, **138**, 301.
1112.   Int J Clin Pharmac Ther Tox 1985, **2**, 59.
1113.   Chemotherapy 1976, **22**, 19.
1114.   Arzneim Forsch 1970, **20**, 538.
1115.   New Engl J Med 1973, **289**, 1063.
1116.   Antimicrob Agents Chemother 1969, **9**, 42.
1117.   J Antimicrob Chemother 1987, **19**, 87.
1118.   Drugs 1986, **32**, 291.
1119.   Clin Pharmacokinet 1981, **6**, 89.
1120.   Clin Pharmac Ther 1976, **20**, 401.
1121.   Therapie 1967, **22**, 521.
1122.   Drugs 1987, **34**, 50.
1123.   Helv Chim Acta 1957, **40**, 395.
1124.   Drugs 1976, **11**, 45.
1125.   Clin Pharmacokinet 1994, **27**, 256.
1126.   Biopharm Drug Disposit 1990, **11**, 607.
1127.   Drugs 1991, **41**, 521.
1128.   Anaestheology 1986, **64**, 72.
1129.   Eur J Clin Pharmac 1984, **27**, 127.
1130.   Clin Pharmacokinet 1982, **7**, 93.
1131.   Toxicol Appl Pharmac 1969, **15**, 269.
1132.   J Pharm Pharmac 1981, **33**, 134.
1133.   Drugs 1991, **41**, 225.
1134.   J Pharm Sci 1974, **63**, 708.
1135.   Drugs 1989, **37**, 628.
1136.   J Med Chem 1987, **30**, 1342.
1137.   Br J Clin Pharmac 1979, **8**, 459.
1138.   J Clin Pharmac 1977, **17**, 231.
1139.   Clin Pharmac Ther 1981, **30**, 404.
1140.   Merck Index 1989, **11th edn.**, 1132.
1141.   J Infect Dis 1985, **152**, 750.
1142.   Clin Pharmacokinet 1983, **8**, 332.
1143.   Drug Intell Clin Pharma 1987, **21**, 459.
1144.   Drugs 1987, **34**, 50.
1145.   Neuropharmacology 1980, **19**, 831.
1146.   J Pharm Sci 1974, **63**, 389.
1147.   Drugs of the Future 1988, **13**, 801.
1148.   Curr Ther Res 1986, **40**, 871.
1149.   Clin Pharmacokinet 1983, **7**, 421.
1150.   Br J Clin Pharmac 1985, **19**, 657.
1151.   Drugs 1985, **29**, 342.
1152.   Analyt Prof Drug Subs 1975, **4**, 319.
1153.   J Analyt Toxicol 1979, **2**, 253.
1154.   Eur J Clin Pharmac 1973, **6**, 15.
1155.   Br J Clin Pharmac 1986, **22**, 61.
1156.   Analyt Prof Drug Subs 1978, **7**, 359.
1157.   Br J Clin Pharmac 1985, **19**, 657.
1158.   J Pharmacokinet Biopharm 1973, **1**, 319.
1159.   Analyt Prof Drug Subs.
1160.   Clin Pharmacol 1990, **30**, 372.
1161.   Anaesth Anaklg Curr Res 1973, **52**, 161.
1162.   J Clin Pharmacol 1990, **30**, 372.
1163.   Clin Pharmacokinet 1979, **4**, 153.
1164.   Drugs 1985, **30**, 6.
1165.   J Pharma Pharmac 1990, **42**, 804.
1166.   Drugs 1976, **12**, 1.
1167.   Clin Pharmac Ther 1986, **40**, 650.
1168.   Eur J Clin Pharmac 1983, **25**, 357.
1169.   Pharmacokinet 1994, **26**, 120.
1170.   Drugs 1984, **28**, 375.
1171.   J Pharm Sci 1973, **62**, 2024.
1172.   Therapie 1986, **41**, 27.
1173.   J Pharm Belg 1972, **27**, 281.
1174.   Br J Clin Pharmac 1983, **15**, 287.
1175.   Scand J Gast 1979, **14**, Suppl 57.
1176.   Clin Pharmacokinet 1987, **13**, 254.
1177.   Drugs 1984, **28**, 292.
1178.   Clin Pharmac Ther 1977, **21**, 721.
1179.   J Antimicrob Chemother 1975, **1**, 39.
1180.   Eur J Clin Pharmac 1982, **23**, 249.
1181.   Eur J Clin Pharmac 1983, **25**, 759.
1182.   Antimicrob Ag Chemother 1987, **31**, 1051.
1183.   Clin Pharmac Ther 1978, **23**, 241.
1184.   Clin Pharmac Ther 1973, **14**, 26.

1185.	Clin Pharmacokinet 1994, **27**, 94.
1186.	J Clin Pharmac 1984, **24**, 446.
1187.	Eur J Clin Pharmac 1978, **14**, 281.
1188.	Clin Pharmacokinet 1980, **5**, 365.
1189.	Clin Pharmacokinet 1979, **4**, 111.
1190.	Endocrinology 1985, **4**, 325.
1191.	Biopharm Drug Disposit 1986, **7**, 47.
1192.	Arzneim Forsch 1973, **23**, 74.
1193.	Eur J Clin Pharmac 1986, **31**, 205.
1194.	Analyt Prof Drug Subs 1988, **17**, 749.
1195.	Clin Pharmacokinet 1981, **6**, 135.
1196.	Drugs 1978, **15**, 409.
1197.	Clin Pharmacokinet 1978, **3**, 97.
1198.	Clin Pharmac Ther 1972, **13**, 279.
1199.	Analyt Prof Drug Subs 1976, **5**, 403.
1200.	Br J Clin Pharmac 1987, **23**, 137.
1201.	Eur J Clin Pharmac 1985, **28**, 73.
1202.	J Pharm Sci 1982, **71**, 633.
1203.	Br Med J 1980, **280**, 825.
1204.	Br J Clin Pharmac 1986, **31**, 205.
1205.	Martindale 1989, **29th edn.**, 765.
1206.	Br J Clin Pharmac 1983, **15**, 287.
1207.	New Engl J Med 1990, **322**, 518.
1208.	Br J Clin Pharmac 1977, **7**, 89.
1209.	Postgrad Med J 1985, **61**, Suppl 3, 64.
1210.	Clin Pharmac Ther 1986, **40**, 29.
1211.	Handbook of Clin Pharm Data 1992, **ed.1**, P-131.
1212.	Drug Intell Clin Pharma 1983, **17**, 736.
1213.	J Pharma Pharmac 1970, **22**, 26.
1214.	Tubercle 1976, **57**, 97.
1215.	Eur J Clin Pharmac 1980, **18**, 423.
1216.	Pharm Res 1990, **7**, 1055.
1217.	Drug Met Dispos 1985, **13**, 25.
1218.	Clin Pharmac Ther 1974, **16**, 376.
1219.	Drugs 1991, **41**, 378.
1220.	Clin Pharmacokinet 1980, **5**, 150.
1221.	Clin Pharmacokinet 1985, **10**, 187.
1222.	J Clin Pharmac 1984, **24**, 343.
1223.	Eur J Clin Pharmac 1984, **27**, 577.
1224.	Clin Pharmacokinet 1984, **9**, 211.
1225.	Br J Clin Pharmac 1976, **3**, 583.
1226.	J Clin Pharmac 1985, **25**, 633.
1227.	Clin Pharmacokonet 1993, **24**, 101.
1228.	Antimicrob Agents Chemother 1989, **33**, 1237.
1229.	Clin Pharmacokinet 1978, **3**, 108.
1230.	Clin Pharmacol Ther 1987, **42**, 449.
1231.	Br J Clin Pharmac 1976, **3**, 583.
1232.	Pharmacotherapy 1994, **14**, 253.
1233.	Clin Pharmacokinet 1991, **20**, 218.
1234.	Drugs 1972, **3**, 314.
1235.	J Pharma Pharmac 1978, **30**, 386.
1236.	Drugs 1985, **30**, 368.
1237.	J Pharm Sci 1984, **73**, 1657.
1238.	J Pharm Sci 1984, **73**, 56.
1239.	J Pharma Pharmac 1975, **27**, 923.
1240.	Br J Clin Pharmac 1978, **6**, 542.
1241.	Martindale 1989, **29th edn.**, 649.
1242.	Clin Pharmacokinet 1993, **24**, 203.
1243.	Clin Pharmacokinet 1993, **24**, 195.
1244.	J Pharma Pharmac 1972, **24**, 525.
1245.	Drugs 1987, **34**, 311.
1246.	J Antimicrob Chemother 1980, **6**, 647.
1247.	Drug Met Rev 1978, **8**, 51.
1248.	Br J Clin Pharmacol 1991, **31**, 143.
1249.	Analyt Prof Drug Subs 1986, **16**, 507.
1250.	J Clin Pharmac 1977, **17**, 379.
1251.	Clin Pharmacokinet 1986, **11**, 18.
1252.	Clin Pharmacokinet 1986, **11**, 372.
1253.	Martindale 1989, **29th edn.**, 310.
1254.	Clin Pharmacol Ther 1991, **49**, 402.
1255.	Clin Pharmacokinet 1980, **5**, 247.
1256.	Eur J Clin Pharmacol 1985, **28**, 97.
1257.	J Pharmacokinet Biopharm 1982, **10**, 281.
1258.	Drugs 1968, **16**, 97.
1259.	J Pharm Sci 1984, **73**, 1128.
1260.	Martindale 1989, **29th edn.**, 305.
1261.	Clin Pharmacokinet 1980, **5**, 274.
1262.	Analyt Prof Drug Subs 1988, **17**, 571.
1263.	Clin Pharmacokinet 1978, **3**, 319.
1264.	Antimicrob Ag Chemother 1976, **9**, 557.
1265.	Clin Pharmacokinet 1985, **10**, 285.
1266.	Clin Pharmacokinet 1982, **7**, 42.
1267.	Clin Pharmacokinet 1976, **1**, 406.
1268.	Br J Pharmac 1988, **94**, 123.
1269.	J Antimicrob Chemother 1982, **10**, 49.
1270.	Clin Pharmac Ther 1989, **3**, 634.
1271.	Clin Pharmacol Ther 1995, **57**, 281.
1272.	Drugs of Today 1979, **15**, 349.
1273.	J Pharma Pharmac 1986, **38**, 888.
1274.	Biopharm Drug Disposit 1990, **11**, 499.
1275.	Clin Pharmacokinet 1987, **12**, 223.
1276.	Eur J Clin Pharmac 1990, **38**, 547.
1277.	Drugs 1987, **33**, 461.
1278.	Drug Met Rev 1983, **14**, 295.
1279.	Chemotherapy 1983, **29**, 322.
1280.	J Clin Pharmacol 1992, **32**, 267.
1281.	Br J Derm 1977, **97**, 237.
1282.	Chromatogr 1981, **226**, 175.
1283.	Can J Hosp Pharm 1977, **30**, 146.

1284. Med Res Rev 1983, **3**, 119.
1285. Proc Nat Acad Sci 1981, **8**, 2545.
1286. Clin Pharmac Ther 1983, **34**, 546.
1287. J Chromatogr 1982, **233**, 417.
1288. Toxical Appl Pharmac 1966, **9**, 31.
1289. J Int Med Res 1983, **11**, 137.
1290. Cancer Res 1971, **31**, 1627.
1291. Clin Pharmacokinet 1987, **13**, 1.
1292. Eur J Clin Pharmac 1978, **14**, 341.
1293. Martindale 1989, **29th edn.**, 652.
1294. J Pharm Pharmac 1971, **23**, 719.
1295. Handbook of Clin Pharm Data 1992, **ed.1**, 131.
1296. Eur J Clin Pharmac 1986, **31**, 397.
1297. Drugs 1985, **29**, 208.
1298. J Int Med Res 1977, **5**, 308.
1299. Drugs 1987, **34**, 222.
1300. Clin Pharmac Ther 1985, **38**, 409.
1301. Antimicrob Ag Chemother 1969, **9**, 267.
1302. Biopharm Drug Disposit 1990, **11**, 351.
1303. Drugs 1981, **22**, 211.
1304. Analyt Prof Drug Subs 1974, **3**, 513.
1305. Eur J Clin Pharmac 1985, **28**, 573.
1306. Drugs 1978, **15**, 429.
1307. Clin Pharmac Ther 1984, **36**, 493.
1308. Drug Research 1988, **38**, 164.
1309. Eur J Clin Pharmac 1981, **20**, 65.
1310. Clin Pharmac Ther 1986, **40**, 444.
1311. Drugs 1981, **21**, 401.
1312. Clin Pharmacol 1995, **35**, 302.
1313. Eur J Clin Pharmac 1979, **16**, 39.
1314. Clin Pharmac Ther 1986, **39**, 313.
1315. Clin Pharmacokinet 1983, **8**, 233.
1316. Clin Pharmac Ther 1973, **14**, 147.
1317. J Pharm Sci 1984, **73**, 261.
1318. J Pharm Sci 1977, **66**, 841.
1319. Clin Pharmacokinet 1983, **2**, 417.
1320. Drug Met Pharmacokinet 1989, **14**, 139.
1321. Clin Pharmacokinet 1984, **9**, 222.
1322. Clin Pharmacokinet 1977, **2**, 230.
1323. Drugs 1990, **40**, Suppl 4, 67.
1324. Clin Pharmacokinet 1980, **5**, 67.
1325. Drug Intell Clin Pharm 1970, **4**, 332.
1326. Anaesthesiol 1983, **58**, 405.
1327. J Clin Pharmacol 1992, **32**, 716.
1328. Clin Pharmacokinet 1985, **10**, 248.
1329. Antimicrob Ag Chemother 1980, **18**, 709.
1330. Br J Clin Pharmac 1989, **27**, 19S – 22S.
1331. Drugs 1977, **13**, 401.
1332. Clin Pharmacokinet 1983, **8**, 202.
1333. Clin Pharmacokinet 1986, **11**, 483.
1334. Drug Met Dispos 1984, **12**, 652.
1335. Arzneim Forsch 1977, **27**, 2143.
1336. Clin Pharmacokinet 1995, **28**, 351.
1337. Proc Nat Acad Sci Usa 1985, **82**, 7096.
1338. Arzneim Forsch 1981, **31**, 486.
1339. Clin Pharmacokinet 1995, **29**, 142.
1340. Int J Clin Pharmac Ther Tox 1985, **23**, 97.
1341. Acta Psychiat Scand 1981, **64**, Suppl 294, 1.
1342. Ivan H.Stockley "Drug Interactions" 2nd Ed. Blackwell Scientific Publication, London. P 14-600.
1343. Clin. Pharmacol. Ther, 1981, **30**, 239–245.
1344. .J AM MED ASSOC, 1998, **279**, 1200-1205.
1345. The lancet, 2000, **356**, 1255–1259.
1346. J Indian Acad Clin Med, 2004; **5(1):** 27-33.
1347. Int J Pharm Pharm Sci, 2012, **Vol 4,** Suppl 4, 698-704.
1348. Eur J Clin Pharmacol, 2007; **64(3):**303-9.
1349. Can. Med. Assoc. J.,2009,**180(7),**713-18.
1350. Clin Pharmacol Ther, 1997 62, 464–475.
1351. Aust Prescr 2012; 35:85–8.
1352. Clin Pharmacol Ther, 2007, 81, 298-304.
1353. Br J Clin Pharmacol, 2004,58(6),569-570.
1354. Br J Clin Pharmacol,2006,61,650-665.
1355. Clin Pharmacol ther 2007, 81(1), 17-18.
1356. Clin Pharmacol ther, 2008, 83(2),213-217.
1357. Clin Pharmacol ther, 2007,81 (1),3-6.
1358. J Clin Pharm Ther, 1999,**24**, 339–346.
1359. Pharmacopsychiatry, 1997; **30**: 94-101.
1360. Planta Med 1998; **64(4):** 353-356.
1361. Br. J. Clin. Pharmacol , 2004,**57**, 6–14.
1362. Exp Clin Endocrinol Diabetes 2000; **108(2),** 100-105.
1363. J R Soc Med, 2011,**104**,292-298.
1364. Nat RevGenet, 2010, **11**, 241-246.

Appendix

Table A.1 Hematological Values

	Conventional units	SI units*
Blood Volume		
RED CELL VOLUME Male Female	20 – 36 ml/kg body weight 19 – 32 ml/kg body weight	0.020 – 0.036 L/kg body weight 0.019 – 0.32 L/kg body weight
PLASMA VOLUME Male Female	25 – 43 ml/kg body weight 28 – 45 ml/kg body weight	0.025 – 0.043 L/kg body weight 0.028– 0.045 L/kg body weight
TOTAL BLOOD VOLUME	70 ± 10 ml/kg body weight	0.070 ± 0.010 L/kg body weight
Complete Blood Count (CBC)		
HEMATOCRIT Male Female Infants (full term cord blood) Children, 3 months Children, 3 – 6 yrs Children, 10 – 12 yrs.	 40 – 54% 38 – 47% 54 ± 10% 38 ± 6% 40 ± 4% 41 ± 4%	Volume fraction 0.40 – 0.54 0.38 – 0.47 0.54 ± 0.10 L/L 0.38 ± 0.06 L/L 0.40 ± 0.04 L/L 0.41 ± 0.04 L/L
HEMOGLOBIN Male Female	13.5 – 18.0 g/dl 12.0 – 16.0 g/dl	2.09 – 2.79 mmol/L 1.86 – 2.48 mmol/L
RED CELL COUNT Male Female	$4.6 – 6.2 \times 10^6$ /μl $4.2 – 5.4 \times 10^6$ /μl	$4.6 – 6.2 \times 10^{12}$ /μl $4.2 – 5.4 \times 10^{12}$ /μl
RED CELL INDICES (1) Mean Corpuscular Volume (MCV) Adults Infants (full term cord blood) Children, 3 months (2) Mean Corpuscular Hemoglobin (MCH) Adults Children, 3 months Children, 1 yr. Children, 3-6 yrs Children, 10-12 yrs. (3) Mean Cell Hemoglobin Concentration (MCHC) Adults & children	 80 – 96 cubic microns 27 – 31 pg 32 – 36%	 80 – 96 fl 106 fl (mean) 95 fl (mean) 27 – 31 pg 29 ± 5 pg 27 ± 4 pg 27 ± 3 pg 27 ± 3 pg Concentration fraction 0.32 – 0.36

Table A.2 Hematological Values (cont.)

Red Cell Diameter		
(MEAN VALUES) Adults (dry films) 6	6.7 – 7.7 µm	
RED CELL DENSITY	1092 – 1100 g/l	
RETICULOCYTES Adults/children Infants (full term cord blood) LEUCOCYTE COUNT Adults Infants (full term, 1st day) Infants, 1 yr Children, 4 – 7 yrs Children, 8 – 12 yrs	0.2 – 2% 2 – 6% $4.5 – 11 \times 10^3/\mu l$ $18 \pm 8 \times 10^3/\mu l$ $12 \pm 6 \times 10^3/\mu l$ $10 \pm 5 \times 10^3/\mu l$ $9 \pm 4.5 \times 10^3/\mu l$	$25 – 85 \times 10^9$ /L 150×10^9 /L $4.5 – 11 \times 10^9$/L $18 \pm 8 \times 10^9$/L $12 \pm 6 \times 10^9$/L $10 \pm 5 \times 10^9$/L $9 \pm 4.5 \times 10^9$/L
DIFFERENTIAL COUNT Adults Neutrophils Lymphocytes Monocytes Eosinophils Basophils	 40 – 75% 20 – 45% 2 – 10% 1 – 6% < 1%	 $2.0 – 7.5 \times 10^9$/L $1.5 – 4.0 \times 10^9$/L $0.2 – 0.8 \times 10^9$/L $0.04 – 0.4 \times 10^9$/L $<0.01 – 0.1 \times 10^9$/L
ERYTHROCYTE SEDIMENTATION RATE (ESR)* **Westergreen Method** Males < 50 yrs >50 yrs females < 50 yrs > 50 yrs **Wintrobe Method** Males Females	 < 15 mm/hr < 20 mm/hr < 20 mm/hr < 30 mm/hr 0 – 9 0 – 20	 < 15 mm/hr < 20 mm/hr < 20 mm/hr < 30 mm/hr
MISCELLANEOUS Hemoglobin A_2 Hemoglobin – F Viscosity Zeta sedimentation ratio	1.5 – 3.5% of total hemoglobin < 2% 1.4 – 1.8 times water 41 – 54%	Mass fraction 0.015 – 0.035 of Total hemoglobin Mass fraction < 0.02 1.4 – 1.8 times water Fraction 0.41 – 0.54

*WHO has recommended the adoption of SI (International system of Units) by the medical community throughout the World.

Table A.3 Liver Function Tests

Blood values	Conventional units		SI units*
BILIRUBIN Conjugated Unconjugated Total Newborns (total)	Serum	Upto 0.3 mg/dl 0.1 – 1.0 mg/dl 0.1 – 1.2 mg/dl 1 – 12 mg/dl	Up to 5.1 µmol/L 1.7 – 17.1 µmol/L 1.7 – 20.5 µmol/L 17.1-205.0 µmol/L
CHOLESTEROL Total Esterified	Serum	150 – 250 mg/dl 65 – 75% of total Cholesterol	3.90 – 6.50 µmol/L Fraction of total Cholesterol : 0.65 – 0.75

Blood values		Conventional units	SI units*
LIPIDS Total Triglycerides Phospholipids Phospolipid phosphorous Free fatty acids	Serum Plasma	400 – 800 mg/dl 10 – 190 mg/dl 150 – 380 mg/dl 8.0 – 11.0 mg/dl < 18 mg/dl	4.00 – 8.00 g/L 3.9 – 6.5 mmol/L 1.50 – 3.80 g/L 2.58 – 3.55 mmol/L <180 mg/L
PROTEINS Total Albumin Globulin Fibrinogen	Serum Plasma	6.0 – 7.8 g/dl 3.2 – 4.5 g/dl 2.3 – 3.5 g/dl 200 – 400 mg/dl	60 – 78 g/L 32 – 45 g/L 23 – 35 g/L 2.00 – 4.00 g/L
PROTHROMBIN TIME		70 – 110% of control	70 – 110% of control
PHOSPHATASES Alkaline Acid	Serum	30 – 120 U/L 0 – 5.5 U/L	0.5 – 2.0 μkat/L 0.90 μKat/L
TRANSFERASES Asparatate amino Transferase (SGOT/AST) Alanine amino Transferase (SGPT/ALT) Gamma glutamyl Transferase (GGT) Cephalin flocculation Thymol turbidity	Serum	10 – 40 U/ml (karmen) At 25^{0}C 10 – 30 U/ml (karmen) At 25^{0}C 5 – 40 IU/1 at 37^{0}C Up to 2 + in 48 hrs 0 – 4 units	8 – 29 U/L at 30^{0}C 4 – 24 U/L at 30^{0}C 5 – 40 U/L at 37^{0}C

*WHO has recommended the adoption of SI (International System of Units) by the medical community throughout the world.

Table A.4

Blood Biochemistry	
Alphal Antitrypsin (serum)	80 – 215 mg/dl
Alpha Fetoprotein (serum)	< 30 mg/ml
Bicarbonate	21 – 28 mEq/L
pH	7.38 – 7.44
Bicarbonate as alkali reserve	55 – 70 vols. Co_2/100 cc
Bicarbonate (serum) as HCO_3	24 – 26 mEq/L
Blood creatinine	1 – 1.5 mg/dl
Blood glucouse (Glucose oxidase method) Fasting PP (2 hours)	 55 – 90 mg/dl < 140mg/dl
Blood sugar (Folin Wu) Fasting PP	 80 – 120 mg/dl < 130mg/dl
Blood sugar (True sugar, Nelson-Somogyi, Modified Folin-Wu) Fasting PP	 60 – 100 mg/dl < 110mg/dl

Serum Calcium	9 – 11 mg/dl
Serum Ionised Calcium	4.5 – 5.5. mg/dl (2.3 – 2.8 mEq/L)
Serum Carcinoembryonic Antigen (CEA)	0 – 2.5 ng/ml
Serum Ceruloplasmin	27 – 37 mg/dl
Serum Chloride	85 – 105 mEq/L
Serum Copper	100 – 128 mg/dl
Serum Gastrin	40 – 200 pg/ml (40 – 200 mg/L)
Serum Immunoglobulins IgG	800 – 1500 mg/dl
IgM	45 – 150 mg/dl
IgA	90 – 325 mg/dl
IgD	0 – 8 mg/dl
IgE	<0.025 mg/dl
Serum inorganic	
Phosphorus	2 – 5 mg/dl
Serum Magnesium	1.5 – 2.5 mEq/L
Serum Potassium	4.0 – 6.0 mEq/L
Serum protein (total)	5.5 – 8.0 gm/dl
Serum albumin	3.0 – 5.0 gm/dl
Serum globulin	1.5 – 3 gm/dl
A/G ratio	More than 1
Serum Sodium	130 – 145 mEq/L
Serum Potassium	3 – 4.5 mEq/L
Serum triglyceride	50 – 150 mg/dl
Serum urea	12 – 40 mg/dl
Blood urea nitrogen (BUN)	6 – 20 mg/dl
Serum uric acid	2.0 – 8 mg/dl (Men)
Serum zinc	100 – 140 mg/dl

Table A.5

Vitamins	
Vitamin A (Serum)	20 – 100 mg/dl
Vitamin C (Plasma)	0.7 – 1.5 mg/dl
Vitamin B_1	5.5 – 9.5 mg/dl
Vitamin B_{12}	200 – 600 pg/ml
Serum Folate	6 – 21 ng/ml
Vitamin D 1, 25 Hydroxy D	20 – 60 pg/ml

Table A.6

Enzymes (Serum)	
Aldolase	0-8 I.U./L (0 – 130 mmol/L)
Amylase	60 – 180 Somogyi units/dl 13 – 53 mmol/L 8 – 32 Wohlgemuth Units/100 cc
Creatine Phosphokinase (CPK) Male Female Lactic dehydrogenase	25 – 90 units/ml 10 – 70 units/ml 60 – 100 units/dl (Wacker)

Table A.7

Blood Gases	
PO_2	80 – 100 mm of Hg (11-13 kPa)
PCO_2	35 – 45 mm of Hg (4.7 - 5.9 kPa)
CO_2 content Venous blood	50 – 60 Vol % (21 – 30 mEq/L)
Arterial blood	45 – 55 vol%
Oxygen saturation Arterial blood Venous blood CO_2 combining power	97% 60% - 85% 55 – 65 vol% (21 – 2.8 mEq/L)
O_2 content Venous blood CO_2 combining power	 11 – 56 vol% 15 – 22 vol%
Whole blood Ammonia (venous)	80 – 100 mg/dl

Table A.8

Cardiovascular Values	
Cardiac output (Fick)	$2.5 – 3$ liters/m^2/min
Circulation time Arm to tongue Arm to lung	 9 – 18 S 4 – 8 S

Table A.9

Pressures	
Left atrium	2 – 12 mm Hg
Right atrium	0 – 5 mm Hg
Left ventricle Systole Diastole	 120 mm Hg 2 – 12 mm Hg
Right ventricle Systole Diastole	 25mm Hg 0 – 5 mm Hg
Pulmonary artery Systole Diastole	 12 – 28 mm Hg 3– 13 mm Hg
Aorta Systole Diastole	 100 – 140 mm Hg 60 – 90 mm Hg
Arteriovenous Oxygen difference	30 – 50 ml/L
Ejection fraction	0.55 – 0.78
End diastolic volume	60 – 90 cc/M^2
End systolic volume	17 – 33 cc/M^2
Systemic vascular Resistance	770 – 1500 dynes/cm^2
Pulmonary vascular Resistance	20 – 120 dynes/cm^2

Table A.10

Hormones	
Plasma ACTH	< 80 pg/ml
Plasma cortisol	5 – 25 µg/dl 8 Am
	3 – 12 µg/dl 4 PM
17 Ketosteroids	7 – 25 mg/day (Men)
4 -15 mg/day (Women) Plasma Angiotensin II	10 – 30 pg/ml 8 Am
Plasma calcitonin	< 50 pg/ml
Plasma Glucagon	50 – 100 pg/ml
Plasma Gonadotropin Male : FSH	5 – 20 miu/ml
LH	5 – 20 miu/ml
Female : FSH	5 – 20 miu/ml
LH	5 – 25 miu/ml
Prolactin	2 – 15 ng/ml
TSH	< 5µ/ml
T_3 Resin uptake	25 – 35%
T_3 Plasma	70 – 190 ng/dl
T_4 Serum	5 – 12 µg/dl

Table A.11

Stool	
Amount	80 – 140 gm/day
Dry weight	< 60 gm/day
	Water 60 – 70%
Alpha$_1$ Antirypsin	0.8 – 1 mg/gm
Fat	< 6 gm/day
Protein Nitrogen	< 1.7 gm/day

Table A.12

Urine	
Volume in 24 hours	1000 – 2000 ml
Sp. Gr.	1010 – 1025
pH	5 – 6.5

Table A.13

Organic Constituents (gm/day)	
Creatine	0.0 – 0.06
Creatinine	1.64
Nitrogen Total	13.20
Undetermined	0.6
Urea	25 – 30
Uric acid	0.5 – 0.8
Urobilinogen	1 – 4 mg/day
Amylase	35 – 260 Somogyi, units/hour
Somogyic Ammonia	30-50 mEq/24 hours

Inorganic Constituents (gm/day)	
Calcium	0.1 – 0.2
Chloride (as NaCl)	9 – 16
Potassium	2
Sodium	4
VMA	< 8 mg/day
Catecholamine	100 mg/24 hours

Table A.14

Cerebrospinal Fluid	
Cell count	0 – 5 lymphocytes/cmm Lympho 60% - 70% Mono 30% - 50% Neutro 1% - 3%
pH	7.3 – 7.7
Pressure	100 – 200 mm of water
Sp.Gr.	1003 - 1008

Table A.15

Organic Constituents	
Glucose	40 – 70 mg/dl
Protein Total Albumin Globulin Al/Gl ratio	 15 – 45 mg/dl 8 – 32 mg/dl 2 – 8 mg/dl 3 : 1

Table A.16

Gastric Juice	
Volume	2 – 3 litres / 24 ours
pH	0.9 – 1.5
Basal fasting volume	30 – 70 ml/hour
Acid output (Basal) Males Females	 1 – 5 mEq/hour 0.2 – 3.8 mEq/hour
Acid output (Maximal) Males Females	 20 – 30 mEq/hour 10 – 25 mEq/hour

Table A.17

Body Fluid (70 kg body wt.)	
Total	50 L
Intracellular Fluid	35 L
Extrcellular fluid	15 L
Plasma	3.5 L
Interstitial fluid	11.5 L

Index

B

C

G

Gabapentin, 74, 183

Gallopamil, 25, 74, 183

Ganciclovir, 25, 74, 183

Gemfibrozil, 25, 74, 183

Gentamicin, 5, 25, 56, 74, 183

Gingko biloba, 202

Glibenclamide, 25, 74, 184

Glibornuride, 74, 184

Gliclazide, 25, 74, 184

Gliquidone, 26, 75, 184

Glutethimide, 5, 26, 54, 75, 184

Glyburide, 75, 184

Glycerin, 75, 184

Glyceryltrinitrate, 26

Glycopyrronium, 26, 75, 184

Glymidine, 26, 75, 184

Gold sodium thiromalate, 5

Gold sodium, 75, 184

Goserelin, 26, 75, 184

Granisetron, 75, 184

Griseofulvin, 56, 75, 184

Guanabenz, 26, 75, 184

Guanadrel, 26, 75, 184

Guanethidine, 5, 26, 75, 184

Guanfecine, 75, 184

Guanoxan, 75, 184

H

Haloperidol, 26, 75, 184

Heparin, 54, 75, 184

Heroin, 51, 56, 75, 184

Hexobarbital, 51, 76, 184, 185

Homatropine, 51, 76, 184

Hydralazine, 5, 6, 26, 76, 184, 185

Hydrallazine, 56

Hydrochlorothiazide, 6, 26, 51, 76, 185

Hydrocortisone, 26, 76, 185

Hydroflumethiazide, 6, 27

Hydroxizine, 27, 76, 185

Hydroxy progesterone, 27

Hydroxychloroquine, 27, 185

Hydroxychloroquine, 76

Hydroxyprogesterone, 76, 185

Hydroxyurea, 27, 76, 185

Hydroxyzine, 27, 76, 185,

Hyoscine, 27, 51, 77, 185

I

Ibuprofen, 27, 51, 77, 185

Idoxuridine, 27, 77, 185

Ifosfamide, 27, 77, 185

Imipenem, 77, 185

Imipramine hydrochloride, 4

Imipramine, 6, 27, 51, 54, 56, 77, 185

Indapamide, 27, 77, 185

Indomethacin, 27, 54, 56, 77, 185

Indoramin, 27, 51, 77, 185, 186

Insulin, 5, 27, 77, 186

Interferon (alfa), 77

Interferon (beta), 77

Interferon, 185, 186

Iodine, 4

Ipratropium, 27, 77, 186

Iprindole, 51, 77, 186

Iproniazid, 28, 77, 186

Isocarboxazid, 28, 77, 186

Isoniazid, 4, 28, 54, 77, 186

Isoprenaline, 28, 51, 78, 186

Isoproterenol, 6

Isosorbide dinitrate, 28, 78, 186

Isosorbide mononitrate, 28, 78, 186

Isosorbide, 28

Isotretinoin, 78, 186

Isoxsuprine, 28, 51, 78, 186

Isradipine, 28, 78, 186

Itraconazole, 28, 78, 186

Ivermectin, 28

K

Kanamycin sulfate, 4

Kanamycin, 5, 28, 54, 78, 186

Kava, 202

Ketaconazole, 28

Ketamine, 28, 78, 186

Ketanserin, 28, 78, 186

Ketazolam, 29, 78, 186

Ketoconazole, 78, 186

Ketoprofen, 29, 78, 186

Ketorolac, 29, 78, 186

L

Labetalol, 29, 78, 186

Lamivudine, 29

Lanatoside C, 29, 78, 186

Latamoxef, 79, 186

Lesuride, 29

Leucovorin, 79, 187

Levallorphan, 51, 79, 187

Levamisole, 29, 79, 187

Levobunolol, 79, 187

Levobutalol, 29

Levodopa, 29, 51, 56, 79, 187

Levolorphan, 29

Levonorgestre, 79, 187

Levorphanol, 56, 79, 187

Lidoflazine, 29, 79, 187

Lignocain, 79, 187

Lignocaine, 29, 51

Lincomycin, 4, 5, 29, 51, 54

Lincornycm, 79, 187

Liothyroine, 79, 187

Liothyronine, 6, 29

Liquorice, 202

Lisinopril, 30, 79, 187

Lisuride, 79, 187

Lithium carbonate, 4, 5

Lithium, 30, 56, 79, 187

Lodoqumol, 79, 187

Lofepramine, 30, 79, 187

Lomefloxacin, 30, 79, 187

Loperamide, 30, 79, 187

Loracarbef, 80, 187

Loratidine, 30, 80, 187

Lorazepam, 30, 51, 56, 80, 187

Lorcainide, 30, 80, 187

Lormustine, 30, 80, 187

Lornoxicam, 30, 80, 187

Lovastatin, 80, 187

Lymecycline, 30, 80, 187

Lysergide, 51, 80, 188

M

Maprotiline, 80, 188

Mazindol, 80, 188

Mebendazole, 30, 80, 188

Mecamylamine, 51, 56, 80

Mecillinam, 30, 80, 188

Meclizine, 30, 80, 188

Medazepam, 30, 80, 188

Medifoxamine, 30, 80, 188

Medigoxin, 80, 188

Medroxy progesterone, 31, 81, 188

Mefenamic acid, 31, 81, 188

Mefenamic, 51

Mefloquin, 31, 81, 188

Mefruside, 31, 81, 188

Melphalan, 31, 81, 188

Menadione, 6

Mepacrine, 31, 51, 54, 56, 81, 188

Mepenzolate, 31, 81, 188

Meperidine hydrochloride, 4

Meperidine, 51, 54, 56, 81, 188

Mephenytoin, 6

Mepivacaine, 31, 81, 188

Meprobamate, 5, 31, 81, 188

Meptazinol, 31, 81, 188

Mepyramine, 31, 81

Mercaptopurine, 31, 81, 188

Mercurials, 5

Mesalazine, 31, 81, 188

Metaraminol, 31, 51, 81, 188

Metbyltestosterone, 82

Metformin, 31, 81, 189

Methadone, 5, 31, 51, 54, 81, 189

Methaqualone, 32, 82, 189

Methazolamide, 6

Methenamine mandalate, 5

N

U

V

W

X

www.ingramcontent.com/pod-product-compliance
Lightning Source LLC
LaVergne TN
LVHW081925160726
843514LV00005B/932